The Evolution
of Medical Genetics

A British Perspective

T0186555

The Evolution of Medical Genetics

A British Perspective

Peter S. Harper

University Research Professor
(Emeritus) in Human Genetics
Cardiff University
United Kingdom

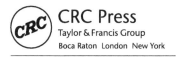

CRC Press
Taylor & Francis Group
Boca Raton London New York

CRC Press is an imprint of the
Taylor & Francis Group, an **informa** business

CRC Press
Taylor & Francis Group
6000 Broken Sound Parkway NW, Suite 300
Boca Raton, FL 33487-2742

© 2020 by Taylor & Francis Group, LLC
CRC Press is an imprint of Taylor & Francis Group, an Informa business

No claim to original U.S. Government works

Printed on acid-free paper

International Standard Book Number-13: 978-0-367-35632-3 (Hardback)
978-0-367-17809-3 (Paperback)

Library of Congress Cataloging-in-Publication Data

Names: Harper, Peter S., author.
Title: The evolution of medical genetics : a British perspective / Peter S. Harper.
Description: Boca Raton : CRC Press, [2020] | Includes bibliographical references and index. | Summary: "This informative new book presents an accessible account of the development of medical genetics over the past 70 years, one of the most important areas of 20th, and now 21st, century science and medicine. Based largely on the author's personal involvement and career as a leader in the field over the last half century, both in the UK and internationally, it also draws on his interest and involvement in documenting the history of medical genetics. Underpinning the content is a unique series of 100 recorded interviews undertaken by the author with key older workers in the field, the majority British, which has provided invaluable information going back to the very beginnings of human and medical genetics. Focusing principally on medically relevant areas of genetics rather than the underlying basic science and technological aspects, the book offers a fascinating insight for those working and training in the field of clinical or laboratory aspects of medical genetics and allied areas; it will also be of interest to historians of science and medicine and to workers in the social sciences who are increasingly attracted by the social and ethical challenges posed by modern medical genetics"-- Provided by publisher.
Identifiers: LCCN 2019024848 (print) | ISBN 9780367178093 (paperback ; alk. paper) | ISBN 9780367356323 (hardback ; alk. paper) | ISBN 9780429340789 (ebook)
Subjects: MESH: Genetics, Medical--history | Genomics--history | History, 20th Century | History, 21st Century | United Kingdom
Classification: LCC RB155 (print) | LCC RB155 (ebook) | NLM QZ 11 FA1 | DDC 616/.042--dc23
LC record available at https://lccn.loc.gov/2019024848
LC ebook record available at https://lccn.loc.gov/2019024849

Visit the Taylor & Francis Web site at
http://www.taylorandfrancis.com

and the CRC Press Web site at
http://www.crcpress.com

Dedication

To all workers in the field of Medical Genetics, past, present and future; in Britain and elsewhere across the world.

Contents

Preface

Why do I feel the need to write a book specifically on the history of medical genetics in *Britain*, rather than on the topic worldwide? There are several reasons, including the following:

First, I have already attempted to cover the field from an international perspective in my earlier (2008) book *A Short History of Medical Genetics*. While writing this I found that I had accumulated a large amount of material on British work and workers which was important, but which could not possibly be included in that book without unjustly omitting contributions from other countries. A second reason is that over the 12-year period from 2003 to 2016 I had been undertaking a series of recorded interviews, totalling more than 100 altogether, with key older scientists and clinicians in human and medical genetics, many of which were, for mostly logistic reasons, with British workers. Fortunately I had been able to make the transcripts available on the Web (www.genmedhist.org/interviews) as I went along, but they contained much material that I felt needed weaving together and synthesising into a more cohesive account; although I have tried to do this in some published papers, it was impossible to do the topic justice without the space and freedom provided by a book. I have quoted frequently from the interviews throughout the following chapters and they are listed in Appendix 2 (Table A2.4), being cited in the text by a number enclosed in square brackets [--].

A final reason, probably the most important, is that, in my opinion at least, Britain has indeed made particularly important contributions to the field of medical genetics, especially if one uses the term in its widest sense, as I have done here, to include both laboratory and clinical aspects, whether research or service orientated. Many of these contributions have been made by people who would not be considered, or consider themselves, as medical geneticists, but it has been this wide-ranging collaborative network, international as well as between UK individuals and groups, that has perhaps been the principal characteristic of British medical genetics, and probably its greatest strength. This is a community whose workers deserve to be remembered as a whole, even if many of them may not have individually made spectacular discoveries. The detailed record provided by the interview series again provides a graphic picture of the excitement felt by these workers in the field and their enjoyment and pride in forming part of it, even when their contribution may only have been a small one.

Although little more than a decade ago there seemed to be a real danger that much of the more recent history of this field would be irretrievably lost, something urgently emphasised in my previous book, this is fortunately no longer the case, at least for Britain; Appendix 2 gives details of the now rich resource of material, both written and oral, that is available to historians and others for detailed and critical analysis, something that has only just begun, but which at least now has an abundance of facts to be based on. I have not attempted a detailed historical approach here, principally because I have been too involved personally, having seen much of modern medical genetics evolve over my own professional lifetime. I have, though, frequently expressed my own opinions throughout this book — perhaps indeed too frequently — so it will be good when historically trained workers study the field more objectively than I have been able to.

I need to note another limitation of this account, which results from my being primarily a clinician and clinical research worker; my emphasis is thus more on the clinical aspects of medical genetics than on the basic science and technology underpinning it. Likewise, I have frequently focused on the people responsible for advances and applications in the field more than on the detailed underlying science, and have also included a number of quotes and other material that some may consider too anecdotal.

Who have I written this book for? First and foremost, for my colleagues and friends working in medical genetics, and perhaps especially for those in allied fields, who are less likely to be familiar with the rich history of genetics in medicine. Equally I have had in mind those in medical genetics outside the UK, who will be familiar with much current British work but probably not with its origins and history. I hope, too, that historians will find the book of interest, since it touches on numerous themes that deserve more detailed study by them. And finally, given the widespread interest in genetics today among the wider public, some general readers should find it of interest and I have tried to write it simply, with them in mind.

I have recorded my principal sources in the text and the appendices, but have drawn extensively on my own experience of more than 50 years in various aspects of medical genetics. I also found of the greatest value the accounts given by those whom I interviewed of their own teachers and mentors, which reach back almost a century to the dawn of genetics and which supplement the incomplete written records from that time.

Acknowledgements

I owe a great debt to many people who have made it possible for me to write this book, though I must emphasise that the opinions expressed and any errors made are entirely my own responsibility.

My first thanks are due to all those who agreed to take part in the recorded interview series and to allow the edited transcripts to be placed in the public domain on the Web. I hope that many readers will take the opportunity to move from the brief quotes from these interviews given in this book to the full versions on www.genmedhist.org/interviews. An increasing number of interviewees are now no longer living, which makes me particularly glad that I was able to capture their memories in a permanent form.

Many workers across the UK have contributed photographs of themselves and of former colleagues. I thank them all, but must apologise to those numerous people whose photographs, for reasons of space, have not in the end been used; also to those, even more numerous, who are not mentioned in the book at all, an indication of how the field has grown in recent years. I am most grateful to Brian Marsh, of the University Hospital of Wales Media Resources Department, for greatly improving the quality of many of the illustrations.

My colleagues and successors in Cardiff, Julian Sampson and Angus Clarke, generously took on the onerous task of reading and criticising a full early draft of the book, making a number of helpful suggestions and correcting some major errors and omissions, while Peter Farndon (Birmingham) and Andrew Wilkie (Oxford) kindly reviewed specific chapters, making valuable comments.

Most of my own historical work has been carried out post-retirement, and has fortunately not required specific grant funding, but I must thank Wellcome Trust for its financial support of a number of areas of my work, notably the series of international workshops mentioned in Appendix 2, and for much general support and encouragement, which was especially valuable in the early stages before the overall project gained momentum. Cardiff University has continued to allow me access to its IT and other facilities, and I am especially grateful to Karen Pierce from Cardiff University libraries and to Peter Keelan, Alan Hughes and Alison Harvey from Cardiff University Special Collections and Archives. Cardiff University also hosted the Genetics and Medicine Historical Network

(Genmedhist) website for the first 12 years of its existence, something now continued by the European Society of Human Genetics.

In putting this book together from a large amount of previously scattered fragments and in the transcription of the recorded interviews I have been helped by a series of able and willing clerical workers, notably Christine Holness. All have given considerably more time to this than they were officially meant to, but equally they have all commented to me how interesting they found the topic, something which encourages me to think that other general readers may also enjoy it.

Taylor & Francis Group have proved helpful and sympathetic publishers and I am especially grateful to them for their tolerance in relation to the large number of illustrations in the book, something that I am sure readers will agree adds greatly to the interest of the book.

Finally, my family have, as always, continued to be supportive and tolerant of my book writing activities, even though they might reasonably have expected these to have ceased some years ago. I am deeply grateful for their support and affection, without which this book would never have been completed.

Cardiff
August 2019

1

Forerunners: Genetics and medicine before World War II

ABSTRACT

The history of genetics in British medicine goes back several centuries, with a long series of articles on familial disorders, as well as of studies into the nature of heredity. The nineteenth century especially saw many detailed reports in the medical literature on hereditary conditions, but no underlying basis for their occurrence could be found until the recognition of Gregor Mendel's work in 1900. After this many of the previously observed families could be interpreted along mendelian lines, in studies by William Bateson and others, so that by 1914 the specific patterns of single gene inheritance were well established, with evidence from genetic disorders playing a major role in genetics overall. The quantitative aspects of normal human variation, originally studied by Francis Galton, likewise became well established and gave a basis for the inheritance of common non-mendelian diseases.

In the twentieth century, despite the initial lack of laboratory approaches, the period between the wars produced a series of highly original studies on human genetics by workers such as JBS Haldane, RA Fisher and others, so that the foundations for future medical genetics were largely in place by the outbreak of World War II.

Human and medical genetics have a long history, far longer than the history of genetics itself as a field of science. Physicians and others have over the centuries recorded familial aspects of disorders in patients under their care, even though most did not attempt any explanation for this. Natural philosophers across Europe from the earliest times, especially during the eighteenth century Enlightenment, speculated on the nature of heredity in animals and plants, and human inheritance was often at the forefront of their interest.

I do not attempt to cover these early aspects here in any detail. I have done so from a worldwide perspective in my earlier book *A Short History of Medical*

Genetics (Harper, 2008), where a fuller range of sources can also be found; others have done so for their own countries and fields of interest. Rushton's valuable book (2009), *Genetics and Medicine in Great Britain, 1600–1939*, gives detailed listings of early clinical reports. Here I give just a few examples that seem to me to be of particular relevance to the field of medical genetics, using the term in the widest sense, and where the contributions have been made by those living and working in Britain. It has always been a surprise to me how early were some of these observations, and how much we can still learn from them, particularly now that we have the detailed scientific knowledge which was lacking to observers and recorders at the time.

WILLIAM HARVEY (1578–1657) AND THE IMPORTANCE OF 'RARE DISORDERS'

William Harvey is now best remembered for his observations on circulation of the blood, but his wide-ranging observations and experimental studies on embryonic development led to his dictum *ex ovo omnia* – 'all things from the egg', as relevant to genetics as to embryology (Figure 1.1). Harvey's most detailed findings were on the developing hen's egg, but as physician to the king (Charles I) he had access to

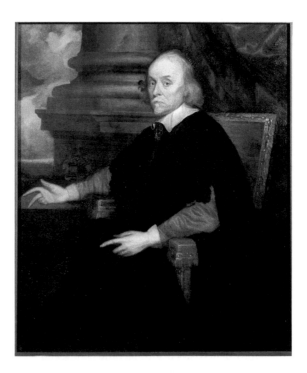

Figure 1.1 William Harvey (1578–1657). (Courtesy of Royal College of Physicians, London.)

deer and other animals killed during royal hunts, and closely examined the fetal roe deer, including the amniotic fluid and membranes.

> I saw long since a foetus the magnitude of a peasecod cut out of the uterus of a doe, which was complete in all its members and I showed this pretty spectacle to our late King and Queen. It did swim, trim and perfect, in such a kinde of white, most transparent and crystalline moysture (as if it had been treasured up in some most clear glassie receptacle about the bignesse of a pigeon's egge, and was invested with its proper coat.

> *Harvey 1651; quoted in Needham J 1931; vol 1, page 139.*

Harvey's practical observations were enhanced by his willingness (like Charles Darwin two centuries later), to talk with and learn from those involved in practical matters, like huntsmen and gamekeepers.

Even more relevant for medical genetics is his often-quoted statement, in a 1652 letter to Dr Vlackweld of Haarlem, Netherlands, on the value of studying rare diseases:

> Nature is nowhere accustomed more openly to display her secret mysteries than in cases where she shows traces of her workings apart from the beaten path; nor is there any better way to advance the proper practice of medicine than to give our minds to the discovery of the usual law of nature by careful investigation of cases of rarer forms of disease. For it has been found, in almost all things, that what they contain of useful or applicable nature is hardly perceived unless we are deprived of them, or they become deranged in some way.

> *Harvey 1652*

A number of mostly younger friends and colleagues of William Harvey, including Sir Thomas Browne and Nathaniel Highmore, continued his approach of direct observation and experiment, despite disruption, especially in London, from the civil war; Oxford was a major centre for these people, before the focus returned to London after restoration of the monarchy. The newly formed Royal Society now became the centre for exchange of ideas, rather than the Royal College of Physicians as previously. Invention and development of the compound microscope by Robert Hooke and others, notably Anton van Leeuwenhoek in the Netherlands, whose drawings of human sperm are especially notable, gave a new dimension, especially for studies of development, but clinical observations of inherited disorders in families also began to appear. One of the clearest of these was that reported by Kenelm Digby (1603–1665; Figure 1.2), who became a naval 'privateer' and during a visit to Algiers was fortunate enough to be given direct

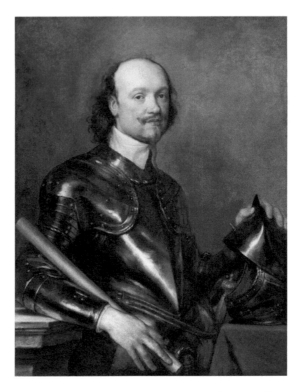

Figure 1.2 Kenelm Digby (1603–1665). (Courtesy of National Portrait Gallery, London.)

access to a family with 'double thumbs' which he described from three members seen by himself and two older generations stated as affected:

> And another particular that I saw when I was at Algiers… was of a woman that having two thumbs upon the left hand; four daughters that she had all resembled her in the same accident, and so did a little child, a girl of her eldest daughter, but none of her sonnes. While I was there I had a particular curiosity to see them, although it is not easily permitted unto a Christian to speak familiarly with Mohametan women; yet the condition I was in there and the civility of the Bassha, gave me the opportunity of full view and discourse with them; and the old woman told me that her mother and grandmother had been in the same manner.
>
> *Digby 1645*

ALBINISM IN CENTRAL AMERICA AND LIONEL WAFER

One cannot always take the accounts of the early British explorers at face value, but there is no reason to doubt that the observation by Lionel Wafer (1660–1705?)

Figure 1.3 Lionel Wafer's book 'A New Voyage and Description of the Isthmus of America' contains the first detailed description of albinism as 'white Indians' (Wafer, 1699).

of 'white Indians' in the isthmus of central America represents true albinism. Wafer, a ship's surgeon originally from Wales, was also one of the 'buccaneering' Caribbean explorers who combined serious observations with occasional piracy when the opportunity arose; a severe leg injury (from exploding gunpowder) gave him the enforced opportunity of living for several months with the local tribes, who seem to have been hospitable, and of making his observations in detail and at first hand, reporting them in a book (Wafer 1699; Figure 1.3), which is accessible in entirety as a facsimile on the internet.

White Indians

There is one complexion so singular among a sort of people of this country, that I never saw nor heard of any like them in any part of the world.

They are white, and there are of them of both sexes; yet there are few of them in comparison to the copper coloured, possibly but one to two or three hundred.

Their bodies are beset all over, more or less, with a fine short milk-white down, which adds to the whiteness of their skins.

Their eyebrows are milk-white also, and so is the hair of their heads and very fine withal.

For they see not very well in the sun, poring in the clearest day; their eyes being weak, and running with water if the sun shines towards them, so that in the day-time they care not to go abroad, unless it be a cloudy dark day.

They are not a distinct race by themselves, but now and then one is bred of a copper-coloured father and mother; and I have seen a child of less than a year old of this sort. But besides that the Europeans come little here, and have little commerce with the Indian women when they do come. These white people are as different from the Europeans in some respects, as from the copper-coloured Indians in others. And besides, where an European lies with an Indian women, the child is always a Mostese or Tawney, as is well known to all who have been in the West-Indies. But neither is the child of a man and women of these white Indians, white like the parents, but copper-coloured as their parents were.

Wafer 1699

Albinism has been recognised since antiquity, but Wafer is probably the first to have described the inheritance pattern that with hindsight is clearly autosomal recessive. It would be another 200 years before this would be confirmed scientifically by Castle (1903). Wafer does, however, give one inconsistency, since he implies that offspring of two affected parents are of the normal 'coppery' colour, whereas one would expect, at least in a small population with a single mutation likely, all to be albino. He gives this as an observation made by someone else and does not distinguish it from the much more frequent situation where just one parent was affected, for which his statement would be correct.

JOHN DALTON (1766–1844)

A noted scientist of the late eighteenth century, ranging widely in his experimental work from meteorology to the properties of gases and other chemicals, and who first proposed a detailed atomic theory, Dalton (Figure 1.4) was the first person to note accurately what would later become recognised as X-linked inheritance, by recording colour blindness in himself and in family members. He spent most of his life in Manchester, and in his 1794 paper to the Manchester Literary and Philosophical Society he described his own anomalous colour vision:

I have often seriously asked a person whether a flower was blue or pink, but was generally considered to be in jest. Notwithstanding this, I was never convinced of a peculiarity in my vision, till I accidentally observed the colour of the flower of the Geranium zonale by candle-light, in the Autumn of 1792. The flower was pink, but appeared to me almost an exact sky-blue by day; in candle-light, however, it was astonishingly changed, not having then any blue in it, but being what I called red, a colour which forms a striking contrast to blue.

Dalton 1798

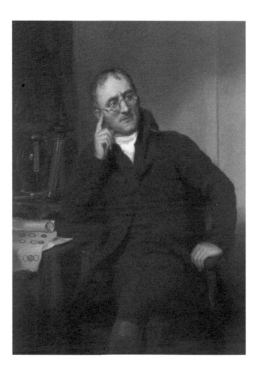

Figure 1.4 John Dalton (1766–1844). First identifier of red-green colour-blindness (he was himself affected). Portrait by Joseph Allen. (Courtesy of Harris Manchester College, Oxford University.)

He analysed his vision by a series of tests, made more rigorous by the fact that he was himself expert in optics. For the colour green, seen by daylight:

> I take my standard idea from grass. This appears to me very little different from red. The face of a laurel-leaf (Prunus Lauro-cerasus) is a good match to a stick of red sealing-wax; and the back of the leaf answers to the lighter red of wafers. Hence it will be immediately concluded, that I see either red or green, or both, different from other people.

His brother was similarly affected and, recognising that it seemed to be confined to males, Dalton obtained an approximate estimate of its frequency by sending strips of coloured thread to his past and present students, finding 3 out of 50 to have red-green colour-blindness, which has also been named 'Daltonism'. His studies have a modern postscript since in his will he left to the Manchester Literary and Philosophical Society not only his papers but his eyes, from which molecular geneticists 200 years later have been able to isolate DNA, which has confirmed a mutation for red-green colour-blindness (Hunt et al. 1995). Fortunately for posterity, the tissue had been allowed to dry, not placed in formalin fixative, so destructive to the preservation of DNA! At the time of this study the possibility of molecular analysis on such preserved tissue was novel, but it has since become commonplace; only 20 years later the use of genetic and now whole genome analysis is revolutionising the entire field of human evolution and anthropology (see Chapter 11).

Mention should be made at this point of another important Enlightenment figure, the English mathematician and nonconformist clergyman *Thomas Bayes* (1702–1761), whose work on probability has become of key later importance in relation to genetic risk estimation. His notes were assembled and presented to the Royal Society of London after his death and a recent very readable book (McGrayne 2012) shows how widely his concepts are now applied. Medical geneticists have used them for over 50 years (see Chapter 6) and they have become very much an integral part of 'genetic thinking'.

JOSEPH ADAMS (1756–1818)

None of those people mentioned so far would seem to have had any concept of genetics playing a direct role in the practice of medicine, which makes Joseph Adams such an important figure for the future field of medical genetics. Adams wrote his book, *A Treatise on the Supposed Hereditary Properties of Diseases* (Figure 1.5), in 1814, not long before he died, so his views reflect his long experience in medical practice as well as his tolerant and humane

(a)   (b)

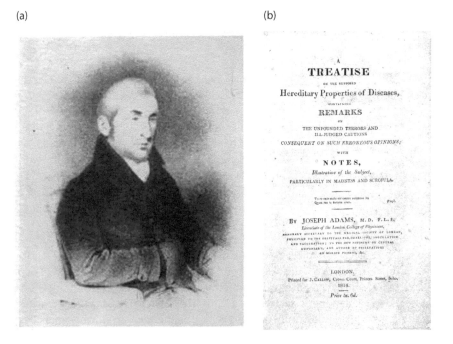

Figure 1.5 **(a)** Joseph Adams (1756–1818) and **(b)** his book (Adams 1814). Adams has been described as the first medical geneticist. (Courtesy of the Royal College of Surgeons, London.)

nature. He distinguished between *disposition*, by which he meant the clear-cut inheritance of a specific disorder, and *predisposition*, where a disorder would occur only in the presence of some environmental factor, which might itself be avoided:

> If the family or hereditary susceptibility is such, that the disease, though not existing at birth, is afterwards induced without any external causes, or by causes which can not be distinguished from the functions of the economy, such a state may be called, a DISPOSITION to the disease.
>
> But if the susceptibility, though greater than is remarked in other families, is so far less than a disposition as always to require the operation of some external cause to induce the disease; this minor susceptibility may be called, a PREDISPOSITION to the disease.

These categories correspond broadly to what we now recognise as mendelian and multifactorial diseases.

He also cautioned (see Chapter 6) against the advising of celibacy if there were a family history of mental illness, on the grounds that this might deprive society of some of those best suited to be parents. Later proponents of eugenics would have done well to heed his advice.

Two valuable articles on Joseph Adams by prominent medical geneticists, Arno Motulsky (1959) and Alan Emery (1989), have been written, while Adams' book itself has been digitised and placed on the website of the Genetics and Medicine Historical Network (www.genmedhist.org/digitalresources).

CHARLES DARWIN (1809–1883)

Although Charles Darwin's own theory of heredity, 'pangenesis', based on the migration of supposed particles ('gemmules') scattered throughout the body to the gonads, proved to be erroneous, his lifelong interest in variation and its causes led him to document a range of human genetic disorders (Darwin 1868, 1890), thanks to his extensive network of correspondents scattered across the world in various parts of the then British Empire. A notable example is given in the second edition of his book *The Variation of Animals and Plants under Domestication*:

> I may give an analogous case, communicated to me by Mr W Wedderburn, of a Hindoo family in Scinde, in which 10 men, in the course of four generations, were furnished, in both jaws taken together, with only four small and weak incisor teeth and with eight posterior molars. The men thus affected have very little hair on the body, and become bald early in life. They also suffer much during hot weather from excessive dryness of the skin. It is remarkable that no instance has occurred of a daughter being thus affected; and

this fact reminds us how much more liable men are in England to become bald than women. Though daughters in the above family are never affected, they transmit the tendency to their sons; and no case has occurred of the son transmitting it to his sons. The affection thus appears only in alternate generations, or after longer intervals.

Darwin 1890

This description can confidently be recognised today as the X-linked disorder hereditary anhidrotic ectodermal dysplasia and emphasises the value of accurate historic descriptions (and illustrations) of genetic disorders, as noted below.

GENETIC DISORDERS RECORDED BY CLINICIANS

A considerable number of nineteenth century British physicians recorded and published observations on familial disorders in patients under their care, and a detailed listing of these can be found in Rushton's book (Rushton 2009). Among these clinicians the early contribution of the London physician Edward Meryon, who gave the first description in 1852 of muscular dystrophy in boys (Meryon 1852) should not be forgotten, although Duchenne's 1862 full description and pictures of what is now known worldwide as 'Duchenne muscular dystrophy' gave more details of the clinical features, pathology and familial nature of this disorder, with its name understandably assigned to Duchenne himself. A valuable book by Alan and Marcia Emery (1995) gives a detailed history of the condition from its initial recognition to recent research on its molecular basis. There must be numerous other genetic disorders where a comparable historical approach would be possible and interesting, but so far my pleas to those who have written theses on such specific disorders to develop and publish their often lengthy historical introductions as fuller historical studies have fallen on deaf ears!

Other inherited disorders documented during the nineteenth century included numerous reports of haemophilia, though the first publications on this were of American families (Otto 1803, Hay 1813). Various forms of hereditary blindness were recorded, including optic atrophy and cataract, some of which later formed part of the *Treasury of Human Inheritance*, collated and analysed by Julia Bell (see below). For skin diseases Jonathan Hutchinson in London took a special interest in inheritance; after his death his papers were shipped to Johns Hopkins Hospital in Baltimore, where they were stored in the library basement; 50 years later, they were assiduously studied by the young Victor McKusick, still a cardiologist at the time (Harper 2012). Table 1.1 lists some of the disorders described by British clinicians that would now be recognised as following mendelian inheritance.

From the descriptions given in these reports and from many others in the medical literature, it can be seen that for the 200 years prior to the recognition

Table 1.1 Some early nineteenth century descriptions of inherited disorders by British clinicians

Disorder	Describer	Date
Aniridia (with microphthalmia)	Cooper	1857
Brittle bones (osteogenesis imperfecta)	Arnott	1833
Cataract, juvenile (numerous reports)	Saunders	1811
Haemophilia (numerous reports)	Osborne	1835
Hypertrichosis ('hairy men of Ava', Burma)	Hamilton	1827
Ichthyosis hystrix (Lambert family). Supposed Y chromosome inheritance disproved by Penrose and Stern (1958)	Machin	1732
Polydactyly	Carlisle	1814
Syndactyly	Thomson	1858

of Mendel's work there had been a near-continuous series of British reports on or relevant to human inheritance and inherited diseases, increasingly numerous in the mid and late nineteenth century; comparable examples could have also been given from France and America, but they do seem especially abundant in Britain and have been assiduously gathered together by Rushton (2009).

'ROYAL MALADIES'

While the British Royal family in the nineteenth century (and subsequently) has not been scientifically inclined, apart from the imported Prince Albert, it has supplied copious case material for discussion and speculation in relation to the occurrence of haemophilia (undoubted) and porphyria (less certain) among its members. This has been well studied and documented by Rushton (2008), though molecular analyses akin to those on John Dalton for colour blindness have so far not been conclusive.

FRANCIS GALTON (1822–1911)

Galton's name is now associated with two very different and largely opposed topics: eugenics, of which he was one of the first and most prominent British proponents, as well as the person who coined the term; and the Galton Laboratory at University College, London, which he endowed and which became the world's foremost centre for human genetics after World War II, under the leadership of Lionel Penrose (see Chapter 2), who was a fervent opponent of eugenics (Figure 1.6). The Galton Laboratory and its achievements are a recurring theme throughout this book, but the widely perceived association of anything bearing Galton's name with eugenics persists, something reinforced by the relatively recent (1989) and confusing name change of the former 'Eugenics Society' to 'Galton Institute' (see below).

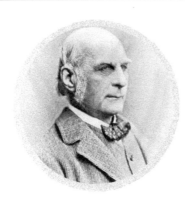

Figure 1.6 Francis Galton (1822–1911). Founder of much of human quantitative genetics and of 'biometry'.

Francis Galton was a half first cousin to Charles Darwin, their shared grandfather being Erasmus Darwin. Born in Birmingham, he started to study medicine, but gave it up and instead read mathematics at Cambridge. With the advantage of an independent income, he embarked on travel, notably to South-west Africa (now Namibia), collecting his experiences into an early 'handbook', *The Art of Travel* (Galton, 1872). He settled down into an established London life, with his scientific work based on quantitative aspects of heredity, statistics, meteorology and a wide range of other topics – including eugenics, to which he gave the name. On his death he endowed what became the 'Galton Laboratory' and the Chair associated with it.

Galton's life has been well described in several biographies (Pearson 1914, Gilham 2001, Bulmer 2003); but what is relevant here is that he made indisputable major contributions to would later become the discipline of human genetics, especially the area of quantitative and statistical genetics known at the time as 'biometry'. Throughout his life he was a compulsive measurer, in a wide range of scientific fields apart from heredity, and his successors, notably Karl Pearson and Ronald Fisher, would provide many of the key contributions to statistics.

Galton, like his cousin Charles Darwin, was unaware of Mendel's work; while he himself formulated a possible system of particulate inheritance, and did not accept Darwin's 'pangenesis', he never developed his own ideas into a satisfactory foundation for heredity, the credit for which belongs entirely to Mendel himself. Nevertheless, Galton's quantitative approach did provide the foundations for the analysis of the genetic basis of normal variation, and in due course for the study of common birth defects and other polygenic disorders, which would be taken forward by Penrose, Falconer, Carter and others (Chapter 2) to give a parallel stream of knowledge that would later, alongside mendelism, underpin much of the practice, as well as the theory of medical genetics.

Among Galton's key contributions were his studies on fingerprints (though he was not their discoverer) and on human height, where he utilised the 1884 London International Health Exhibition to set up a booth to measure the large number of visitors, obtaining widespread biometric data on more than 9000 individuals. His analysis of human intelligence was flawed, though, by his failure to take into account the major biases resulting from social and educational factors. Outside the genetic field he, along with Robert Fitzroy (former captain of HMS Beagle, on which Charles Darwin had voyaged), pioneered the field of meteorology and weather forecasting, while his 'study of the efficacy of prayer', in which he showed no increased longevity of the monarchy despite being prayed for weekly by millions across the country (Galton, 1872), proved to be a let-down for both royalty and clergy.

Mendel and mendelism

It seems irreverent to write on the history of genetics without any mention of Gregor Mendel, but by no stretch of the imagination could he be called British, though he did attend the Great Exhibition in London in 1851, but it is not known if he visited Galton's 'measuring booth'. His most notable 'connection' with Britain was his lack of connection with Darwin, which might have had a profound effect on both men and on science generally had it occurred.

Both Darwin and Galton had struggled, and largely failed, to come up with a convincing mechanism for heredity, despite their valuable contributions, so it is not surprising that when a satisfactory theoretical basis finally became available from Mendel's work (Mendel 1866), many of these early observations rapidly fell into place; the numerous family reports of rare disorders, involving a wide variety of different systems and specialists, now could be looked on as examples of a major general principle rather than just as curiosities. Conversely, examples from human disease provided much of the initial evidence confirming the existence and universality of mendelism. Perhaps surprisingly, this process of acceptance was much more rapid in Britain than for most other European countries, where much of the renewed interest in Mendel was from botanists and plant breeders, rather than physicians. Most of the credit for this progress is due to the energy and collaborative work of William Bateson who, more than anyone else worldwide, established both the universal application of mendelian inheritance and its importance in medicine.

WILLIAM BATESON (1861–1926)

The often-told story of Bateson's recognition of mendelism in 1900, while reading of its rediscovery on a train journey between Cambridge and London to lecture there and rewriting his text as a result, was included in Bateson's biography by his wife (Bateson B 1928a) (Figure 1.7). It is almost certainly no more than a story, but it shows how he, along with others, was receptive to a theory of heredity that could provide a new and unifying explanation for the many facts that had been accumulating since Mendel had published his original unrecognised paper 30 years before.

William Bateson was at the time primarily a zoologist, who had worked on anatomical variation in various species (Bateson W 1894) and had also made major explorations in Russian central Asia (Bateson B 1928b). Back in Cambridge he was finding difficulty in attracting interest or funding for his animal breeding work (a recurrent theme in this book for Cambridge workers over the following century), but after becoming aware of Mendel's work he realised the importance of establishing its applications outside Mendel's domain of plants.

Bateson was tireless in his efforts to promote mendelism, in Britain and internationally; his wider activities included the foundation of the *Genetical Society* (now *Genetics Society*) (Figure 1.8) in 1919; he was also the first to use the

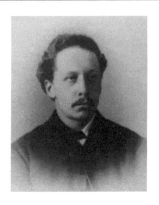

Figure 1.7 William Bateson (1861–1926). Pioneer of mendelian inheritance and collaborator with medical workers on numerous inherited disorders. (Courtesy of the John Innes Archive, Norwich.)

William Bateson was born in Cambridge and studied zoology there, making links with William Brooks at the Chesapeake Bay marine biology station attached to Johns Hopkins University. He then traveled widely in central Asia, analysing variation in the marine life in the various lakes there, work that would later inspire the famous Russian geneticist Nikolai Vavilov to work with him in Britain. Back in Cambridge he continued his work on the inheritance of anatomical variation, making him well prepared to recognise the importance of Mendel's principles when these were rediscovered in 1900. Cambridge University persistently refused to create an established department for him, and he was largely dependent on his wife Barbara in organising his breeding experiments. This lack of support led him to move to the new John Innes Horticultural Institution as its first director, remaining there up to his death in 1926.

word 'Genetics' for the field, a term that has worn well now for over a century. In a 1905 letter unsuccessfully suggesting that a bequest be used to establish a new Chair, he stated:

> If the Quick fund were used for the foundation of a Professorship relating to Heredity and Variation, the best title would, I think, be the Quick Professorship of the study of Heredity. No simple word in common use quite gives this meaning. Such a word is badly wanted, and if it were desirable to coin one, 'Genetics' might do.
>
> *18th April, 1905; letter [probably draft] in John Innes Archive.*

Like Harvey 250 years earlier, Bateson was well aware of the value of rare abnormalities, whether anatomical or physiological. As he states in his 1909 book *Mendel's Principles of Heredity*:

> Treasure your exceptions! When there are none, the work gets so dull that no one cares to carry it further. Keep them always uncovered and in sight. Exceptions are like the rough brickwork of a growing building which tells that there is more to come and shows where the next construction is to be.
>
> *Bateson 1909*

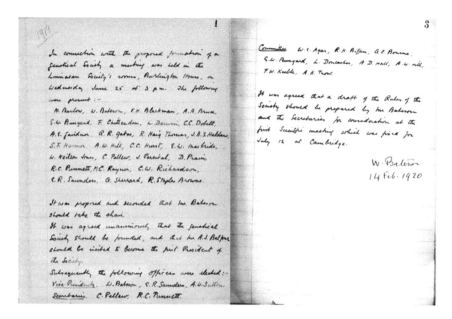

Figure 1.8 Foundation of the Genetical Society, minutes of the inaugural meeting 1920. Bateson was the first Secretary. (Courtesy of the John Innes Archive.)

Despite a somewhat gruff nature, reflected in most photographs of him (Figure 1.7 is the most genial that I could find), Bateson seems to have been a good communicator and collaborator, and soon established links with several London-based medical men; this not only provided ample evidence for the operation of mendelian inheritance, but generated a widespread interest in the topic among London medical circles. As early as 1906 he was invited to lecture on genetics to the London Neurological Society (see Chapter 4). Fortunately, much of Bateson's correspondence has been preserved in the archive of the John Innes Centre (now near Norwich, previously at Merton, outside London).

The best known of Bateson's medical collaborations was with the physician Archibald Garrod, whose interest in chemical abnormalities in disease had led him to study alkaptonuria, in which accumulation of the pigment homogentisic acid occurred in tissues and urine. After Garrod had published his 1901 paper showing occurrence of the disorder in sibs and frequent consanguinity among parents, Bateson wrote to him suggesting that this might be an example of mendelian recessive inheritance; Garrod was able to cite this in his fuller 1902 article and Bateson likewise cited Garrod in a paper with his colleague Elizabeth Saunders, also in 1902. Thus alkaptonuria became the first example of mendelism in human disease, being followed by albinism and by brachydactyly as an example of dominant inheritance, both of these observations coming from the American group of Castle (Castle 1903, Farabee 1905).

Garrod was able to use alkaptonuria as the foundation for his fundamental concept of 'inborn errors of metabolism', brought together in his book and Croonian lecture series under this title (Garrod 1908, 1909) and rightly placing him as the founder of human biochemical genetics.

Despite his fundamental discoveries, Garrod was not really interested in genetics in its own right. The most valuable collaborator for Bateson over the next decade was the ophthalmologist Edward Nettleship (see Chapter 4), who not only provided him with a wealth of detail on inherited eye disorders but corresponded with him widely on inheritance in general (though professing not to understand genetics). Nettleship even gave up his ophthalmologic practice to work on inherited eye disease and his contributions were recognised by the volume dedicated to him in Julia Bell's *Treasury of Human Inheritance* (see below) being given the title of the 'Nettleship Memorial Volume'.

By 1909 Bateson had sufficient material on human mendelian inheritance to bring together as a chapter in his book *Principles of Mendelian Heredity* (Bateson 1909). Non-lethal dominantly inherited disorders, likely to be multigenerational, are prominent in this, especially those affecting skin and eye; it is interesting that Bateson placed Huntington's disease as uncertain, the archived correspondence showing this to be mainly due to most affected individuals in previous generations being no longer living, with the diagnosis unconfirmed. This would prove to still be a problem 70 years later when the first genetic linkage studies on the condition were being done (see Chapter 12).

Although Bateson recognised a special category of 'sex limited' disorders, and the general field of sexual dimorphism had been studied for many years, by Darwin among others, the role of the sex chromosomes in human disease would not be recognised until the work of Wilson (1911) in America, though they had already been discovered in insects by Nettie Stevens in 1905. Bateson was, and for a long time remained sceptical about chromosomes generally. In relation to haemophilia, it was Nettleship again who helped him to avoid a serious error by insisting that the condition never passed from male to male, whereas Bateson had originally thought that half the male offspring of affected men were affected.

Bateson's early zoological work had focused on discontinuous structural variation, and his views on this had, even before the rediscovery of Mendel's work, brought him into conflict with Galton's followers Karl Pearson and Walter Weldon, who opposed any suggestions of particulate inheritance, including mendelism. The controversy deepened as the evidence for mendelian disorders increased, becoming personal when Weldon died suddenly and Bateson was blamed for this by his widow. It was partly to try to resolve this polarised situation that the London Royal Society of Medicine decided to have a debate on heredity and disease in November 1908, an event not seen previously in the world, and which had major consequences for what in the future would become medical genetics.

THE ROYAL SOCIETY OF MEDICINE 'DEBATE ON THE INFLUENCE OF HEREDITY AND DISEASE'

The Royal Society of Medicine had recently been formed in 1907 by a merger of a number of the principal London medical societies, including the London Neurological Society to which William Bateson had given his address in 1906

(Bateson 1906). Most of its members were practicing clinicians in various branches of medicine, and thus had extensive experience of families with unusual disorders in their particular field, though the subtitle of the event, 'with special reference to tuberculosis, cancer and diseases of the nervous system' indicates that they were also considering more common conditions. The meeting was held in weekly sessions over four successive weeks of November 1908 and was published in full in the Society's proceedings (Royal Society of Medicine 1909). A century later (2008) an anniversary meeting was held at the Royal Society of Medicine to mark the event.

The text shows that the views expressed by participants were pragmatic and sober (reflecting the recent death of Weldon during the preceding controversy). Bateson in particular was careful to emphasise that mendelian patterns should not be expected to be found in all disorders and that for common diseases the influence was likely to be on predisposition. Nevertheless the information presented by clinicians from various specialties strongly confirmed that Mendelian inheritance applied to numerous disorders across all systems.

The meeting effectively ended the conflict between 'mendelians' and 'biometricians', and it was left to RA Fisher, Pearson's successor in the Galton Chair, to point out that quantitative inheritance was entirely compatible with particulate mendelian inheritance, and that the conflict between the two groups had been largely unnecessary (Fisher 1918). We still see echoes of this division today, though, with some workers on common disease genetics tending to regard any focus on rare mendelian disorders as less relevant. Medical geneticists, though, have always recognised that the two categories each form essential parts of the overall whole picture of genetic disease; in this they are lineal descendants of Archibald Garrod a century earlier, and indeed of Joseph Adams two hundred years ago.

THE TREASURY OF HUMAN INHERITANCE

Following the Royal Society of Medicine debate, a further important step was the decision of Karl Pearson, the principal proponent for those favouring continuous rather than mendelian inheritance, and newly appointed as the first 'Galton Professor of Eugenics', to launch the *Treasury of Human Inheritance*, under the auspices of the Galton Laboratory. His idea was to publish the raw pedigree data on a range of human genetic disorders, leaving it to others to form opinions on the theoretical basis of their inheritance. Pearson had been bruised by the debates with Bateson and the increasingly successful supporters of mendelism.

> For a publication of this kind to be successful at the present time, it should, as I have indicated above, be entirely free from controversial matter. The Treasury of Human Inheritance therefore contains no reference to theoretical opinions.

> *Pearson 1912*

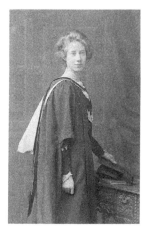

Figure 1.9 Julia Bell (1879–1979), principal author of the *Treasury of Human Inheritance*. For details of Bell's life and work see Bundey (1996) and Harper (2006).

While some of the initial sections were little more than a catalogue, the development of the *Treasury* was taken on as what would become her life's work by Julia Bell (Figure 1.9), who combined a thorough search of the world literature (something still possible at that time) with a detailed quantitative analysis of family data (Bell J, 1931–1947). While she followed Pearson's injunction to avoid 'theoretical opinions', it was clear from the data that most of the conditions studied did indeed follow mendelian inheritance, and after Pearson had retired, to be succeeded as Galton Professor and general editor of the *Treasury* by Ronald Fisher and even later by Lionel Penrose, she was able to state her conclusions on this clearly.

I have written elsewhere about the importance of Bell's work (Harper 2006), while a valuable article on her life has been written by Sarah Bundey (1996), but the lasting value of this monumental work makes the *Treasury* a permanent memorial for Julia Bell, reflecting not only her persistence over a period of 50 years, outliving three successive Galton Professors, but her combination of mathematical and clinical skills, not to mention her clarity of writing.

GH HARDY AND THE HARDY WEINBERG EQUILIBRIUM

Gregor Mendel himself built a mathematical approach into his experimental work, as did Francis Galton, but not all the early geneticists were mathematically

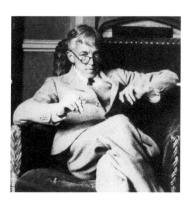

Figure 1.10 GH Hardy (1877–1947). Cambridge mathematician and co-originator of the 'Hardy-Weinberg equilibrium'. (Courtesy Professor Anthony Edwards.)

inclined. William Bateson's skills in this area did not extend much beyond the mendelian ratios, nor did those of Thomas Hunt Morgan in America. A question that arose at the 1908 Royal Society of Medicine 'Debate' (see above) was why, if a disorder or trait followed dominant inheritance, did it not increase in relation to the normal allele in the general population?

Bateson and his colleague (and later successor in Cambridge) Reginald Punnett were unable to answer this; it is surprising that Karl Pearson did not, as he easily could have. Fortunately Punnett had as a friend the brilliant Cambridge mathematician GH Hardy (1877–1947; Figure 1.10), who, as related by Punnett (1950), not only produced the solution but was persuaded, reluctantly, to write a brief note on the topic that was published in the American journal *Science*; the initial part is given below. Despite its brevity, Hardy's paper identifies the key factors that relate gene and genotype frequencies, and their stability over time.

To the Editor of Science: I am reluctant to intrude in a discussion concerning matters of which I have no expert knowledge, and I should have expected the very simple point which I wish to make to have been familiar to biologists. However, some remarks of Mr. Udny Yule, to which Mr. R.C. Punnett has called my attention, suggests that it may still be worth making.

In the Proceedings of the Royal Society of Medicine (Vol. I., p. 165) Mr. Yule is reported to have suggested, as a criticism of the Mendelian position, that if brachydactyly is dominant "in the course of time one would expect, in the absence of counteracting factors, to get three brachydactylous persons to one normal."

It is not difficult to prove, however, that such an expectation would be quite groundless. Suppose that Aa is a pair of Mendelian characters, A being dominant, and that in any given generation the numbers of pure dominants (AA), heterozygotes (Aa), and pure recessives (aa) are as p:2q:r. Finally, suppose that the numbers are fairly large, so that the mating may be regarded as random, that the sexes are evenly distributed among the three varieties, and that all are equally fertile. A little mathematics of the multiplication table type is enough to show that in the next generation the numbers will be as

$$(p + q)^2 : 2(p + q)(q + r) : (q + r)^2,$$

or as

$$P_1 : 2q_1 : r_1, \quad \text{say}$$

The interesting question is - in what circumstances will this distribution be the same as that in the generation before? It is easy to see that the condition for this is $q^2 = pr$. And since $q_1^2 = p_1 r_1$, whatever the values of p,q and r may be, the distribution will in any case continue unchanged after the second generation.

Hardy 1908

At the same time and independently, what became known as the 'Hardy-Weinberg equilibrium' was set out by Wilhelm Weinberg in Germany (Weinberg 1908). Unlike Hardy, who was, according to Punnett, totally uninterested in genetics, Weinberg was a physician with a strong interest in all aspects of heredity. He also proposed the 'Weinberg method' for correcting for ascertainment bias in pedigree analysis by deducting the proband.

JBS HALDANE AND HUMAN GENETICS

The life of John Burdon Sanderson Haldane (1892–1964), known universally as 'JBS', was a remarkable one, even without genetics forming part of it, but it is fair to say that no other single person contributed as much worldwide in advancing the field of genetics in the period between the two world wars and extending up to 1960 (Figure 1.11). Many of his main contributions were based on human genetic disorders, even though he was himself not medically trained (indeed he admitted that he had no formal biological training or degree whatsoever). Some of these contributions are listed in Table 1.2.

Haldane also had a gift for expressing himself clearly and simply in articles for the general public on genetics and other topics, notably in his regular pieces for the Communist party newspaper, the *Daily Worker*. Always controversial and often inconsistent over political matters, he brought the field of genetics into the public eye in a way that has probably not been seen since. Despite this he was apparently a hopeless lecturer, according to some of his London University students, several of whom I was able to interview (see Appendix 2).

Haldane's early career was passed in the Cambridge biochemistry department headed by Frederick Gowland Hopkins, giving him a clear appreciation of the relationship of enzymes to genetics, but his ideas found fullest expression in the remarkable scientific environment of University College, London, where

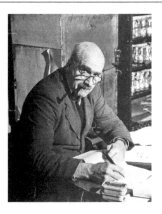

Figure 1.11 JBS Haldane (1892–1964). (Courtesy of Professor Peter Kalmus.)

Born in Oxford, son of the renowned physiologist John Scott Haldane, JBS Haldane studied Classics at Oxford, but had already begun his first experiments in genetics at home with his work on genetic linkage (then termed 'reduplication') in mice. He was severely wounded in World War I, and in 1923 joined the new Cambridge biochemistry department under Frederick Gowland Hopkins, also linking with Bateson's John Innes Institute. In 1933 he moved to University College, London, in a succession of Chairs, and remained based there (with an interruption from joining the International Brigade in the Spanish civil war) until 1957, when he moved to India for the last years of his life, which were shortened by colorectal cancer. Haldane's active political life as a communist party member was somehow combined with dangerous war-related submarine physiology research for the government during World War II. He eventually left the Party, after much prevarication, following the Russian suppression of genetics by Lysenko and Stalin. The biography by Clark (1968) gives a fascinating account of his colourful, contradictory, but scientifically highly important life and career.

Table 1.2 JBS Haldane: some contributions to human genetics

Mutation rate of a human gene (haemophilia), 1935
First human gene linkage (haemophilia, with Julia Bell), 1937
Use of linked markers in genetic prediction (1937)
Modifying genes in human inherited disorders (1941)
Selective advantage of sickle haemoglobin against malaria (1949)

workers at the Galton Laboratory (Julia Bell, RA Fisher, Lionel Penrose), and allied departments (Hans Grüneberg, John Maynard-Smith), as well as Lancelot Hogben at the neighbouring London School of Economics, gave full scope for interaction and debate, making it hard at times to assign a contribution to one person in particular. In my own interviews with a number of students of these workers during this period (see Appendix 2), an indication can be obtained of the atmosphere of this unique circle.

Haldane's special skill was to combine the data collected by others on human inherited disorders with his own mathematical abilities so as to extract every possible fragment of information on genetic problems that must at that time have seemed intractable, such as mutation rate (haemophilia and tuberous sclerosis) and genetic linkage (haemophilia again; see Chapter 12). He also laid the foundations for the 'formal analysis' of genetic disorders and, along with Fisher (see below), and Sewall Wright in America, for population genetic analysis. He predicted (1936) the future use of genetic linkage data for the presymptomatic testing of genetic disorders and suggested selective advantage as the reason for maintaining genetic polymorphism in sickle cell disease.

Two other British workers who, alongside Haldane, made major contributions to advancing genetics in the inter-war period were Ronald (RA) Fisher (Figure 1.12a) and Lancelot Hogben (Figure 1.12b). Both were highly skilled mathematically, and their work ranged over a wide variety of topics and species, including human genetics, though neither was medically trained. While they were no longer alive at the time of my recorded interview series, I was able to interview a number of their former students (see Appendix 2); their character, as with Haldane, emerges more clearly, perhaps, from these interviews than it might have done from direct interviews during their lifetime, though the numerous anecdotes have doubtless evolved over the years! It is interesting too, how these various students have reflected their mentors' characteristics and are often fiercely loyal to their reputations. Good biographies also exist, though those of Haldane (Clark 1968) and Hogben (Hogben and Hogben 1998) focus mainly on their wider life. Clark's book contains a complete bibliography of Haldane's remarkably varied writings. Fisher's biography is by his daughter Joan (Box 1978), herself a scientist.

Fisher, after some years based at the Rothamsted Agricultural Station, followed Karl Pearson in the Galton Chair at University College London (UCL) and in theory was a supporter of eugenics, though he quarrelled with the British Eugenics Society, whose policies he considered were unsound scientifically. Many of his statistical methods have continued in use for experimental analysis until

(a)

(b)

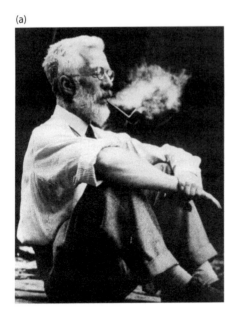

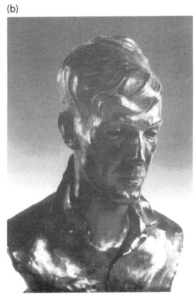

Figure 1.12 Two key figures in the inter-war period alongside JBS Haldane, Ronald A Fisher and Lancelot Hogben. Valuable accounts of their lives are given by Joan Box (1978), Fisher's daughter, and in an autobiography of Hogben edited by his children (Hogben and Hogben, 1998). **(a)** RA Fisher (1890–1962). (Courtesy of Dr Joan Box.) **(b)** Lancelot Hogben (1895–1975). Sculpture by Henry Meyerowitz, Capetown. (Courtesy University of Birmingham.)

the present, though his most original contribution was the formal demonstration, mentioned above, that mendelian and quantitative inheritance were compatible with each other. His mouse breeding work at the Galton Laboratory identified some of the first mutants that were later studied in detail by others such as Mary Lyon and her Harwell colleagues, while he also started a 'serum unit' that would be developed after the war by Robert Race as the Medical Research Council (MRC) Blood Group Unit (see Chapters 2 and 12).

Hogben was more broadly biologically orientated, working both on cytogenetics and on physiological topics, and later (in Birmingham) on the epidemiology of malformations. He was strongly opposed to eugenics, his influence, along with that of Penrose and Haldane, helping to ensure that it was kept out of the mainstream of British human genetics, thus allowing this to develop relatively 'uncontaminated' after the war.

EDINBURGH AND EARLY GENETICS

Edinburgh has a long and illustrious history in genetics, beginning a century ago in 1921 with the creation of the University's Institute of Animal Genetics, whose first Director Francis Crew (1886–1973) was medically trained but also had a lifelong interest in poultry breeding. After World War II he became Professor of

Public Health and Social Medicine in Edinburgh University. During the 1930s the Institute developed an international reputation, with workers such as Conrad Hal Waddington, pioneer of developmental genetics and epigenetics (see Chapter 11), and for a time JBS Haldane, Julian Huxley and Lancelot Hogben. All these people, including Waddington, were also major public and political figures outside the field of genetics, making a remarkable range of cultural contributions through their writing, lecturing and other public activities.

As described below, Edinburgh was the location for the ill-fated Seventh International Genetics Congress in August 1939, and during the war it gave refuge to such outstanding workers as Hermann Muller after his escape from Russia, Guido Pontecorvo from fascist Italy and Charlotte Auerbach from Berlin, who discovered chemical mutagenesis during this time (Auerbach and Robson 1946). But genetics research was badly disrupted by the war, with Crew himself in the forces and Waddington in London for war work unrelated to genetics.

Looking ahead a little, after the war the genetics departments became partly merged, under Waddington's leadership, with the newly created Agricultural Research Council's (ARC) genetics unit, and contained workers such as Douglas Falconer in quantitative genetics and Mary Lyon in mouse genetics, both of whom would have a major, if indirect influence on human and medical genetics (Falconer 1960). Falconer has written a valuable and amusing historical review of these early times (Falconer 1993) and the wise, even if unintended policy of the research council units in appointing able people and then leaving them alone, is apparent.

> No one 'directed' our work. The ARC itself seemed to take no interest in what we did, or what we achieved. Waddington, nominally our director, left us free to do what we each thought best. This was a wise policy, and it worked; I do not think that any of us wasted much time in doing the wrong things. And the freedom was greatly appreciated.

> *Falconer 1993*

The second world war had major disruptive effects on all scientific research unconnected with the war effort, including genetics, but the effects on Haldane, Fisher and Hogben illustrate graphically its impact on the careers and personal lives of people who were already established and well-known scientists in genetics.

Haldane had already, in 1936, left for Madrid to fight in the Spanish Civil War; it is not clear how much actual fighting he did (he was now nearly 50 and had been severely wounded in World War I), but on his return he found that the University authorities were trying to force him to resign. Ignoring this he not only continued working but became responsible for a programme of dangerous submarine research for the government, involving the effects of high pressure and oxygen deprivation, in which he involved his wife and some members of his

UCL unit, including Hans Kalmus, pioneer of sensory genetics, for whom he had earlier found a post as a Jewish refugee from Prague.

Fisher, like Haldane, found his Galton laboratory closed because the mouse stocks were considered a hazard in the event of bombing; he was even arrested, and a female assistant manhandled while trying to force an entry to his own unit. Moving to Cambridge, he was able to continue blood group research there, which moved back to London under Robert Race at the end of the war as already mentioned, while Fisher remained in Cambridge and continued his mouse genetics research.

Hogben, who was on Nazi death lists on account of his opposition to eugenics and Nazi policies generally, was invited in 1940 to address the Norwegian Genetics Society, but the morning after his lecture his return to Britain was prevented by the German invasion of Norway, which had begun overnight. He and his daughter managed with difficulty, as recounted in his autobiography, published by his children (Hogben and Hogben 1998), to cross into neutral Sweden, where they found refuge with fellow geneticist Otto Dahlberg, also a staunch anti-eugenicist, but he was unable to move further except by entering Russia, by now an ally, and travelling via the Trans-Siberian Railway to Japan (not yet in the war) and then America, eventually returning to Aberdeen to find that his university post had been abolished in his absence!

It is good to reflect on these, and worse, experiences affecting the geneticists of these troubled times; those of us making our careers in post-war western Europe can consider ourselves fortunate indeed to have avoided such traumas (so far at least) and I have tried to put some of this on record in a recent article (Harper 2017).

EUGENICS IN THE UK

In a book focusing on genetics and medicine after World War II, and on contributions from Britain, the early and international aspects of eugenics cannot be dealt with in any detail. Fortunately, historians have analysed the subject fully (though until recently at the expense of almost ignoring the rest of human and medical genetics), while I have tried to assess its significance for modern medical genetics in my own *Short History of Medical Genetics* (2008). The book of Kevles remains the clearest and most balanced account overall. The archives of the UK *Eugenics Society* (founded in 1907 as the *Eugenics Education Society*), are now kept at the Wellcome Library and have been partly digitised.

We have seen that Francis Galton coined the word 'eugenics'; he considered the most important aspect to be encouraging those of high intelligence to have larger families (so-called positive eugenics) more than discouraging the less talented. His views, in contrast with his counterparts in America, who stressed 'negative eugenics', especially in relation to the segregation and later the sterilisation of the 'feeble minded', received very little political or wider social support. (A bill to enforce sterilisation of the mentally handicapped was rejected by Parliament in 1931 and subsequently.) His principal followers in the early twentieth century, such as Karl Pearson and subsequently RA Fisher, were more concerned with theoretical aspects, leading to considerable feuding, especially in relation to the more 'campaigning eugenics' approach pursued by the Eugenics Society, under the leadership of Leonard Darwin, youngest son of Charles Darwin, whose influence deserves more critical attention than it has so far received. The book of Pauline Mazumdar (1992) gives a full account of the evolution and decline of the Eugenics Society. Although she notes its low profile as a 'minor learned society' following its name change to 'Galton Institute', it still acts as a focus for the political aspects of eugenics, involving issues of class and race, that have dogged the whole topic from its inception. It is of interest that the topic of eugenics has attracted people from both 'left' and 'right' of the political spectrum. To my knowledge, neither the UK Eugenics Society nor its successor has ever formally disowned or apologised for the abuses committed 'in the name of eugenics' that it was associated with during the first half of the twentieth century.

THE MEDICAL RESEARCH COUNCIL HUMAN GENETICS COMMITTEE

Although the various MRC Units relating to genetics were only established in the post-war years, as described in the next chapter, there was strong interest from the MRC considerably earlier. In early 1932 it established a 'Human Genetics Committee' which met a total of 14 times between 1932 and 1939, assessing grant proposals on a wide range of human and medical genetics topics. The committee's minutes are archived with other MRC material at the British National Archives, Kew, London (see Appendix 2). The committee was an impressive one; chaired by JBS Haldane (who apparently forget to turn up at one meeting); members also included Lancelot Hogben, RA Fisher, Julia Bell, Lionel Penrose and Edward Cockayne (dermatologist and author of the book *Genetic Disorders of the Skin*). John Fraser Roberts was soon co-opted to further strengthen the clinical expertise, while A Bradford Hill, chief statistician at MRC, was also invited to attend. There was not a hint of eugenics and the evaluation of applications was rigorous.

The committee seems to have lapsed with the outbreak of war in 1939 but its very existence at this early time is an indicator of the high ranking of human genetics in British science during the 1930s; nothing equivalent existed in America or elsewhere in the world. And the work of the committee provided firm foundations for the resumption of sound human genetics research once the war was over, as well as for the subsequent development of medical genetics.

Thus by the end of the 1930s, as we have seen, human genetics as a science, and genetics as a whole, had developed strong foundations, to which British workers, many but not all of them medical, had made special contributions. The close links between scientists and clinicians, and the institutional support of bodies like the MRC and the Royal Society of Medicine, held real promise for fruitful applications of genetics to medicine in the near future. But sadly, the world as a whole was on the edge of a precipice that would destroy most of these hopes until peace and sanity could to some extent begin to return at the end of the war.

It is ironic that the Seventh International Genetics Congress, successor to the ill-fated congress that should have been held in Moscow two years previously, now took place in Edinburgh in August 1939, on the very eve of World War II. Francis Crew was organiser, with the President's chair left empty, as the previously elected President, Nikolai Vavilov, had been arrested in Russia and it was not known whether he was even still alive. The Congress had to finish early, with many delegates anxious to return home before the outbreak of war made travel difficult or impossible. Its final act was to issue what has become known as 'The Geneticists' Manifesto'. Organised by Hermann Muller, who was working in Edinburgh after fleeing Stalin's Russia, along with Haldane and Crew, the 'Manifesto', responding to a somewhat naive question posed to the Congress on 'genetic improvement', stated clearly that this was dependent on the resolution of more urgent social and economic problems, including racism, economic inequality and deprivation, the position of women, contraception, abortion and education of the population, as well as the prevention of war (Anon 1939).

In this defiant spirit the international genetics community made it clear to the world at large that it saw genetics as part of future progress not only in science, but for society as a whole.

Not all Congress delegates had a safe return; some of the Polish delegation, their country now invaded and divided by both Germany and Russia, remained in Edinburgh for the rest of their lives. The ship *Athene*, carrying many of the American delegation, was torpedoed and sunk a few days after the end of the Congress, though fortunately most passengers were rescued by another ship also carrying participants. And so international links and collaborations in genetics were largely destroyed or suspended for the next six years.

REFERENCES

Adams J. 1814. *A Treatise on the Supposed Hereditary Properties of Diseases.* London: Callow.

Anon. 1939. Men and Mice at Edinburgh. Reports from the Genetics Congress. *J Hered.* 30: 371–4.

Arnott A. 1833. Thirty one fractures in one and the same individual. *London Medical Gazette.* 12:366.

Auerbach C, Robson JM. 1946. Chemical production of mutations. *Nature.* 157:302.

Bateson B. 1928a. *William Bateson, FRS, Naturalist: His Essays and Addresses, together with a Short Account of His Life.* Cambridge: Cambridge University Press.

Bateson B (ed.). 1928b. *Letters from the Steppe.* London: Methuen.

Bateson W. 1894. *Materials for the Study of Variation.* Cambridge: Cambridge University Press.

Bateson W. 1906. An address on mendelian heredity and its application to man. *Brain.* 29:157–79.

Bateson W. 1909. *Mendel's Principles of Heredity.* Cambridge: Cambridge University Press. (Reprinted as part of The Classics of Medicine Library by Leslie B. Adams Jr., Birmingham, AL, 1990.)

Bateson W, Saunders E. 1902. Experimental studies in the physiology of heredity. *Reports to the Evolution Committee, Royal Society.* 1:133–4.

Bell J. 1931. Hereditary optic atrophy (Leber's disease). In: Pearson K (ed.). *Treasury of Human Inheritance*, vol. 2, part 4. London: Cambridge University Press; 325–423.

Bell J. 1934. Huntington's chorea. In: Fisher RA (ed.). *Treasury of Human Inheritance*, vol. 4, part 1. London: Cambridge University Press; 1–67.

Bell J. 1947. Dystrophia myotonica and allied diseases. In: Penrose LS (ed.). *Treasury of Human Inheritance*, vol. 4, part 5. London: Cambridge University Press; 343–410.

Bell J, Haldane JBS. 1937. The linkage between the genes for colour-blindness and haemophilia in man. *Proc R Soc Lond B*. 123:119–50.

Box JF. 1978. *R. A. Fisher: The Life of a Scientist*. New York: Wiley.

Bulmer W. 2003. *Francis Galton: Pioneer of Heredity and Biometry*. Baltimore: Johns Hopkins University Press.

Bundey S. 1996. Julia Bell (1879–1979): Steam boat lady, statistician and geneticist. *J Med Biol*. 4:8–13.

Carlisle A. 1814. An account of a family having hands and feet with supernumerary fingers and toes. *Phil Trans*. 104:94–101.

Castle WE. 1903. Note on Mr Farabee's observations. *Science*. 17:75–6.

Clark RW. 1968. *JBS: The Life and Work of JBS Haldane*. Oxford: Oxford University Press.

Cooper W. 1857. Microphthalmos. *Royal London Ophthalmic Hospital Reports*. 1:110–6.

Dalton J. 1798. Extraordinary facts relating to the vision of colours: With observations. *Memoirs of the Literary and Philosophical Society of Manchester*. 5:28–45.

Darwin C. 1868. *The Variation of Animals and Plants under Domestication*. London: John Murray.

Darwin C. 1890. *The Variation of Animals and Plants under Domestication*, 2nd ed. London: John Murray.

Digby K. 1645. *Two Treatises: In the One of which, The Nature of Bodies, In the other, The Nature of Man's Soule, Is Looked Into: In Way Of Discovery Of The Immortality of Reasonable Soules*. London: John Williams; 266.

Duchenne GBA. 1868. Recherches sur la paralysie musculaire pseudo-hypertrophique ou paralysie myo-sclérosique. *Arch Gén Méd*. 11:5–25, 179–209, 305–21, 421–33, 552–8. (From translated works by Poore GV 1883. Selections from the Clinical Works of Dr Duchenne de Boulogne. London:New Sydenham Society.)

Emery AEH. 1989. Joseph Adams (1756–1818). *J Med Genet*. 26:116–8.

Emery AEH, Emery MLH. 1995. *The History of a Genetic Disease, Duchenne Muscular Dystrophy or Meryon's Disease*. London: Royal Society of Medicine Press.

Falconer DS. 1960. *Quantitative Genetics*. Edinburgh: Oliver and Boyd.

Falconer D. 1993. Quantitative Genetics in Edinburgh: 1947–1980. *Genetics*. 133:137–42.

Farabee WC. 1905. Inheritance of digital malformations in man. *Papers of the Peabody Museum*. 3:69–77.

Fisher RA. 1918. The correlation between relatives on the supposition of mendelian inheritance. *Trans R S Edinb*. 52:399–433.

Galton F. 1872. Statistical inquiries into the efficacy of prayer. *Fortnightly Review.* 12:125–35.

Galton F. 1898. A diagram of heredity. *Nature.* 57:293.

Garrod A. 1901. About alkaptonuria. *Lancet.* 2:1484–6.

Garrod A. 1902. The incidence of alkaptonuria: A study in chemical individuality. *Lancet.* 2:1616–20.

Garrod A. 1908. The Croonian Lectures on inborn errors of metabolism. *Lancet.* 2:1–7, 73–79, 142–8, 214–20.

Garrod AE. 1909. *Inborn Errors of Metabolism.* London: Henry Frowde, Oxford University Press, Hodder & Stoughton.

Gilham NW. 2001. *Sir Francis Galton: From African Exploration to the Birth of Eugenics.* Oxford: Oxford University Press.

Haldane JBS. 1935. The rate of spontaneous mutation of a human gene. *J Genet.* 31:317–26.

Haldane JBS. 1947. The mutation rate of the gene for haemophilia, and its segregation ratios in males and females. *Ann Eugen.* 13:262–71.

Haldane JBS. 1948. The formal genetics of man. *Proc R Soc London B.* 153:147–70.

Haldane JBS, Penrose L. 1935. Mutation rates in man. *Nature.* 136:432.

Hamilton A. 1827. Hairy men; white Negroes. *London Medical Repository and Review.* 5:266–7.

Hardy GH. 1908. Mendelian proportions in a mixed population. *Science.* 28:49–50.

Harper PS. 2006. Julia Bell and the Treasury of Human Inheritance. *Hum Genet.* 116:422–32.

Harper PS. 2008. *A Short History of Medical Genetics.* New York: Oxford University Press.

Harper PS. 2012. Victor McKusick and the history of medical genetics. In: Dronamraju K, Francomano C (eds.). *Victor McKusick and the History of Medical Genetics.* New York: Springer, pp. 145–161.

Harper PS. 2017. Human genetics in troubled times and places. *Hereditas.* 155:7.

Harvey W. 1651. *Exercitationis de Generatione Animalium.* London. (Translated by Robert Willis. Sydenham Society, 1847.)

Harvey W. 1652. *Letter to Dr. Vlackweld, Haarlem.* Reprinted in Willis R (ed.). 1848. The Works of William Harvey. London: Sydenham Society; 616.

Hay J. 1813. Account of a remarkable haemorrhagic disposition, existing in many individuals of the same family. *N Engl J Med.* 2:221–5.

Hogben A, Hogben A (eds.). 1998. *Lancelot Hogben, Scientific Humanist: An Unauthorised Autobiography.* Woodbridge, Suffolk, UK: Merlin Press.

Hunt DM, Dolai KS, Bowmaker JK, Mollon JD. 1995. The chemistry of John Dalton's colour-blindness. *Science.* 267:984–8.

Kevles DJ. 1985. *In the Name of Eugenics: Genetics and the Uses of Human Heredity.* New York: Knopf.

Machin J. 1732. An uncommon case of distempered skin. *Philos Trans R Soc.* 37: 299–300.

Marie J. 2004. *The Importance of Place: A History of Genetics in 1930s Britain.* PhD thesis in history and philosophy of science, University College, London.

Mazumdar PMH. 1992. *Eugenics, Human Genetics and Human Failings.* London: Routledge.

McGrayne SB. 2012. *The Theory That Would Not Die.* New Haven: Yale University Press.

Mendel G. 1866. Versuche über Pflanzen-hybriden [Experiments on plant hybrids]. In: *Proceedings of the Natural History Society of Brünn (Verhandlung des Naturforscheden Vereines in Brünn).* 4:3–47.

Meryon E. 1852. On granular and fatty degeneration of the voluntary muscles. *Medico- Chirurgical Transactions.* 35:73–84.

Motulsky AG. 1959. Joseph Adams (1756–1818): A forgotten founder of medical genetics. *Arch Intern Med.* 104:490–6.

Needham J. 1931. *Chemical Embryology.* Volume 1. Cambridge: Cambridge University Press.

Osborne J. 1835. Account of a haemorrhagic diathesis existing in a family, and also a peculiar appearance of the iris belonging to a family. *Dublin Journal of Medicine and Chemical Sciences.* 7:32–5.

Otto JC. 1803. An account of an haemorrhagic disposition existing in certain families. *Medical Repository.* 6:1–4.

Pearson K (ed.). 1912. *Treasury of Human Inheritance*, vol. 1. London: Dulau.

Pearson K. 1914. *The Life, letters and labours of Francis Galton.* Cambridge: Cambridge University Press.

Penrose LS, Stern C. 1958. Reconsideration of the Lambert pedigree (ichthyosis hystrix gravior). *Ann Hum Genet.* 22(3):258–83.

Punnett RC. 1950. Early days of genetics. *Heredity.* 4:1–10.

Royal Society of Medicine. 1909. The influence of heredity on disease, with specific reference to tuberculosis, cancer and diseases of the nervous system. *Proceedings of the Royal Society of Medicine.* pp. 9–142.

Rushton AR. 2008. *Royal Maladies: Inherited Diseases in the Ruling Houses of Europe.* Victoria, British Columbia: Trafford Publishing.

Rushton AR. 2009. *Genetics and Medicine in Great Britain, 1600–1939.* Bloomington, IN: Trafford Publishing.

Saunders JC. 1811. *A Treatise on some Practical Points Relating to Diseases of the Eye.* London: Longman, p. 134.

Stevens NM. 1905. *Studies in Spermatogenesis with Especial Reference to the Accessory Chromosome.* Publication No. 6. Washington, DC: Carnegie Institute of Washington.

Thadani KI. 1921. The 'Bhudas' of India - a case of sex-linked inheritance. *J Hered.* 12:87–8.

Thomson J. 1858. On the comparative influence of the male and female parent upon progeny. *Edinburgh Medical Journal.* 4:501–4.

Wafer L. 1699. *A New Voyage and Description of the Isthmus of America.* London: James Knopton.

Walker A. 1839. *Intermarriage.* New York: Langley.

Weinberg W. 1908. Über den nachsweis der vererbung beim menschen. *Jahreshefte des Vereins für Vaterländische Naturkunde in Württenberg, Stuttgart.* 64:368–82.

Wilson EB. 1911. The sex chromosomes. *Mikrosk Anat Entwicklungsmech.* 77:249–71.

2

The founders of post-war British medical genetics

ABSTRACT

Human genetics became a specific field of scientific research soon after the end of World War II, with the appointment of Lionel Penrose as head of the London Galton Laboratory. Together with a remarkable series of other workers at University College London, Penrose's unit became the focus for those from Britain and many other countries wishing to train in human genetics, who in turn provided the foundation for specifically medical genetics research in their own units. Parallel to this, a series of Medical Research Council units was founded, largely to understand the genetic risks of radiation, a topic of special concern following the development of nuclear weapons. Two of these, at Edinburgh and Harwell, pioneered techniques for studying human chromosomes and were responsible for discovery of the first chromosome disorders from 1959 onwards. MRC units at Oxford and Institute of Child Health, London, initiated systematic clinical and family studies of genetic disorders, led by Alan Stevenson and John Fraser Roberts. Elsewhere, the Paediatric Research Unit at Guy's Hospital, London under Paul Polani and the Liverpool Medical Genetics Institute under Cyril Clarke developed clinically orientated research that established medical genetics as a well-defined part of both paediatric and adult medicine.

For Britain, as for almost all of the rest of Europe, World War II marked an enforced break in medical research, apart from that directly related to the war, and genetics was no exception. There were small islands of genetic progress, such as Charlotte Auerbach's discovery of chemical mutagenesis (see below), but even though most British scientists, such as JBS Haldane, Conrad Waddington and Max Perutz, were co-opted into war-related research, rather than sent to the battlefield as in the previous world war, their work was mostly on topics far removed from genetics.

Some, notably Haldane, undertook dangerous submarine physiology; others, such as Francis Crew and John Fraser Roberts, went directly into the army or civil defence forces. Hans Kalmus, originally from Prague and now at University College London, thanks to Haldane's efforts to find posts for Jewish refugees, was co-opted by Haldane into the submarine research; he was also stimulated to write his popular (Pelican) book on genetics in 1942, as a response to a fellow London air-raid watcher who had complained to him while they were on night watch together that he could never understand the subject. Some others, such as Paul Polani (later at Guy's Hospital), and Ursula Mittwoch (later with Penrose at the Galton Laboratory), were interned as 'enemy aliens' in the Isle of Man internment camp, as was chemist and future molecular biologist Max Perutz, who has left a memorable account of this chapter of events in his essay *Enemy Alien* (Perutz 1998). Being a young girl did not make Ursula Mittwoch, recently arrived from Berlin with her family, exempt, as can be seen in my interview with her:

UM: 1940. Well that was a cue to intern certain aliens, certain foreigners.

PSH: Oh yes.

UM: OK. Now my parents had been exempt from internment because at the beginning of the war they went before a tribunal and they were exempt. Well, I hadn't been before a tribunal because I wasn't 16 and then of course I was 16 just before and so that was bad luck.

PSH: Oh dear.

UM: So I went to the Isle of Man and my younger sister was jealous, she wanted to, she liked to travel but she had to stay at home and I went off for about 9 weeks and then, you know, they brought this sort of category of, I don't know, children, teenagers or whatever and they brought them back. But it didn't do my schooling any good.

PSH: I had no idea that women were sent to the Isle of Man as well. I imagined it was just men who were involved with that.

UM: Far more men went than women, but it depended to a certain extent, people who lived on the south coast were more likely to be interned than those who lived in London. Anyway neither of my parents were interned. You know the aliens, they got certain categories. Those who were interned immediately. Those free of internment and then there were the in-betweens. So my parents were exempt from internment altogether. And I was the intermediate one. Of course I hadn't been before a tribunal, but I thought it was logical, I didn't protest against it.

PSH: Everyone I have spoken to has been amazingly tolerant of this process. People like Paul Polani and Max Perutz seem to have been, to my mind, extraordinarily tolerant of what they were put through.

UM: Oh I don't know. There was a war on and people didn't know what they know now and so on, and officials had to do their jobs.

Interview with Ursula Mittwoch 02/03/2004 [07]

In America there was less of a discontinuity, with research able to carry on in a limited way. In much of continental Europe, of course, human genetics had hardly begun to exist when war broke out, while in Russia, where it was well developed, it had already been virtually destroyed by Stalin. Even in Scandinavia the strong early developments in classical genetics, both human and more generally in agriculture, had to struggle against a local 'fifth column' of Nazi supporting eugenicists, with only neutral Sweden able to continue after other Scandinavian countries had been invaded and occupied. Nazi eugenics, already largely discredited across most of Europe, was able to continue its abuses unchecked throughout the period of the third Reich.

But when the war was over and normal scientific life could begin to resume, was genetics, especially human genetics and the nascent medical genetics, fundamentally different from what was being carried out before the war? Or did those already in genetics just pick up the threads and continue to develop their work?

So far as Britain is concerned, there was indeed a new start after the war. None of the major pre-war workers, apart from Ronald Fisher, had been proponents of eugenics, in contrast to many in America; Penrose and Hogben had been outspoken in their opposition to it, while the Eugenics Society had lost most of its influence.

Nevertheless, human genetics in post-war Britain might have remained under suspicion as still connected with eugenics and the Nazi abuses had it not been for the pivotal influence of one man, Lionel Penrose, and his followers, both British and from other countries. I make no excuses for emphasising his role here, as the person who, more than anyone else, was responsible for determining the shape of British human genetics and, though less directly, what would over the coming decades become medical genetics.

A FRESH START: PENROSE AND THE GALTON LABORATORY

Penrose had already in the 1930s become a major figure in British human genetics, as we have seen in Chapter 1; his now classic 'Colchester study' (Penrose 1938) on a hospital population of mentally handicapped people, had been supported by the MRC and he was a member of its Human Genetics Committee (Figure 2.1). But when World War II shut down all research and other academic work other than that directly related to the war, Penrose, who was a Quaker and pacifist, chose to stay in Canada, where he had been visiting with his family; here he became Director of Psychiatric Research for the province of Ontario and remained there, based in London, Ontario, for the next six years. This was something that upset some British colleagues, including those at Colchester (see page 50), but in 1945 he was nonetheless appointed Galton Professor of Eugenics at University College London, in succession to RA Fisher. JBS Haldane was apparently the key influence, having remarked:

> I think that you and I are the British people under 60 who have contributed most to human genetics, and therefore one of us should have the chair. As you have specialised on man and I have not, your claim is somewhat greater.

Kevles 1985, p. 213

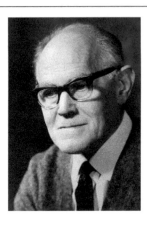

Figure 2.1 Lionel Sharples Penrose (1898–1972). (Courtesy of Shirley Hodgson.)

Lionel Penrose was born into a Quaker family in London and, as a pacifist, served in the Friends Ambulance Unit during the first world war. After attending Cambridge University and qualifying in medicine, he married fellow student Margaret Leathes and decided to train in psychiatry. In 1930 he was appointed by the Medical Research Council to undertake a detailed study of the mentally handicapped patients at the Colchester Institution, which took seven years to complete, being published in 1938 as the now classical 'Colchester Study'. After spending the war years in Canada he returned to Britain in 1945 as Galton Professor of Eugenics (later Human Genetics) until retirement in 1965 (at that time compulsory aged 67 at London University), when he moved his mental handicap research to Harperbury Hospital, continuing it there up to the time of his death. Sadly, no scientific biography of Penrose has yet been written; the small book compiled from the symposium to mark the centenary of his birth (Povey, 1998) best captures the spirit of the man and the environment of the Galton Laboratory.

Penrose was determined from the outset to remove all vestiges of eugenics from the Galton Laboratory, though it took him until 1963 to change the title of his Chair from 'Professor of Eugenics' to 'Professor of Human Genetics'. *Annals of Eugenics* became *Annals of Human Genetics* in 1954, and ties with the Eugenics Society were dissolved. The unit focused exclusively on human genetics research (Penrose's predecessor RA Fisher had done numerous mouse studies) and the only direct continuity with pre-war work was Julia Bell's *Treasury of Human Inheritance*, which continued till 1958, with Julia Bell herself outliving Penrose as well as his predecessors.

Penrose gave his inaugural lecture on January 21, 1946, using as a paradigm for human genetics the disorder phenylketonuria (Penrose 1946). Although discovered by the Norwegian chemical pathologist Asbjörn Fölling (Fölling 1934), Penrose had found several affected individuals in his Colchester study population and actually suggested the name 'phenylketonuria'; he used the disorder to show how human genetics might develop, including possible future therapies, which he lived to see realised. He also showed as a fallacy the possibility of preventing the disorder by sterilising heterozygous carriers for this recessively inherited disorder:

> The frequency of carriers of the gene is double the gene frequency, because the gene may be on either one of a pair of chromosomes. Hence, the frequency of carriers in this country is

of the order of 1 in 100. To eliminate the gene from the racial stock would involve sterilising 1% of the normal population, if carriers could be identified. Only a lunatic would advocate such a procedure to prevent the occurrence of a handful of harmless imbeciles. Sterilisation of the affected imbeciles would do no good, except in the very rare cases where they might be expected to have offspring. The attempt to reduce the frequency of the genes by assuming close relations of affected cases to be carriers and sterilising them necessarily involves many errors. Such a plan would leave far the largest reservoir of genes -that in the general population -untouched.

In spite of the alleged interest taken in the subject of hereditary disease in Germany, no search for phenylketonurics has been reported there. If such a search had been instituted, a curious situation might have arisen; for, up to the present time, no phenylketonuric of Jewish origin has been discovered though cases of German, Irish, Italian, Slavonic, and Dutch origin were found in the USA. Moreover, there were no cases found among American negroes. This ... is a somewhat refreshing change from that presented by Tay-Sachs disease (the infantile form of amaurotic idiocy), whose incidence is almost confined to Jewish communities. A sterilisation programme to control phenylketonuria confined to the so-called Aryans would hardly have appealed to the recently overthrown government of Germany.

Penrose 1946

In addition to his inaugural lecture, Penrose gave a highly critical address in 1949 to the Eugenics Society itself; although titled 'the Galton Laboratory: its work and aims' it also was an indictment of much of what the Eugenics Society had previously been doing (Penrose 1949).

Penrose's own core group of workers at the Galton Laboratory was not large, but included, at various times, Cedric (CAB) Smith as statistician, James Renwick in genetic linkage analysis (see Chapter 12), Sylvia Lawler, Harry Harris (later to return as Penrose's successor), Elizabeth (Bette) Robson, Ursula Mittwoch (interview [07]) and Hans Kalmus, founder of the field of sensory genetics. Some of these are shown in Figure 2.2.

But what made the Galton such a unique centre during the 1950s and 1960s was the constant stream of visiting workers and research students coming from all over the world for periods varying from a few months to several years, some of whom are listed later in Table 9.1. For Americans, including Arno Motulsky, Victor McKusick, Barton Childs and Orlando J Miller, it became almost a 'rite of passage' to spend a period of time at the Galton, in much the same way as the next generation would see a flow in the reverse direction, in particular to Victor McKusick's unit in Baltimore. American visitors in particular found the stimulating yet relaxed atmosphere a refreshing contrast to scientific centres in

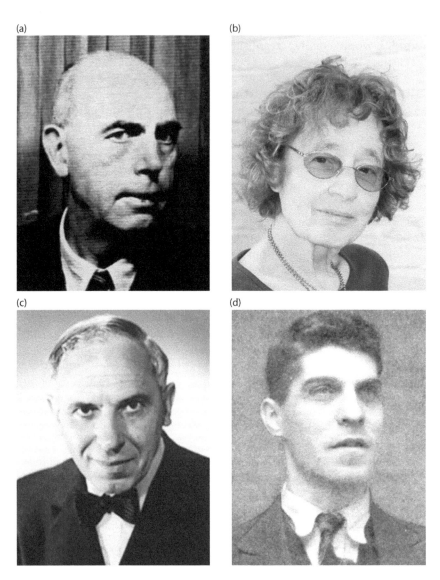

Figure 2.2 Early post-war workers at the Galton Laboratory. **(a)** Cedric AB Smith (1917–2002), key mathematician and statistician at the Galton Laboratory. This rare photograph comes from the website *squares.net* which also contains interesting details on his life written by Newton Morton and Steve Jones. **(b)** Ursula Mittwoch (born 1924), early worker on human sex differentiation. (Courtesy of Ursula Mittwoch and Genetics and Medicine Historical Network.) **(c)** Harry Harris (1919–1994) Successor to Penrose and among the first to study inherited variation in enzymes. (Courtesy of University of Pennsylvania Archives.) **(d)** Hans Kalmus (1906–1988) Pioneer of sensory genetics at the Galton Laboratory and one of the numerous refugees from Nazi controlled Europe who enriched British science. The photograph is taken from the rear cover of his book, *Genetics* (Pelican), which he wrote while on night patrol watch during the war (see Page 32).

their own country, as recounted by Barton Childs, from Johns Hopkins Hospital, who spent a year there in 1952:

> The opportunity at The Galton Laboratory in the early 1950's was unique. The breadth and depth of the Galtonians' grasp of genetics and human biology, and the lack of structure that allowed a student (like me) time for reading and contemplation, provided the wherewithal to go on in whatever direction seemed compatible with temperament and interests. Those were leisurely days, but leisure did not mean waster, it might mean thoughtful. I was conscious of great privilege in participating in life at The Galton. Am I an old fool in wishing there could be more such opportunities today? I hope not.

The same was true for Arno Motulsky a few years later, in 1957–1958:

> Intellectual life was very different for someone used to the task-driven atmosphere of an American medical school. One could spend one's time reading, studying, writing, talking, arguing and soaking up the intellectual atmosphere of human genetics. The building's inside temperature in winter became quite cold and we sometimes wore an overcoat when working at the desk.

Both these quotations are taken from the centenary celebration of Penrose's birth in 1998 (Povey 1998). An interview with Sue Povey in 2008 [71], herself one of the key later members of the Galton Laboratory, gives a valuable account of the generation of workers there, mainly involved in gene mapping, who followed Penrose.

Many of the future continental European leaders in the field also did their initial training at the Galton and absorbed much of Penrose's philosophy. These hugely important international links are described further in Chapter 9. Likewise, a number of future medical geneticists across Britain started their career there under Penrose's influence.

Penrose and his wife also provided hospitality to a number of workers who needed it, such as Herman vanden Berghe, from Leuven;

> … when I got there the first day, he asked me, where do you stay? I said well, for the moment I am looking along Tottenham Court Road to see if I can find a small room here and then he said 'no, no'. I said why not? And he said 'you stay with me. I have a large home with 14 bedrooms. There is only one condition. You have to play chess with me every night'. I stayed with him and played chess......
> But we would be sitting there over this chess board and he would be talking genetics, teaching genetics to me and we would have one game and then after an hour or two hours he would say 'By the way, I am taking your queen'.

Interview with Herman Vanden Berghe 01/06/2007 [66]

Renata Laxova [55] and her family arrived in more traumatic circumstances from Brno after the Russian invasion of Czechoslovakia and were likewise welcomed by the Penroses, as she describes in her autobiography (Laxova 2001) and in a memorable article, written after Penrose's death and quoted in Chapter 9.

The reputation and primacy of the Galton Laboratory during these post-war years cannot be attributed to any special ability of Penrose to organise or to communicate. As Paul Polani noted (see later in this chapter), 'you had to pick pearls as they dropped out of his mouth'. Any organisation was due not to Penrose himself but to his highly efficient (and also protective) departmental secretary and assistant Helen Lang-Brown, who gained the affectionate label of 'the Cerberus'. Such unsung heroines of many famous academic departments deserve recognition and attention from historians. Male research students apparently found that the best way to avoid this barrier and have an unscheduled meeting with Penrose was to place some comfortable chairs inside the vestibule of the men's toilet and have a discussion there!

A further important factor was the existence of a circle of outstanding people at University College who were not formally part of the Galton Laboratory but who linked closely with it, thus expanding the range of laboratory and theoretical areas available to those research students not deciding to do a project directly with Penrose himself. Key people in this respect included JBS Haldane, already mentioned in Chapter 1, until his departure for India in 1957; Hans Grüneberg (genetics of mouse malformations, see Chapter 4), John Maynard Smith (evolutionary biology), Hans Kalmus (Figure 2.2d), like Grüneberg a refugee from fascism, and Charles Dent (metabolic physician at nearby University College Hospital), with whom Charles Scriver from Montreal mainly worked while attached to the Galton lab [56].

The Medical Research Council's Blood Group Unit, which grew out of Fisher's pre-war Serum Unit, begun at the Galton Laboratory in 1935, was directed by Robert Race between 1946 and 1973 and later by his colleague and wife Ruth Sanger; it was also a key element for the long running gene mapping research programme (see Figure 2.3 and also Chapter 12) that was central to much of the Galton Laboratory work. This unit has recently been well documented historically (Bangham 2014) and there is extensive archival material on the unit at the Wellcome Library and on its website (see Appendix 2). Its exceptionally collaborative attitude gave great encouragement to numerous younger workers in the field, especially clinicians (including myself), with potentially valuable family material.

One area that was virtually unrepresented at the Galton Laboratory up to 1960 was human or mammalian cytogenetics, which largely developed elsewhere, as described later in the chapter. Those who did try to

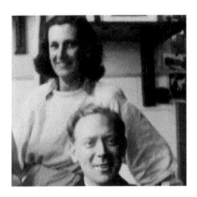

Figure 2.3 Robert Race (1907–1984) and Ruth Sanger (1918–2001), photograph 1947. (Courtesy of Wellcome Library.)

establish this, such as Ursula Mittwoch and Joy Delhanty (see interviews [07] and [25]), were hampered in the early years by lack of equipment and inadequate facilities.

My interview with Anthony Searle [19], later one of the key Harwell geneticists along with Mary Lyon and Bruce Cattanach, provides a good example of these wider links, in his case with Haldane and Grüneberg; he came as an older student to University College London in 1946, after four years in a Japanese prisoner-of-war camp.

> …. he [Haldane] suggested it would be a very interesting possibility to study the population genetics of cats because of the fact, and this is where the Lyon hypothesis comes in, they had a sex-linked gene for yellow or orange coat colour, and the heterozygote could easily be distinguished because it was a tortoiseshell, and so he took me out, of course I knew nothing about the genetics of cats, and we went around local streets near University College London and he would tell me tabby, striped tabby, blotched tabby and so on and of course tortoiseshells and various other easily distinguishable visible genotypes. And then after that, … I had the job of examining hundreds of dead cats you see, which had been killed by the various wildlife … 'rescue centres'. So-called animal rescue centres who had the job of killing off all the stray cats.
>
> PSH: That's a good sample.
> AS: And as a result I was able to show, and this is my first paper, 'Gene frequencies in London's Cats' [Searle, 1949] and this is 50 years, no, more than that, 55 years ago, published in the *Journal of Genetics*. And that was, as I say, almost due entirely to JBS Haldane. ….it was one of Haldane's ideas, one of the first papers on this sort of thing, mammalian population genetics, and so lots of people all over the world started looking at their cat population and I was able to show that they mated more or less at random which, you see, certainly it wouldn't be so if you tried it on dogs of some breed or other.
>
> *Interview with Anthony Searle 11/10/2004 [19]*

Searle went on to earn a PhD at UCL with Hans Grüneberg, who he found 'straightforward' but 'very pedantic'; this time the work was on mouse mutants:

> I felt a safer bet was Grüneberg, you see, the great mouse geneticist who had already written a book about mouse genetics, which amazed me that so much was known on the genetics of mice. And so I decided for that reason to work with him, but the most people in a group I suppose was the Penrose group. It was much bigger and we used to meet up with them and various geneticists, the

ones with Grüneberg and so on, we'd all meet up together. So it was obviously a very good group to be in with lots of interesting people there really, and so then I did my degree on zoology with genetics as a special subject.

Caroline Berry (see Chapter 3), who later developed clinical genetics in Paul Polani's unit, earned a PhD with Grüneberg too, on a more anthropological topic:

CB: We dug up the skulls at St Ninian's [Shetland]. I feel, looking back, it wasn't really a very nice thing to do.
PSH: When you say you dug up the skulls, was this the human skulls or the mouse skulls?
CB: I did all humans, you see. Sam [her husband RJ Berry] did the mice and I did the humans.
PSH: I got the wrong end of the stick. I thought you were doing the mouse craniums.
CB: Oh no no no. I did the humans. It was all human.
PSH: Right. You know I had forgotten about St Ninian's. You probably wouldn't be allowed to do that now would you? It wouldn't get through an ethical committee or anything would it?
CB: And we stacked them all up in somebody's barn. You know, thinking back I wonder what they thought.

Interview with Caroline Berry 14/10/2004 [20]

My interview series contains numerous examples of the influence and character of this remarkable group of workers, who collectively played such a large role in shaping post-war human genetics, and in training many of the first medical geneticists. Penrose in particular inspired a deep loyalty among those who had worked with him, whether they were from Britain or from other European countries. As Jean Frézal (Paris) put it simply when I interviewed him in France:

PSH: ...which person in your career has had the biggest influence on the development of your work? Can you identify one person, especially?
JF: Penrose.
PSH: That's very interesting.
JF: Penrose. I was very influenced by Penrose's spirit you know.
PSH: So many people who I have talked with have named Penrose in this way. He was a very inspirational person.
JF: Absolutely.

Interview with Jean Frézal 22/04/2005 [44]

Other pioneers across continental Europe deeply influenced by Penrose included Jan Mohr (Oslo and Copenhagen [51]), Herman Vanden Berghe (Leuven [66]) and Marco Fraccaro (Pavia [09]), so that his influence was Europe-, indeed worldwide (Harper 2017).

The work of Penrose and his colleagues, including that of JBS Haldane, was largely theoretical in nature, with a strong mathematical emphasis; in part this was because there was little laboratory-based experimental research relevant to genetics that was feasible at the time. It is salutary to remember that in 1950 almost nothing was known about human chromosomes; the techniques were still inadequate even to determine the correct number. Enzymes were recognised, but there was no concept of how they might be related to heredity beyond Garrod's original 'one gene, one enzyme' proposal, though Harry Harris's subsequent work at both the Galton Laboratory and King's College London identified the extensive genetic variation in them. The gene itself remained a theoretical concept, with no general acceptance that it was composed of DNA rather than protein, which was widely considered to be the most likely primary material for inheritance. Even after the double helix was recognised, the idea that DNA and human genes might be directly analysed in an individual seemed a remote prospect.

For Penrose's Galton Laboratory of the 1950s and 1960s there was no element of clinical or other genetic services, even though the ultimate goal of much of the research was the understanding and alleviation of human inherited diseases. As Penrose himself had stated firmly in his presidential address to the Third International Human Genetics Congress, remembering the recent abuses of eugenics:

> At the moment we are only scratching the surface of this great science and our knowledge of human genes and their action is still so slight that it is presumptuous and foolish to lay down positive principles for human breeding. Rather each person can marvel at the prodigious diversity of the hereditary characters in man and respect those who differ from him genetically.
>
> *Penrose 1967*

It can thus be seen that for those medically trained workers who would go on to become the first medical geneticists in many UK centres, their emphasis would likewise be primarily on research and only later service. But the 'spirit' of Penrose in those early years would help to ensure that, in both the UK and internationally, medical genetics practice would have both a sound scientific and ethical basis.

RADIATION, CHROMOSOMES AND EARLY MEDICAL GENETICS RESEARCH

The early post-war development of medical genetics received a powerful stimulus from concern about the genetic and other risks of atomic radiation. This concern was worldwide, voiced notably by Hermann Muller, based on his research on radiation-induced mutation in Drosophila. After his enforced moves from America successively to Germany, Russia and Edinburgh, he was now back in America, and was tireless in warning against the dangers of radiation, being given further influence by receiving the Nobel Prize in 1946 for his work (Carlson 1981).

The initiation of the American-Japanese study of atomic bomb survivors (Neel 1994) was the first practical result of these concerns, but it was clear that much wider research on genetics, and especially human genetics, would be needed if the dangers of radiation, whether from atomic fallout or from increasing medical use, were to be understood and avoided.

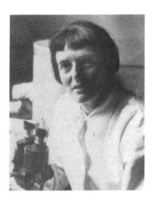

Figure 2.4 Charlotte Auerbach (1899–1994), discoverer of chemical mutagenesis.

The gravity of the situation was well recognised in Britain by both scientists and politicians; with Britain developing its own nuclear weapons, and with increasing medical diagnostic and therapeutic use of radiation, the Medical Research Council (MRC) was the obvious body to be involved alongside the physicists in the biological and medical aspects of the work. The sound foundations laid by pre-war workers in human and wider genetics meant that work could resume immediately, once wartime disruption was over. Research had in fact already begun during the war, since Charlotte Auerbach (Figure 2.4), a refugee from Nazi Germany, had studied with Muller during his time in Edinburgh; she subsequently discovered the mutagenic effects of chemicals such as nitrogen mustards in Drosophila, though the work was initially kept secret and only published after the war was over (Auerbach and Robson 1946).

Although some information on the human effects of radiation could be obtained from theoretical studies of mutation rate, such as those by Haldane (1935) and by Penrose (1956), this was limited, and it was clear from the outset that, unless there were further disasters such as the Japanese atomic explosions, the data would have to come from experimental work. The MRC therefore initiated a series of new units in which various aspects of radiation hazard were addressed, using information both from human diseases and from mutation studies on experimental species. De Chadarevian (2006 and in press) has given a detailed account of the background to this, emphasising the extent to which the development of human genetics overall was dependent on the dangers of radiation. Here I cover only the cytogenetics aspects, and only briefly since I have already written a more detailed account in an earlier book (Harper 2006).

Table 2.1 shows the main genetics research units sponsored by the Medical Research Council that evolved over the coming decades; a remarkable amount of their work proved to be directly relevant to the development of medical genetics, even though this was largely unintended. The two main centres involved were Edinburgh, with its extensive pre-war record under the Agricultural Research Council of basic genetics research, and Harwell, near Oxford, where the main UK research nuclear reactor had been built. In addition, two other more clinically orientated units were also created, one at Oxford, under Alan Stevenson, to give more extensive estimates on the frequency of mendelian disorders; the other in London, under John Fraser Roberts, to provide information on the genetics of common diseases.

Table 2.1 Medical Research Council (MRC) units related to the development of medical genetics

Name	Location	First director	Dates
Clinical Effects of Radiation Unit (now Human Genetics Unit)	Edinburgh	Michael Court-Brown	1956–present
Radiobiology Research Unit (now Mammalian Genome Unit)	Harwell	James Loutit (TC Carter head of genetics section)	1954–present
Clinical Genetics Research Unit	Institute of Child Health, London	J Fraser Roberts (succeeded by Cedric Carter)	1947–64 1964–82
Clinical and Population Genetics Research Unit	Oxford	Alan Stevenson	1958–74
Blood Group Unit	Lister Institute, London	Robert R Race (succeeded by Ruth Sanger)	1946–95
Blood Group Reference Unit	Lister Institute, London	Arthur Mourant	1946–65
Animal Breeding Unit (ARC) and successors	Edinburgh	Francis Crew	1945–present

The Edinburgh MRC Human Genetics Unit

Originally entitled the 'MRC Clinical Effects of Radiation Unit', this was opened in 1956, with Michael Court Brown as its first director. Court Brown was a medically trained radiotherapist who had previously shown a link between radiation treated ankylosing spondylitis and subsequent leukaemia. It was a clinically orientated unit, with its own beds at the adjacent Western General Hospital, but from the genetics perspective its key early step, noted in its first annual report, was the appointment of a young biologist, Patricia Jacobs, to develop techniques for studying human chromosomes from cultured bone marrow. She was able to do this by combining the bone marrow culture method devised by Laszlo Lajtha of Oxford with the mammalian cytogenetics of Charles Ford at nearby Harwell.

Jacobs was officially meant to be applying this to patients with radiation-induced leukaemia, but these were few, so she had spare time and accepted the suggestion of John Strong, clinical endocrinologist at Western General Hospital, to study the marrow of a patient with Klinefelter syndrome, a condition in which the possibility of a chromosome abnormality had already been raised because of their female chromatin positive pattern. The discovery of an XXY chromosome constitution (Jacobs and Strong 1959) was one of the three initial and essentially simultaneous reports of human chromosome abnormalities. The story is told in full in interviews with Patricia Jacobs [06] and with her technician Muriel Lee [12], as well as in my book *First Years of Human Chromosomes* (Harper 2006).

Further discoveries by Patricia Jacobs around this time included the independent identification of trisomy 21 as the basis of Down syndrome, which had been published shortly before by the Paris workers (Lejeune et al. 1959), and the presence of an abnormal chromosomal fragment in chronic myeloid leukaemia (1960), also detected just beforehand by Nowell and Hungerford in Philadelphia (1960). In subsequent years other sex chromosome abnormalities were discovered, including the XXX and XYY syndromes (Figure 2.5).

Although I have described Patricia Jacobs' discovery in more detail elsewhere, I cannot resist quoting here from my 2004 interview with her, and separately with her technician Muriel Lee:

> I looked at the Klinefelter and the preparations were really very bad, even though I had practiced. And I thought there were 47 chromosomes and there were two Xs and a Y, and remember we couldn't separately identify any of them, couldn't even tell the Y. But I did and I couldn't believe it. And this was not the perceived wisdom of what Klinefelters were in that day and age. There were two kinds of Klinefelters, called chromatin positive and chromatin negative and nobody had clearly made any distinction between them except in their sex chromatin body; and everybody assumed that they were sex-reversed females, so everybody expected them to be XX and I thought I could see 47 chromosomes. And I thought I could see something that was compatible with being a Y, which means there were 5 acrocentrics rather than 4. So I thought, well that's very funny. .... I went on holiday and I asked my technician to prepare a tray of slides with the Klinefelter in it

(a)   (b)

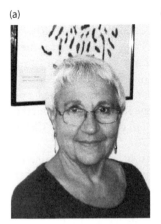 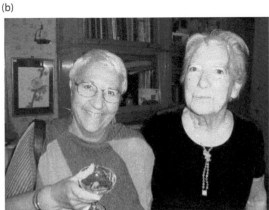

Figure 2.5 **(a)** Patricia Jacobs (born 1934). (Courtesy of Patricia Jacobs.) **(b)** Two discoverers of trisomy 21. Patricia Jacobs with Marthe Gautier at the 2009 celebration dinner in Paris to mark the 50th anniversary of the discovery of trisomy 21.

and lots of other things in it too, and I would come back and score them blind, and I did. I came back from my holiday and I scored them blind and I thought, well that's funny because there seemed to be two that seemed to have 47 chromosomes, not just one as I had expected. So I said to her, I've got two that I really think might have 47 chromosomes and she broke into a big grin, because she had put two from the Klinefelter's in the tray. So I thought, well that may be true. So that's it. So we told Michael Court Brown, who saw the significance of it. We didn't. I mean I was 22 years old or something and I knew nothing about how the Y wasn't supposed to do anything, because we were all supposed to be like Drosophila and it didn't have any effect whatsoever on sex, and he seemed to think it was very important …and I remember it clearly. He said well you had better go and write it up.

Interview with Patricia Jacobs,13/02/2004 [06]

Seen from Muriel Lee's perspective, as an even younger technician:

PSH: Do you remember when about was it that you came up with something that was clearly abnormal?

ML: Well, the first real abnormal was the Klinefelter that I can remember, and that was really, we had got the sample from Professor Strong and we did all the technique and then Pat actually looked at it and she thought that there were 47 chromosomes, but as I said the preps weren't really ideal at that time and so she thought that but she wasn't absolutely certain. So she asked me, she was going away for a few days and she asked me if I would put in some ones that I knew to be normal and just put this in and mark them all so that just a, b, c or whatever, so she didn't know what they were. So she was looking at them blind, just a tray of slides. So I did that, and she came out and she was quite excited. She said I think we've actually got two with 47 chromosomes. And I said, well that's right because I put in two. So she was quite impressed with that. She has always been quite impressed with that.

PSH: So you did that without telling her?

ML: So that was a real test. Yes. I thought that would be a real test, you know, if she could see it in two slides.

Interview with Muriel Lee, 26/05/2004 [12]

Some important general points emerge from this story: first, how very young both Patricia Jacobs and Muriel Lee (then Brunton) were – in their early 20s – yet their seniors left them free to work as they considered best, though being available if needed, especially for general interpretation and the writing of papers, which rarely carried the names of supervisor or head of unit. The value of a good technician (sadly they are now an endangered species) is also shown here, and more so when one reads the full interview transcripts. I am sorry not to have interviewed more of these technicians, essential to most important discoveries and often surviving longer for historians to interview, being mostly female and younger than the main investigator. A final point, as I have already mentioned, is the value of the freedom which the MRC gave in those days to unit directors in following important scientific leads far beyond the unit's primary remit.

The other key discovery relating to medical genetics that involved the MRC radiation units at this time was the chromosomal basis of Turner syndrome. On this occasion it was the Harwell unit, whose genetics group, including outstanding workers such as Charles Ford, Mary Lyon (see Chapter 11), Anthony Searle and Bruce Cattanach, had evolved as an offshoot from that in Edinburgh and maintained close links with it after the move to Harwell.

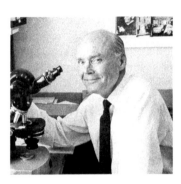

Figure 2.6 Charles E Ford (1912–1999). A key member of the Harwell mammalian cytogenetics group, Ford's development of techniques for studying mammalian chromosomes (principally in the mouse), was essential for the subsequent collaborative work with Patricia Jacobs and Paul Polani on human chromosome abnormalities. (Photo courtesy of Dr K Madan.)

Charles Ford in particular (Figure 2.6) had developed techniques for studying mammalian chromosomes, but was not especially interested in human chromosomes until after Tjio and Levan's recognition in 1956 that 46 was the correct human chromosome number, a finding that he and John Hamerton rapidly confirmed (Ford and Hamerton 1956). This caught the attention of Paul Polani (Figure 2.7), who had already been studying Turner syndrome patients and strongly suspected that their chromatin negative nature indicated an XO chromosome complement, a conclusion which was initially met with scepticism by Penrose and most others.

Polani managed (with some difficulty, see interview [01]) to persuade Ford to analyse bone marrow chromosomes from a series of Turner patients (Ford et al. 1959) that Polani had previously studied for their sex chromatin status (Polani et al. 1954). The results not only confirmed Polani's earlier hypothesis that they might be XO chromosomally, but completely overturned current thinking on the mechanism of sex determination in mammals, showing, as did Patricia Jacobs' simultaneous Klinefelter study (Jacobs and Strong 1959), that presence or absence of the Y chromosome is the critical factor in this, not the number of X chromosomes as in Drosophila. Patients with a range of rare sex chromosome anomalies would continue to be vital for research into the mechanisms of mammalian sex determination for the next 50 years, culminating in the isolation of the Y chromosome SRY gene by Peter Goodfellow and colleagues, as described in Chapter 11.

Polani and Ford also had a series of Down syndrome patients planned for study but, as with Jacobs, found themselves forestalled by the Paris group. They were

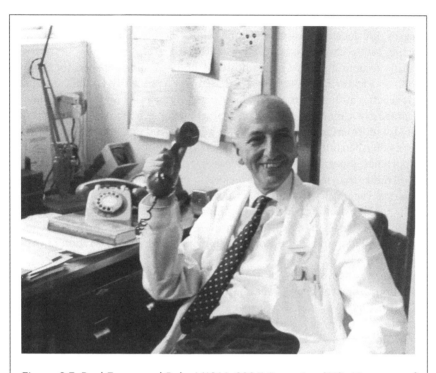

Figure 2.7 Paul Emmanuel Polani (1914–2006) (interview [01]). (Courtesy of the Paediatric Research Unit, Guy's Hospital, London.)

Born in Trieste, at that time part of the Austro-Hungarian Empire but subsequently in Italy, Polani received a thorough education in biology, including considerable genetics, in Siena and Pisa, where he qualified in medicine. He and his family were strongly anti-fascist, so he came to Britain to gain postgraduate experience, only to find that war had broken out on the day of his arrival in 1939. Since his Italian qualification was recognised in Britain, he was able initially to work as a ship's surgeon, but when Italy joined the war he was interned as an 'enemy alien' in the Isle of Man detention camp before being sent to the Evelina Children's Hospital, London, where he was its sole resident medical officer for the whole duration of the war.

Here he made close links with paediatricians at nearby Guy's Hospital, where he was given a research post, initially to work on kernicterus, at that time a major cause of neonatal brain damage. Recognising his research abilities, the children's charity 'The Spastics Society' funded a major institute for Polani, in which he focused on genetic and developmental causes of disability, especially chromosomal disorders, as well as creating a centre for genetic services (see Chapters 3 and 4). Polani remained at Guys Hospital for his entire career and was able, at the age of 90, to open the new 'Polani Research Laboratories' named in his honour.

able, however, to identify from a number of patients born to younger mothers, a case of translocation Down syndrome, whose mother, a balanced translocation carrier, had 45 chromosomes (Polani et al. 1960).

This dramatic series of chromosomal findings, all published in 1959 and 1960, and featuring principally UK-based workers, firmly established human cytogenetics at the forefront of human genetics generally; up to then it had been regarded as a 'Cinderella' area by many other human geneticists, not just in Britain but also in America and France. But the advances did much more than this: they also established human chromosome analysis as being of medical and diagnostic importance, especially when non-invasive techniques allowing it to be done on blood rather than marrow were developed in 1960 by Moorhead and by Nowell in America. Paediatricians and endocrinologists began to be interested in genetics, while the demand for genetic counselling and interpretation of chromosomal results gave rise to an increasing number of clinicians becoming involved in the work of genetics units, who would form many of the first generation of clinical geneticists.

From the scientific viewpoint of the MRC, the results on human chromosomes emerging from their units may not have been exactly what they had been expecting, but they had shown that at last there was a laboratory indicator for genetic damage, which had been conspicuously lacking until then. Both as a body, and at the level of individual units, MRC and their unit directors deserve great credit for supporting lines of work that must at the time have seemed only tenuously related to their primary remit.

The later development of UK clinical cytogenetics as a diagnostic service is described in Chapter 10 and occurred mainly outside the MRC, whose human cytogenetics research remained concentrated in its Edinburgh unit, later renamed the 'MRC Human Population Cytogenetics Unit' and finally the 'MRC Human Genetics Unit'. Although the Harwell unit reverted to its mouse genetics role, its subsequent research would remain highly relevant to human and medical genetics, with pioneering contributions in such areas as X chromosome inactivation, comparative genetics and genetic imprinting.

Paul Polani and Guy's Hospital London

Among the key figures of early UK human chromosome research, Paul Polani alone was not part of one of the MRC radiation research units, though closely linked through his collaboration with the Harwell workers. His strongly clinical background, along with the consistent support from his Guy's Hospital base and generous funding from medical charities (notably the Spastics Society) gave him the freedom to develop not only his chromosomal research, but also his broad vision for genetics in medicine, resulting in what was to become probably the outstanding medical genetics unit in the country.

Although Polani had already acquired a considerable knowledge of basic genetics before the war in Italy, he was able to build on this by linking closely with Penrose in the post-war years.

Well, in practice I spent all my spare time at the Galton, shall we say 'sitting at his feet' if you like, but I mean you had to do that, because Penrose was not a man that was given to a great deal of effusion, so you had to pick pearls as they happened to drop out of his mouth.

Interview with Paul Polani, 12/11/2003 [01]

Polani, like Penrose, inspired great loyalty and affection among his colleagues, as can be seen in the interview with Caroline Berry, who initially joined him at Guy's Hospital on a purely ad hoc basis to develop genetic counselling services, but who became one of the UK's first NHS-based clinical geneticists and took on the clinical leadership of the unit from Polani.

PSH: What was your impression of Paul Polani at that time?
CB: When I went to visit the unit, which at that stage was in Keats' house, a sort of private department at Guys, he was a great enthusiast. I remember he showed me around the department and it was awfully interesting and exciting and he said 'here we breathe genetics', and we did.
PSH: He still is an enthusiast isn't he?
CB: Yes, yes.
PSH: It makes such a difference.

Interview with Caroline Berry [20]

Martin Bobrow, his successor, was equally clear about both Polani's personal qualities and his organisational abilities:

PSH: Did you have much interaction with Paul himself?
MB: Paul came in all the time. Paul was a regular part of the department, still goes in occasionally but I reached very, very early agreement with Paul that he had free access. I did it with care, but I was confident, and proven right, that he was someone who would always be helpful and never be a problem and that's exactly how it was. He would occasionally sort of shuffle into the room and after a few minutes of polite pleasantries he would very tangentially mention that I had really upset someone somewhere and this is what I might do about it. He was just incredibly helpful. Really, really supportive.
PSH: I mean that is really very unusual isn't it?
MB: It is. Mostly keeping your predecessor in the department with you is a really dumb idea, but it was absolutely the right thing to do then. He was wonderful.
PSH: I have interviewed Paul himself. He was the first person I went to see. I was amazed at his vitality still, but also talking with other people, everybody seems to have not just respect for Paul as a scientist and an organiser, but a very real affection going along with it, which seems to have lasted right the way through. It's quite remarkable.

MB: Absolutely. Wonderful man. Wonderful man. A man of deep principle, fantastic depth of humanity, really just an excellent chap.

PSH: And also a very practical organiser, at least in appointing and encouraging good people who would do things well.

Interview with Martin Bobrow 01/11/2004 [24]

A series of able more recent colleagues and successors, building on Polani's foundations, has ensured that the Unit continues to flourish today as one of the UK's leading medical genetics centres. Some of its more recent contributions are mentioned in Chapter 3 and later chapters.

The Institute of Child Health, London, Clinical Genetics Research Unit

Although the finding of human chromosomal abnormalities may have been the area of greatest excitement during the late 1950s and the 1960s, the MRC was encouraging other areas too. The pre-war work of John Fraser Roberts on family studies and genetic risk estimates has already been mentioned in Chapter 1, and a very small clinical genetics research unit was established in 1947 to allow him to continue this, based at the Institute of Child Health, London, where he was joined by Cedric Carter, who continued the unit after Roberts retired in 1964. This low-key but meticulously thorough work on the frequency of a series of common disorders and the genetic risks to family members provided the foundations for risk estimation and genetic counselling generally for the next 40 years. In particular, the 'empiric risk' studies on non-mendelian disorders allowed satisfactory genetic counselling to be given even when no chromosomal abnormality or specific mendelian pattern could be recognised. A series of general principles also emerged from this work, including the observation that the risk for offspring is greater when the parent is of the more rarely affected sex, and the relationship of recurrence risk to the frequency of the disorder. The location of this unit as part of London's Great Ormond Street Hospital, the major UK referral centre for rare disorders and specialist paediatric skills, also attracted the attention of those interested in congenital malformations and dysmorphology generally, a topic pursued further in Chapter 4.

As well as starting Britain's first genetic counselling clinic at Great Ormond Street Hospital in 1946 (see Chapter 6), Roberts took over the genetics clinic that had emerged from Penrose's pre-war Colchester Study, Penrose having been deemed unacceptable because of his wartime pacifism, as recounted by Marcus Pembrey:

Then the war came and the superintendent of the Eastern Counties Hospital decided that Penrose had not played his part properly in the war and he physically, this is what Laurie Smith said, [Penrose's Colchester assistant] ... he physically barred his entrance to the hospital when he came back after the war. He was sent off without actually even collecting some of the things he wanted to collect ... So what happened was that when Penrose left, they found John Fraser Roberts, who had an impeccable war record, to take over the clinic.

Interview with Marcus Pembrey 19/09/2006 [62]

Pembrey subsequently took over both this clinic, and also later editions of Roberts' book, *An Introduction to Medical Genetics*, discussed in Chapter 9.

It is of interest that both Carter and Penrose, highly influential men, were quiet, shy and reticent people, not always easy to communicate with, as mentioned above for Penrose (Figure 2.8).

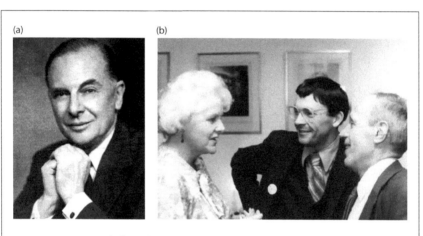

(a) (b)

Figure 2.8 **(a)** and **(b)** John Fraser Roberts and Cedric Carter, Founders of medical genetics at the Institute of Child Health, London. Photo with Kathleen Evans (Chapter 6) and Nick Dennis. (From Witness Seminar Clinical Genetics in Britain [Harper, Jones and Tansey 2010], courtesy Tilli Tansey.)

(a) John Fraser Roberts (1899–1987) (Photo c1964, courtesy Marcus Pembrey.) was born into a farming family in North Wales; his interest from an early age in sheep breeding, especially the badger-faced strain (Haldane would later irreverently call him 'old badger face') led him to an agriculture degree at Bangor, from where he moved to the Edinburgh Animal Breeding Research Unit under Frank Crew (see Chapter 3). Becoming increasingly interested in human quantitative genetic traits such as intelligence, he trained in medicine at Edinburgh and was appointed Director of the Mental Handicap Research Unit at Stoke Park, Bristol, where in 1940 he wrote the first edition of his book *An Introduction to Medical Genetics* (Roberts, 1940). He had already been part of the MRC Human Genetics Research Committee (see Chapter 1) and, after interruptions from serving in World War II (and previously in World War I) he was made director of the new MRC Clinical Genetics Research Unit in 1957 at the Institute of Child

Health, London and Great Ormond Street Hospital, London, where he had already started a genetic counselling clinic in 1946. Here he embarked on his long series of family studies of common disorders, continued by his successor Cedric Carter, which laid the foundations for accurate genetic risk estimates in non-mendelian conditions. After 'retiring' from the MRC in 1964 he transferred to Paul Polani's new centre at Guy's Hospital, and continued in genetic counselling there for many years. Colleagues remember John Fraser Roberts as a courteous, 'gentlemanly' person who related well to patients and families, and who was meticulous as to the facts and figures in his work (see interviews with Caroline Berry [20] and Marcus Pembrey [62]).

(b) Cedric O Carter (1917–1984), colleague and successor to John Fraser Roberts at the Institute of Child Health, was probably the single person who most influenced the development of medical genetics as a clinical specialty during these early years of the late 1960s and 1970s. While Penrose was the undoubted academic leader and principal university influence, the Department of Health looked more to Carter when considering future NHS posts and developments in medical genetics. His base at London's Institute of Child Health, adjacent to Great Ormond Street Hospital, Britain's premier children's hospital, must have helped, but one wonders also if his support for eugenics, virtually alone in this among the post-war medical genetics community, may have also been an unspoken factor in the minds of those health policy makers who saw the 'prevention' of genetic disorders mainly in financial terms. A further major contribution was Carter's key role in the founding of the Clinical Genetics Society in 1970, discussed in Chapter 9. It is sad that he died soon after his retirement, at a time when he might have had much more to contribute through his writing and the analysis of his studies.

Cedric Carter, a very different character to Penrose but equally quiet, can perhaps best be judged from descriptions by his colleagues at the Institute of Child Health. The atmosphere of the unit came as a considerable culture shock to those coming to work there from outside London, such as John Burn, Cedric Carter's final research student, who moved from acute paediatrics in Newcastle:

To then go into this quiet little corridor where everyone just sat and read books and chatted now and again, it was a dramatic change of pace. So we were on the – I think it was the 2nd floor – of the Institute of Child Health and Cedric, his door was always open and he was always facing his desk, you could see it from the side. Michael Baraitser had just arrived. Michael was a neurologist of South African extraction … he was a very, a true intellectual, rather like David Gardner-Medwin, who had a huge influence on me. I had never met people who were so embroiled in academe. They were attracted just to the pure knowledge and joy of learning. And Michael was a tremendous reader and polymath and he knew the literature.

Interview with John Burn (22/09/2014 [100]

Michael Baraitser himself found the situation even more confusing:

I was a South African coming to this very English situation, Queen's Square [Institute of Neurology], then to Cedric, an ex-Oxfordian, scholarly man, actually a very clever man, … and so it was a very strange situation for me, a rather open South African, to come into this very closed, esoteric, very strange situation. He used to sit in his office The door would be open but he rarely came out of the office except on a Tuesday morning when we went through the patients of the week. …But everything Cedric did was good, even though his great interest was only, as you say, normal variation; he would like to have spent his whole life with his Gaussian curves and his multifactorial rules. But we went onto the ward and he was extraordinarily good. If I look back now at misdiagnoses, he made very few. He really was a superb clinician, although it wasn't his great love.

Interview with Michael Baraitser 01/03/2005 [33]

Cedric Carter's reticence also impacted on his patient- and family-related work in genetic counselling (see Chapter 6), where he saw his role as largely limited to risk estimation, with little communication at the emotional level.

Cedric would do genetic clinics and he would allocate, rather like a GP, about 12 minutes to each family and then dismiss them and tell them that he'd write a letter to their doctor. And I mean the idea of actual counselling really hadn't permeated.

Interview with John Burn [100]

Norman Nevin's experiences, 20 years earlier, were similar [26]:

NN: I can remember vividly attending Cedric's counselling clinics.
PSH: Tell me about them.
NN: Well Cedric's counselling clinics were certainly very brief and to the point. Now let's say for example there's been a family who had had a child with cystic fibrosis. All the counselling involved was taking the pedigree, usually on a card and deciding what the inheritance was and then giving a risk of 1 in 4 and that was it. Very brief but one saw a lot of patients with single gene disorders through that particular clinic.
PSH: I mean Cedric was always very interested in genetic counselling but it struck me that he was a man of very few words and, would I be right that in terms of the family on the receiving end, he wasn't really a very receptive…
NN: What I was going to say was in fact that there was no empathy that developed between Cedric and the family and indeed it was always very brief.

Interview with Norman Nevin 04/11/2004 [26]

The theme of communication in genetic counselling is taken up again in Chapter 6.

The key research contributions of Carter and Fraser Roberts were their large scale and meticulous family studies of common disorders, in particular childhood malformations such as cleft lip and palate, neural tube defects and pyloric stenosis, none of which showed mendelian inheritance, but where practical 'empiric risk estimates', invaluable for genetic counselling, could be worked out, which have remained useful up to the present. Important general principles emerged too, notably the Gaussian 'normal' distribution of risk, the concept of 'threshold' for risk producing an actual disorder and (Carter's own particular contribution, as noted by Michael Baraitser), the recognition that risk to offspring is greater when the affected parent is of the more rarely affected sex.

> I asked him once, I don't know why I asked him, how he would like to be remembered. We were talking about various things and he said he would like to be remembered for formulating some of the laws of multifactorial inheritance. I think he did formulate the rule which said, the risk to the unusual sex, in a multifactorial scenario, was greater to offspring. And it has become known as the Carter law. He was very shrewd and I'm pleased he will be remembered for that.
>
> *Interview with Michael Baraitser [33]*

This body of knowledge, put alongside the consequences of Mendelian inheritance, would form the practical foundations for much of medical genetics, including genetic counselling, for the next 50 years.

Cedric Carter had a number of plans for continuing his academic work following his retirement, including a book on genetic counselling, but these never came to fruition, since he died soon afterwards.

> And then the sad thing of course was that he decided in his retirement he would keep fit, and he ran this half marathon and whether it was to do with it or not, I rather suspect it was, he was unwell during the night, felt particularly unwell in the morning and died from a coronary. So he never had a retirement.
>
> *Interview with Marcus Pembrey [62]*

The MRC Clinical and Population Genetics Research Unit

The other MRC unit that was clinically orientated towards medical genetics was the Clinical and Population Genetics Research Unit, based in Oxford and headed by Alan Stevenson (1909–1995) (Figure 2.9), primarily a public health epidemiologist, previously working in Belfast as Professor of Social Medicine, where he had undertaken surveys of a number of mendelian disorders (see interview with Norman Nevin [26]). A good account of his life and early work in Northern Ireland has recently been given by Morrison (2018). Interviews with several people who had worked in the unit, together with discussion at a 'Witness Seminar' in 2008 (Harper et al. 2010), has left me with the feeling that this unit should have worked well and provided leadership for the development of medical genetics across Britain, not just Oxford, but that it never really did so. Stevenson seems not to have been an easy colleague and, according to John Edwards, who worked in the unit at its beginning, had antagonised much of the university establishment, including George Pickering, the Regius Professor of Medicine (best remembered today for his views on the polygenic nature of hypertension and his dispute with Richard Platt of Manchester on this topic). The upshot was that the new unit ended up on the periphery of the city and isolated from the main academic departments. The MRC may not have been entirely happy either, since they closed the unit when Stevenson retired in 1974. Yet some extremely able people worked there, notably Peter Pearson and Martin Bobrow, both of whom made important contributions to cytogenetics, especially in the area of chromosome banding, while clinical and genetic counselling aspects were developed by Clare Davison and Richard Lindenbaum, including a series of peripheral genetic counselling clinics. Stevenson and Davison also wrote one of the first books on genetic counselling (Stevenson et al. 1970), which included the use of Bayesian calculations in risk estimation, as discussed in Chapter 6.

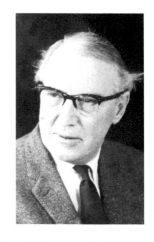

Figure 2.9 Alan Stevenson (1909–1995). (Courtesy of Alun Evans and Patrick Morrison.)

Both Bobrow and Nevin, in my interviews with them [24;26], spoke warmly of Stevenson as a person, despite difficulties from his cyclothymic nature. After closure of the unit Pearson and Bobrow both moved to Chairs of Human Genetics in the Netherlands; Pearson to Leiden, while Bobrow went to Amsterdam, after some time working with Walter Bodmer, who had come to a new basic genetics Chair in the biochemistry department. Lindenbaum remained in Oxford as an NHS clinical geneticist (see Chapter 3).

These details of local difficulties may seem parochial, but they show how deep and long-lasting such personal and seemingly trivial problems can be, often resulting in intractable difficulties for the next generation or even longer, as Martin Bobrow found when attempting to persuade Oxford University to set up an academic medical genetics department after Stevenson had retired:

MB: Two things happened at about that time; one was I had a series of discussions with people in Oxford about the possibility of establishing an academic medical genetics department and basically just met with a blank wall. There was no interest in doing that whatsoever. I foresaw the isolation of this little clinical department as being a major problem out on the Churchill site, which was a pretty non-academic site at that stage, but there were just other pressures and other people had louder voices and there was no support for that.

PSH: Can I just ask, in terms of geography were you then split between the university site for your research and the Churchill for your clinical work?

MB: Yes that's correct. I was doing virtually half and half.

PSH: It is interesting, that the two most unreceptive places over those years for academic medical genetics were I suppose Oxford and Cambridge.

MB: Yes, and I happen to have beaten my head against both! I know, I can show you the scars.

Interview with Martin Bobrow [24]

Cyril Clarke and Liverpool: The birth of 'Genetics in Medicine'

While all of the three London centres described above were led by medically trained people, none of these saw their role in genetics as forming part of regular medical practice; Fraser Roberts and Carter gained their medical degrees mainly to ensure acceptance by their medical colleagues. Even Paul Polani, who had essentially run London's Evelina Children's Hospital, both the medical and surgical aspects, throughout the war, did not continue to practice general children's medicine after beginning his medical genetics research. All three were concerned principally to increase our understanding of the biological and especially the genetic basis of human inherited disorders. They were remarkably successful in achieving this, and in providing the foundations on which the next generation of medical geneticists would develop the field, but their work was not seen by clinicians generally as affecting their regular practice, nor would it be widely so for the next 30 years or more.

The single founding centre that unequivocally aimed to set genetics at the heart of medical practice and thinking was that of Cyril Clarke in Liverpool, which not only made its own outstanding research contributions, but also strongly influenced the character of British medical genetics by training many of the next generation of clinical geneticists who would lead their own centres around the country.

Undeterred by not being a paediatrician, an obstetrician, or an immunologist, Clarke and a series of research fellows, notably Ronald Finn, showed that not only was the disorder due to the destruction of fetal red blood cells by maternal antibodies, usually related to a previous pregnancy, but that this could be prevented by maternal immunisation to destroy fetal red blood cells crossing the placenta, that might otherwise stimulate antibodies in the mother (Finn et al. 1961).

First proposed in 1960, this resulted in the virtual elimination of rhesus haemolytic disease of the newborn worldwide within five years, a remarkable achievement whose completeness has meant that it has largely been forgotten; it remains one of the key examples of therapy for genetic disorders. Clarke fortunately

(a) (b)

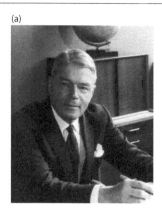
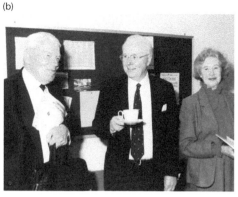

Figure 2.10 **(a)** Cyril A Clarke (1907–2000). (Photo gift of Clarke.) **(b)** Cyril and Féo Clarke (with Liverpool colleague Richard McConnell [see Chapter 4] in centre) at the opening of the Wales Institute of Medical Genetics, Cardiff. (Photograph by author.)

Cyril Clarke came late to genetics, any early academic possibilities for his career having been disrupted by the war. Having obtained a substantive (consultant) hospital medical post in Liverpool, he became intrigued by the possibilities that genetics might offer medical practice, largely as a result of his longstanding interest in breeding and studying genetic variation in butterflies. These possibilities were increased when his friend and colleague Philip Sheppard was appointed to the Liverpool University Chair of genetics, and Clarke decided to tackle the serious and at that time common problem of rhesus haemolytic disease, a classic example of maternal-fetal genetic interaction.

brought all the key papers on the topic together, along with commentaries, in a valuable book (Clarke 1962).

Clarke went on to make a series of wider research contributions to medical genetics with his colleagues, including the book *Genetics for the Clinician* (Clarke 1962), while continuing to practice general internal medicine until his retirement, something that would now be impossible. He then became President of the Royal College of Physicians of London. Like Paul Polani, he had an irrepressible enthusiasm and also was helped greatly by the active involvement of his wife Frieda (Féo), as was Victor McKusick with his wife Anne, all four being close and lifelong friends despite being on opposite sides of the Atlantic.

It was the close link with McKusick that enabled Clarke to provide the detailed further training, in both clinical and laboratory genetics, that was largely absent from his own unit, for the succession of clinicians who wished to take up medical genetics as a career (see Chapter 8). Ironically, Clarke himself was never fully persuaded that this should be regarded as a separate specialty, maintaining the view that genetics should be a part of medical practice overall, something which is only now, 50 years on, beginning to become a reality.

REFERENCES

Auerbach C, Robson JM. 1946. Chemical production of mutations. *Nature*. 157:302.

Bangham J. 2014. Blood groups and human groups: Collecting and calibrating genetic data after World War Two. *Stud Hist Philos Biol Biomed Sci*. 47 (Pt A):74–86.

Carlson EA. 1981. *Genes, Radiation, and Society: The Life and Work of H. J. Muller*. Ithaca, NY: Cornell University Press.

Clarke CA. 1962. *Genetics for the Clinician*. Oxford: Blackwell Scientific Publications.

Clarke CA. 1975. *Rhesus Haemolytic Disease. Selected Papers and Extracts*. Lancaster: MTP Medical and Technical Publishing Co. Ltd.

De Chadarevian S. 2006. Mice and the reactor: The 'Genetics Experiment' in 1950s Britain. *J History Biol*. 39:707–735.

De Chadarevian S. (in press). Heredity under the microscope: chromosomes and the human genome. Chicago: University of Chicago Press.

Finn R, Clarke CA, Donohoe WT. et al. 1961. Experimental studies on the prevention of Rh haemolytic disease. *Br Med J*. 1:1486–1490.

Fölling A. 1934. Über ausscheidung von phenylbrenztraubensäure in dem harn als stoffwechselanomalie in verbindung mit imbecillität [The excretion of phenylpyruvic acid in the urine, an anomaly of metabolism in connection with imbecility]. *Zeitschrift für Physiologische Chemie*. 227:169–176. (English translation reproduced in Harper PS, ed. 2004. *Landmarks in Medical Genetics*. Oxford: Oxford University Press.)

Ford CE, Hamerton JL. 1956. The chromosomes of man. *Nature*. 178:1020–1023.

Ford CE, Jones KW, Polani PE, de Almeida JC, Briggs JH. 1959. A sex chromosome anomaly in a case of gonadal dysgenesis (Turner's syndrome). *Lancet*. 1:711–713.

Haldane JBS. 1935. The rate of spontaneous mutation of a human gene. *J Genet*. 31:317–326.

Harper PS. 2006. *First Years of Human Chromosomes*. Oxford: Scion Press.

Harper PS. 2017. Some pioneers of European human genetics. *Eur J Hum Genet*, doi: 10.1038/ejhg.2017.47.

Harper PS, Reynolds LA, Tansey EM 2010. *Clinical Genetics in Britain: Origins and Development*. London; Wellcome Centre for the History of Medicine at UCL.

Jacobs PA, Strong JA. 1959. A case of human intersexuality having a possible XXY sex-determining mechanism. *Nature*. 183:302–303.

Kalmus H. 1948. *Genetics*. London: Pelican Books.

Kevles DJ. 1985. *In the Name of Eugenics: Genetics and the Uses of Human Heredity*. New York: Knopf.

Laxova R. 1998. Lionel Sharples Penrose, 1898–1972: A personal memoir in celebration of the centenary of his birth. *Genetics*. 150:1333–1340.

Laxova R. 2001. *Letter to Alexander*. Cincinnati, OH: Custom Editorial Productions.

Lejeune J, Gautier M, Turpin R. 1959. Etude des chromosomes somatiques de neuf enfants mongoliens. *CR Acad Sci*. 248:1721–1722,

Moorhead P, Nowell P, Mellman W, Battips D, Hungerford D. 1960. Chromosome preparations of leukocytes cultured from human peripheral blood. *Exp Cell Res.* 20:613–636.

Morrison PJ. 2018. Medical myths and legends. *Ulster Med J.* 87:102–108.

Muller HJ. 1927. Artificial transmutation of the gene. *Science.* 66:84–87.

Neel JV. 1994. *Physician to the Gene Pool.* New York: Wiley.

Nowell PC. 1960. Phytohemagglutinin: An initiator of mitosis in cultures of normal human leucocytes. *Cancer Res.* 20:462–468.

Penrose LS. 1938. *A Clinical and Genetic Study of 1280 Cases of Mental Defect.* Medical Research Council. London: His Majesty's Stationery Office.

Penrose LS. 1946. Phenylketonuria: A problem in eugenics. *Lancet.* 1:949–953.

Penrose LS. 1949. The Galton laboratory; its work and aims. *Eugen Rev.* 41(1):17–27.

Penrose LS. 1956–1957. Mutation in man. *Acta Genet Stat Med.* 6(2):169–182.

Penrose LS. 1967. Presidential address: The influence of the English tradition in human genetics. In: Crow JF, Neel JV (eds.). *Proceedings of the Third International Congress of Human Genetics.* Baltimore: The Johns Hopkins University Press, pp. 13–25.

Perutz MF. 1998. Enemy alien. In: Perutz MF (ed.). 2003. *I Wish I'd Made You Angry Earlier: Essays on Science, Scientists and Humanity,* 2nd edn. Cold Spring Harbor, NY: Cold Spring Harbor Laboratory Press, pp. 73–106.

Polani PE, Hunter JF, Lennox B. 1954. Chromosomal sex in Turner's syndrome with coarctation of the aorta. *Lancet.* 2:120–121.

Polani PE, Briggs JH, Ford CE, Clarke CM, Berg JM. 1960. A Mongol girl with 46 chromosomes. *Lancet.* 1 721–724.

Polani PE, Briggs JH, Ford CE, Clarke CM, Berg JM. 1960. A Mongol girl with 46 chromosomes. *Lancet.* 1: 721–724.

Povey S (ed.). 1998. *Penrose: Pioneer in Human Genetics. Report on a Symposium Held to Celebrate the Centenary of the Birth of Lionel Penrose.* London: Centre for Human Genetics at University College.

Roberts JAF. 1940. *An Introduction to Medical Genetics.* London: Oxford University Press.

Searle AG. 1949. Gene frequencies in London's cats. *J Genet.* 49(3):214–20.

Stevenson AC, Davison BC, Oakshott MW. 1970. *Genetic Counseling.* Philadelphia: Lippincott.

Tjio J-H, Levan A. 1956. The chromosome number of man. *Hereditas.* 42:1–6.

3

A new medical specialty: The spread and growth of medical genetics

ABSTRACT

During the 1960s and 1970s medical genetics spread progressively across Britain from its initial foci, with first university and later National Health Service posts created in regional universities and medical teaching centres, usually with an associated cytogenetics laboratory. By 1980 most centres had a genetic counselling service and varying degrees of medical genetics research and, though progress was uneven across the UK, medical genetics had become a distinct community of clinical and laboratory workers. This chapter looks at the progress and problems encountered by these centres and their early staff, based largely on a series of recorded interviews with many of the founders. The first generation of medical geneticists came from a variety of medical backgrounds but progressively developed a common identity as the specialty of medical genetics became more clearly defined.

By the early 1960s medical genetics had become a recognised and established field of research in a limited number of UK centres, mainly in London and in the series of MRC units described in Chapter 2. But there had been little involvement so far from the medical schools and universities, with the notable exceptions of Cyril Clarke's Department of Medicine in Liverpool and Guy's Hospital School of Medicine in London, the location for Paul Polani's Paediatric Research Unit. The concept of genetic services as a major area of medical practice was likewise still largely undeveloped, for the simple reason that there was little that could be offered as backup to genetic counselling.

This began to change rapidly after 1960 when chromosome analysis proved to have real diagnostic value for congenital malformations and for patients with suspected sex chromosome abnormalities; it had also become technically simpler and could be performed on peripheral blood rather than bone marrow (Moorhead et al. 1960), which greatly increased the demand for its service use. These laboratory advances, described in Chapter 10, in turn created an increased demand for genetic counselling as well as for skilled medical diagnosis to ensure that scarce laboratory resources were used selectively, something that remains as important today as 50 years ago. The interview with pioneer cytogeneticist David Harnden [08] gives an early example of this; he stresses that while there was a high yield of abnormal results from samples sent by an experienced clinical geneticist like John Edwards, samples from general paediatricians showed few abnormalities. In addition, these early developments had all been in research laboratories, often related to radiation biology; the MRC and other research funders could not be expected to continue supporting the rapidly increasing service developments, having already gone well beyond their radiation-related remit in allowing their units to pursue human cytogenetics research on a broad front.

Fortunately for the development of medical genetics, the 1960s were a time of academic expansion, especially in regional medical teaching centres, while from the 1970s the National Health Service (NHS) was also favouring the planned regional development of specialist services. Equally important, the two sectors were often willing at this time to be flexible as to whether the lead organisation for clinical and laboratory posts was academic or NHS based, something that greatly assisted a progressive expansion. It must be said too that the leaders of medical genetics at the time were not only able, often outstanding people scientifically and clinically, but also proactive, energetic, and opportunistic in seeking and obtaining funding. In the initial years Cedric Carter (see Chapter 2) had a particularly important role in linking with the Department of Health in recommending new NHS clinical geneticist posts and possible candidates across the country, much as Penrose had done a few years earlier with the MRC for academic positions.

Needless to say, this happy situation did not last, and for some centres it never existed. From the 1980s onwards, universities and the NHS hit successive financial constraints, while both became progressively narrower and more rigid in their targets and demands, which increasingly diverged from each other. This damaging and short-sighted trend affected medicine as a whole but was especially harmful to the close links between academic and service activities which had developed for medical genetics; it deserves a full and critical historical study. Fortunately though, by this time a network of clinical and laboratory medical genetics centres had evolved across the country; it had developed deep roots and an ability to withstand financial and political pressures that might easily have destroyed the field had they occurred a decade earlier.

Some European countries (e.g.: Germany, Belgium and Netherlands) created a series of carefully planned institutes of human genetics, with new buildings and a full complement of academic and support staff. By contrast, developments in Britain during the 1960s and 1970s were mostly piecemeal, ad hoc, and financially modest; the single exception, Edinburgh, and its disastrous aftermath, is considered later in this chapter. In general, the pattern (insofar as any pattern existed) was for incremental development to occur around a single original founder, who might have been either university or NHS based. This process of 'accretion', while usually unspectacular, was frequently more secure than when services were based solely on research funding, though this, especially when from medical charities, could provide a valuable transition.

This process of development depended on the existence of sufficient workers, some medically trained, some with a laboratory background (a few with both), who had sufficient experience of human and medical genetics to initiate and develop the new centres around the country and thus to form the 'first generation' of medical geneticists in Britain. Who were these people and what was their background? This chapter attempts to give a picture of some of them in the setting of their own centres and I have taken a largely geographical approach, since unlike some countries, there was no single point of origin. In contrast to the largely London-based 'founders' described in Chapter 2, medical genetics in Britain overall has from the outset had a remarkably 'flat' staffing structure and an equitable geographical distribution, contrasting strongly with the more hierarchical patterns often seen in continental Europe.

Some readers may question the space given in this chapter to workers who may individually not have made major research contributions, but I think that they would be missing the point that I am trying to make, which is that UK medical genetics has largely been a collective and cooperative development, and would not have got so far if it had simply been individual people working in isolation. This has been very much in line with the spirit and aims of the UK National Health Service generally, but not at all helped by the more commercially driven models imposed on it in more recent times.

Finally, I have myself been part of this working community and have seen it evolve over a period of more than 50 years. These people deserve to be remembered, even though this account can only be a personal and fragmentary one. In particular I have not tried to describe people or developments involving the past 10–15 years, so apologies are due to those who do not feature in this inevitably brief survey of medical genetics across Britain. I should also add that I have not usually consulted with current workers in the various centres in writing these accounts, which are at times critical, though I hope not unfair.

Given the major contributions of Scotland to early human and medical genetics, it seems appropriate to begin there and to progress steadily southwards. For the benefit of readers from outside the UK I have included a series of maps (Figure 3.1) showing the principal centres initiated at different times.

It can be seen from these maps that, leaving aside the original founding centres and MRC units, the majority of new developments occurred in the 1970s and 1980s, and that the pattern by the end of the 1980s was for each regional specialist centre (usually also containing a medical school) to contain a medical genetics unit also. These 'centres' might initially only contain a single consultant medical geneticist, with a variable degree of laboratory provision, mainly cytogenetic, but at least they provided a focus around which services could and did grow and, to a variable extent, University- and grant-supported research activity also.

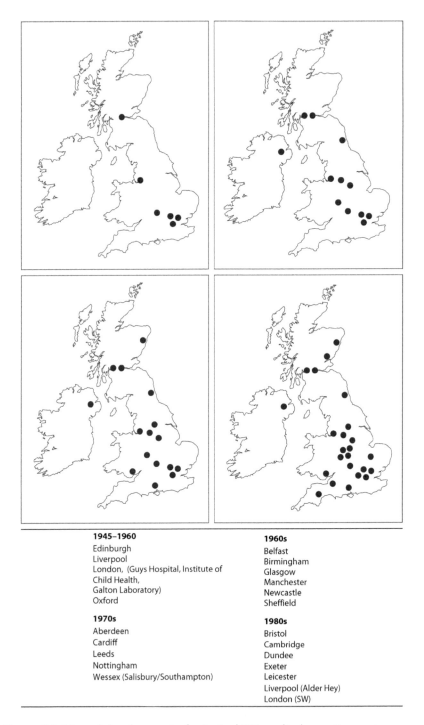

1945–1960	1960s
Edinburgh	Belfast
Liverpool	Birmingham
London, (Guys Hospital, Institute of	Glasgow
Child Health,	Manchester
Galton Laboratory)	Newcastle
Oxford	Sheffield
1970s	**1980s**
Aberdeen	Bristol
Cardiff	Cambridge
Leeds	Dundee
Nottingham	Exeter
Wessex (Salisbury/Southampton)	Leicester
	Liverpool (Alder Hey)
	London (SW)

Figure 3.1 Map of development of principal UK medical genetics centres over four decades.

ABERDEEN

Aberdeen, small in size but possessing one of the four ancient Scottish universities, has a longstanding history in genetics dating back to the 1930s, when geneticist and anti-eugenicist Lancelot Hogben (see Chapter 1) held the Chair of Zoology there. His tenure was cut short by World War II, after he was marooned in Sweden following a lecture in Oslo which coincided with the Nazi invasion of Norway, his misadventures being graphically described in an autobiography published by his children (Hogben and Hogben 1998). Medical genetics was initiated in 1966 by Alan Johnston (Figure 3.2) as an NHS-based adult physician, who was succeeded by John Dean (Figure 3.3a), also from an adult medicine background, while Neva Haites (Figure 3.3b), originally from medical biochemistry, introduced clinical molecular genetics. During the 1980s and 1990s Sheila Simpson built up a comprehensive genetics and wider service

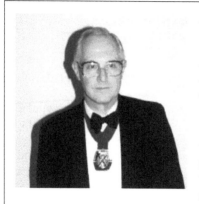

Figure 3.2 Alan William Johnston (1928–2012), first Aberdeen medical geneticist. Interview 24/09/2008 [74]. (Courtesy of Alan Johnston and Genetics and Medicine Historical Network.)

After qualifying in medicine from Cambridge and University College Hospital London, Alan Johnston began training in adult internal medicine and was advised to do a research year with Victor McKusick in Baltimore, possibly more for his cardiology than his genetic interests. He was one of the first British trainees with McKusick, working on the preparation of what would become 'Mendelian Inheritance in Man' and on a range of other clinical genetics projects, especially X-linked disorders, as well as linking with Malcolm Ferguson-Smith (see below) on cytogenetic topics.

On returning to London he made close contacts with the nearby Galton Laboratory, notably for a landmark study of the X-linked lysosomal disorder Fabry disease Johnston et al. 1966). However there was no permanent clinical genetics post available in London or elsewhere, so he had to take an NHS consultant physician's post in Aberdeen and to continue his genetics interest from there. Despite the isolation, he was able to play an important role in the formation of the Clinical Genetics Society and to be involved with the Royal College of Physicians in its Clinical Genetics Committee and its policies for training clinical geneticists (Chapter 9).

Aberdeen-trained clinical geneticist Peter Turnpenny has written a valuable obituary for the Royal College of Physicians (munksroll.rcplondon.ac.uk/details/6560).

(a)   (b)

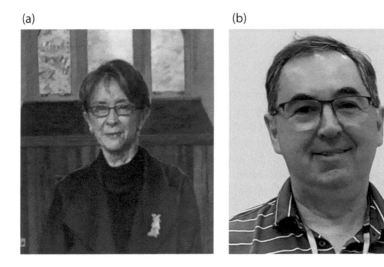

Figure 3.3 Medical genetics in Aberdeen. **(a)** Neva Haites. (Courtesy of Neva Haites.) **(b)** John Dean (Courtesy of John Dean).

for families with Huntington's disease, which had proved to have a particularly high prevalence in the region.

The Aberdeen health region (Grampian)'s relatively small population (c 500,000) has limited its scope for expansion, but this has been mitigated by the Scottish Health Department's wise insistence on a 'consortium' approach for new developments that involves all of the four principal Scottish centres, including Dundee, the least developed of the four in terms of medical genetics, though with a cytogenetics unit (originally headed by Michael Faed) and now also a clinical genetics service (David Goudie).

GLASGOW

Glasgow has much the largest area and population as a Scottish health region (c 3,000,000) and its university also has a long tradition in genetics, dating back to 1951, when Guido Pontecorvo (1907–1999), an Italian Jewish refugee from fascism, and pioneer in fungal and later somatic cell genetics, was appointed, becoming Professor in 1955, and building a flourishing department before moving to the Imperial Cancer Research Fund (ICRF) in London in 1968.

Medical genetics owes its beginnings and its prominence in Glasgow very largely to one individual, Malcolm Ferguson-Smith. Figure 3.4. As the unit developed it moved to the purpose-built Duncan Guthrie Institute of Medical Genetics at Yorkhill Hospital (Figure 3.5a), a prototype for the new pattern of medical genetics units integrating research and service.

In 1987 Malcolm Ferguson-Smith was appointed to the Chair of Pathology in Cambridge, which carried with it the remit to develop medical genetics services (which until then had been extremely backward), along with much else.

(a) (b)

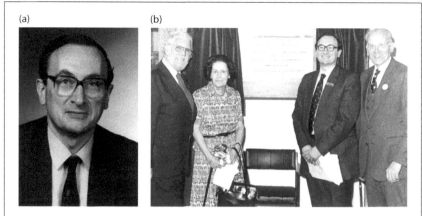

Figure 3.4 **(a)** Malcolm Ferguson-Smith (born 1931). Interview 05/12/2003 [03]. (Photos courtesy of Malcolm Ferguson-Smith.) **(b)** Malcolm Ferguson-Smith with Victor McKusick (Baltimore) at the opening of the Duncan Guthrie Medical Genetics Institute.

Born and brought up in Glasgow, where his father was a dermatologist, (who discovered the familial tumour multiple self-healing epithelioma), he qualified in medicine in 1955, entered pathology and, influenced by Douglas Lennox, began work on the sex chromatin and Klinefelter syndrome, though he was still developing his cytogenetics techniques when the initial papers on its chromosomal basis appeared at the beginning of 1959 (see Chapter 2). At this point he moved to Baltimore to set up for Victor McKusick what was in effect the first diagnostic chromosome laboratory in the United States, working with more clinically orientated Fellows such as Alan Johnston and Alan Emery. Returning to Glasgow after three years, he continued his work on the chromosomal basis of sex determination, making the discovery that the X chromosome has a pairing region with the Y that led later to isolation of the male determining gene *SRY* (see interview [98] with Peter Goodfellow).

As well as developing his cytogenetics research and broadening it into human and comparative gene mapping, he was able progressively to develop a clinical and laboratory genetics service for the West of Scotland region, being one of the first units systematically to develop prenatal chromosome diagnosis, largely the responsibility of his wife Marie Ferguson-Smith. The Glasgow unit was also well placed to take part in the multicentre studies of prenatal screening and preconceptional prevention of neural tube defects (see Chapter 10), which had a particularly high frequency in the West of Scotland.

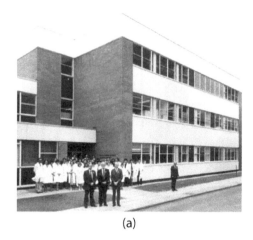

(a)

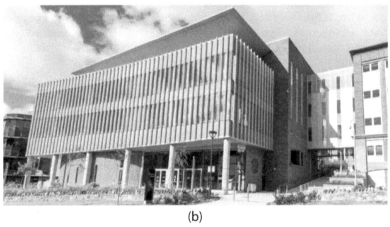

(b)

Figure 3.5 Early purpose-built medical genetics centres in Scotland. **(a)** The Duncan Guthrie Institute of Medical Genetics at Yorkhill Hospital, Glasgow, was the model for the new integrated medical genetics centres starting to develop across Britain. (Courtesy of Malcolm Ferguson-Smith.) **(b)** The MRC Human Genetics Unit at Western General Hospital, Edinburgh; also home initially for the University Department of Human Genetics.

He describes the somewhat unorthodox background to this in his 2003 interview [03]:

> I remember one evening at home in 1986 the telephone rang, 'This is Richard Adrian from Cambridge, we have just appointed you Professor of Pathology' and I roared with laughter. I said 'This must be a mistake. I haven't applied for any job in Cambridge. I didn't even know there was one'. I pulled myself together when he identified himself as Vice Chancellor of the University and

responded politely to the effect that I would certainly be glad to consider it. So Marie and I went down to see Richard Adrian and Marie said 'What on earth do you want to appoint my husband for?' Richard Adrian was quite taken aback by this! Anyway by this time I had realised that the Department of Pathology wasn't just a place that did post mortems and routine surgicals. It was a huge research department of over 400 people, not 40 scientists, and was one of the top pathology departments in the country.

Although the move was a big personal break, Malcolm Ferguson-Smith was able to take several key staff with him, notably John Yates and Nabil Affara, and to ensure that Cambridge at last had a flourishing medical genetics unit. After 'retiring' in 1998 he moved his base to the Cambridge Veterinary Medicine School and was able to play an important wider role in the inquiry into the epidemic of bovine spongiform encephalitis (BSE), as well as returning to one of his old interests, comparative cytogenetics and genomics, with which he continues to be involved to the present.

In terms of wider Glasgow activities, two especially deserve mention: first is the MSc degree course in medical genetics for those planning to enter the field, which has been the starting point for numerous present-day medical geneticists both in Britain and other countries. Second is the popular introductory textbook *Essential Medical Genetics*, initially edited by J Michael Connor, Ferguson-Smith's Glasgow successor, and Malcolm Ferguson-Smith himself.

Other important activities have included the Scottish Muscle Network under Douglas Wilcox, and contributions to dysmorphology from John Tolmie, who sadly died young in a mountaineering accident. In the wider neural tube defect field, Margaretha van Mourik, social worker and genetic counsellor in the unit, played a major role in both support and research.

Recent years have seen academic aspects of medical genetics diminish in Glasgow, and the main research focus is now where it began under Pontecorvo, the university genetics unit headed by Darren Monckton, making important contributions to basic genetics research on myotonic dystrophy and DNA instability.

EDINBURGH

The early years of Edinburgh genetics up to World War II have been outlined in Chapter 1; while this research may have been basic or agriculture orientated, it was to prove highly relevant to subsequent human and medical genetics. The founding of the MRC Clinical Effects of Radiation Unit, now the MRC Human Genetics Unit, was likewise central to the development of human cytogenetics internationally, as has been told in Chapter 2.

Together with the university's creation in 1968 of a new Human Genetics Department, strongly supported by Frank Crew, now professor in the Medical School, this promised well for the future development of human and medical genetics, especially when a purpose-built new Institute (Figure 3.5b) was created to house them both on the campus of the Western General Hospital. This promise has been amply fulfilled in terms of research by the continued success of the MRC unit, currently headed by Wendy Bickmore (see also the recorded interviews with former Directors H John Evans [04] and Nicholas Hastie [11]), but sadly this was not the case for the University Department. A combination of University politics and internal personal rivalries created difficulties from the outset; despite the appointment of an outstanding medical geneticist, Alan Emery (see Figure 3.6 and interview [48]), to the Chair, with other able workers such as David Brock (human biochemical genetics; Figure 3.7) and Charles Smith (statistical genetics), who between them produced much important work, the University decided to close the department in 1983, following Alan Emery's decision to take early retirement.

To lose the only full university department of human genetics in the UK was a major blow to human and medical genetics across the whole country, not just in Edinburgh; while the MRC unit was not directly affected, this unhappy event contributed to a general distancing between basic scientists and more clinical research workers that could and should have been avoided. Part of this saga can be

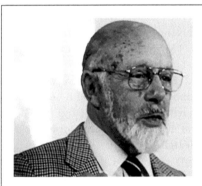

Figure 3.6 Alan EH Emery (born 1928). Recorded interview 10/08/2005 [48]. (Photo courtesy of Alan Emery.)

Alan Emery was born into a poor family in Lancashire but gained a scholarship to study medicine at Manchester University, qualifying in 1960. Continuing in adult medicine he went to Baltimore for three years, working with Victor McKusick at the time when he was changing from cardiology to medical genetics. Emery's research was on X-linked muscular dystrophies and he was responsible for delineating Emery-Dreifuss muscular dystrophy at this time (Emery and Dreifuss 1966). On his return to Manchester he set up a medical genetics unit, but in 1968 was appointed to the new Chair of Human Genetics in Edinburgh (see above), where he remained until 1983, muscular dystrophies continuing to be his main field of interest. In 1989 he became Director of the European Neuromuscular Centre and created a network of research groups and small international workshops on a range of muscular dystrophies that continues to flourish.

He has been a prolific author in a number of fields, not just medical genetics, as well as an artist and published poet, his most notable genetics books being the long-running *Elements of Medical Genetics*, first published in 1968, as well as his major textbook *Principles and Practice of Medical Genetics* with American co-editor David Rimoin.

Born and educated in Capetown, South Africa, David Brock spent time working in organic chemistry in Oxford (under Hans Krebs) and in America, before moving to Edinburgh to join first the Animal Breeding Research Unit and then in 1968 the new University Human Genetics Department. Here, despite the problems of the Edinburgh Department mentioned above, he and his group made some outstanding advances, including the use of amniotic fluid and later serum alphafetoprotein for the prenatal diagnosis and screening of neural tube defects (Brock and Sutcliffe 1972, Brock et al. 1974), and later the carrier detection and prenatal diagnosis of cystic fibrosis, with several major books on these and other human biochemical

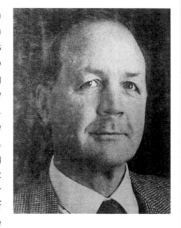

Figure 3.7 David JH Brock (1936–2004). (Photo courtesy of The Scotsman.)

genetics topics. He was also central to the successful consortium development of molecular genetic diagnosis across Scotland.

Following the break-up of the Human Genetics Department, he was the principal person responsible for the rescue of Edinburgh human and medical genetics in the university and NHS, and for the regrouping and renaissance of those involved in a new Molecular Medicine Centre, opened in 1994. After his retirement he took up his old wider interests in farming and other outdoor pursuits and it is sad that, dying aged only 68, he did not have longer years for this. I was also sorry not to have had the opportunity of interviewing him for my recorded interview series.

witnessed in the recorded interview with Alan Emery, but there must be a range of written records that tell the wider story; it is important that they are preserved and archived so that a full and impartial history, however uncomfortable, can be recorded, So far there seems to have been no attempt to create an archive for either the MRC Human Genetics Unit or the University Department of Human Genetics, despite this having been recently done for other aspects of Edinburgh genetics and repeatedly suggested by myself and others.

At the time when Edinburgh medical genetics was threatened with disintegration in the early 1980s, Scottish medical genetics as a whole was fortunate to have a valuable ally in the Scottish Health Department. Rosalind Skinner (Figure 3.8) had previously worked in the University Human Genetics Department and had been married at the time to Alan Emery. Moving into Public Health Medicine, she found that genetic services were part of her remit, and she was able to help them to recover and move forward, a major and lasting achievement being the Scottish Molecular Genetics Consortium, a model that was denied the rest of

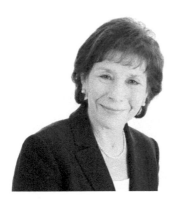

Figure 3.8 Rosalind Skinner, the key person in the Scottish Health Department responsible for planning the later development of medical genetics in Scotland. (Courtesy of Rosalind Skinner.)

the UK for another decade because of the introduction of the damaging NHS 'internal market'. With health matters increasingly devolved after 2000, wise policies within the Scottish Health Department have ensured that Scotland has remained at the forefront of genetic and genomic services as well as basic human genetics research.

It has to be said, though, that clinical genetics has remained a somewhat subsidiary part of the overall medical genetics scene in Edinburgh and until recently, with some notable exceptions, such as Veronica van Heyningen's work on the molecular basis of aniridia and Adrian Bird's separate Wellcome Trust–funded unit, has been undervalued in terms of its potential value for collaborative clinical-laboratory research.

NEWCASTLE

Passing South from Edinburgh into England, the distance is not far until Newcastle on Tyne is reached, a centre that provides a further element in the history of British medical genetics, mostly relatively recent, but with foundations laid in the 1960s by a non-medical worker, Derek Roberts, with the unusual background of human geography (Figures 3.9 and 3.10).

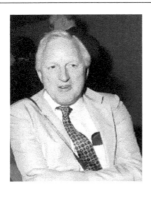

Figure 3.9 Derek Roberts (1925–2017). Recorded interview [02] (2/10/2003).

Derek Roberts started his career as a geographer, with a special interest in human population variation, his undergraduate career having been delayed by the war, in which he lost an arm. Between 1949 and 1963 he worked in Oxford with evolutionary anatomist Wilfred le Gros Clark, doing extensive field work with Nilotic populations in Sudan and linking with blood group geneticists. In 1960 he spent a year in Michigan with James Neel, which reinforced his human genetics interests. He also formed part of an informal Oxford grouping of workers from different departments, including the neighbouring Harwell unit, who had a common interest in genetics and held weekly meetings to discuss the latest developments.

After a short spell in Alan Stevenson's new MRC unit in Oxford he was appointed to a lectureship in human genetics in Newcastle in 1965, developing first a blood group and then a cytogenetics laboratory, and undertaking numerous genetic studies of different populations, including that of Tristan da Cunha after its evacuation. With increasing pressure for medical genetics services and genetic counselling, for which he felt unsuited without a medical qualification, he was able to facilitate an NHS appointment for John Burn (see below), the unit being then able to evolve progressively into a major service and academic medical genetics centre.

John Burn provides a further example of someone who was the first of their family to go to university, thanks to high quality state education. Born and brought up in an industrial mining village near Durham, he won a medical school place at nearby Newcastle University, where he did an intercalated year in human genetics with Derek Roberts. After a range of clinical posts, mainly paediatric, he decided on medical genetics as a career and went to London in 1980 to work with Cedric Carter, who was close to retirement. Here he met with Marcus Pembrey and Michael Baraitser, as well as Robin Winter (see below) and became part of the small group that started the Dysmorphology Club and who helped to establish clinical dysmorphology as a scientific and clinical field in Britain, as described in Chapter 4.

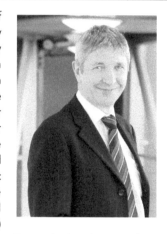

Figure 3.10 John Burn (born 1952). Recorded interview [100] (22/09/2014). (Courtesy of John Burn.)

Returning to Newcastle in 1984 as the first NHS-based consultant clinical geneticist, he progressively built up a flourishing medical genetics service across the Northern health region, with strong support from both clinicians and management, linking with others working in genetic fields and achieving the establishment of the Newcastle Centre for Life, which gave facilities not only for laboratory genetics research but for clinical workers and especially for public education and interaction. When Derek Roberts retired, John Burn was appointed to a chair and to the clinical directorship of the Centre for Life, while Tom Strachan, previously in Manchester, became its scientific director.

At a wider UK level, and across continental Europe, he has made important contributions to health policy in relation to genetics and medicine, acting as a much-needed counterbalance to the often unwise and unrealistic proposals emerging periodically from the English health department over the past two decades.

His own interests have gradually changed from dysmorphology to cancer genetics (see Chapter 4) and he is now much involved in therapeutic trials for the prevention of colorectal cancer, illustrating the increasing involvement of medical geneticists in this wider area.

(a)   (b)   (c)

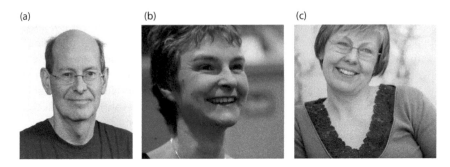

Figure 3.11 Some major contributors to Newcastle medical genetics. **(a)** Tom Strachan, responsible for the development of molecular genetics research at the Newcastle Centre for Life, and previously in Manchester. **(b)** Judith Goodship, clinical geneticist and researcher on inherited cardiac disorders. **(c)** Kate Bushby, developer of services and research for inherited neuromuscular disorders.

Newcastle's major achievements in the area of genetics and medicine show what can be achieved in a regional centre if it values and nurtures its talent, avoids disruptive rivalries and is prepared to 'think big'; fields in which it has made important contributions outside mainstream medical genetics (Figure 3.11) include mitochondrial genetic disorders and their prevention, also muscular dystrophies and allied neuromuscular disorders. It provides a salutary lesson for some of the older traditional academic centres that have failed to make full use of the talent available to them.

MANCHESTER

Manchester's early start in medical genetics came from medicine, not basic genetics, with Alan Emery founding a medical genetics unit there after his return from Johns Hopkins Hospital. After Emery's move to Edinburgh in 1968, Rodney Harris, also from an adult medicine background and with expertise in immunogenetics research, was appointed (Figure 3.12).

Over the next 30 years Harris oversaw the unit's development into a large, comprehensive and flourishing department, becoming very much the model for the integrated development of laboratory and clinical genetics services together with academic aspects. It was one of the first centres to introduce human molecular genetics as part of laboratory genetics services, under Andrew Read (see Figure 3.13, Box) and Tom Strachan (who later moved to Newcastle), becoming one of the two reference laboratories for NHS molecular genetics in England. It also started the first UK MSc degree in genetic counselling under Lauren Kerzin-Storrar (see Chapter 6), who had trained as a genetic counsellor at the Sarah Lawrence College in America.

Rodney Harris was succeeded in 2001 by Dian Donnai (see Figure 3.14), one of the founders of clinical dysmorphology, who had already been involved with this field internationally, as described in Chapter 4.

Rodney Harris's activities provide an outstanding example of the value of building the collaborative service and research networks that have been such an

(a)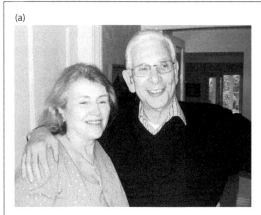

(b)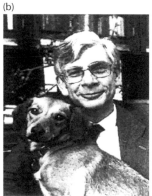

Figure 3.12 Rodney Harris (1932–2018). Recorded interview 07/03/2006 [59]. **(a)** Rodney and Hilary Harris. (Courtesy of Rodney Harris and Genetics and Medicine Historical Network.) **(b)** Rodney Harris and his 'hearing dog'. (Courtesy Hilary Harris.)

Rodney Harris was born in Liverpool and trained in medicine at Liverpool university, where he worked with Cyril Clarke, who encouraged him to learn immunogenetics, sending him to van Rood in Leiden to learn HLA techniques. After returning to Liverpool he was offered a substantive clinical academic post in Manchester in 1968 to develop transplantation immunology and also to run the then small medical genetics unit just vacated by Alan Emery.

Harris's interests moved progressively away from immunology into wider medical genetics as the Manchester department steadily grew, and he also became much involved with policy development at both the Department of Health, where he was advisor on medical genetics for some years, following Cedric Carter, and at the Royal College of Physicians, where he led the College's Medical Genetics Committee (see Chapter 9) and coordinated a series of reports on clinical genetics services, teaching of genetics to medical students, and other areas, which greatly influenced developments, not just in the UK but internationally. He also led a successful major initiative of the European Society of Human Genetics on the development of genetic services across Europe.

important and characteristic feature of UK medical genetics as it has developed over the past 50 years. It should perhaps be mentioned, too, that he achieved this contribution despite severe deafness, which led to his 'hearing dog' being a familiar feature at genetics meetings! (Figure 3.12b).

In addition to the Medical Genetics Department, based at St Mary's Hospital, Manchester, a longstanding inherited metabolic disorders unit, founded by George Komrower (1911–1989) and continued by Edward Wraith (1953–2013),

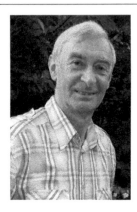

Born in Gloucester, England, Andrew Read's initial field of work was in organic chemistry and nucleic acid structure, first in Cambridge and then Warwick, but links with Edinburgh colleagues led him to molecular genetics. Already based in Manchester at the time, he joined Rodney Harris's department in 1977 and played a key role in introducing DNA-based technology into both research and service activities in the 1980s. His books with Tom Strachan (*Human Molecular Genetics*) and with Dian Donnai (*The New Clinical Genetics*) have had a major influence worldwide and illustrate his longstanding involvement in teaching. Likewise, his influence in policy development of molecular genetics services greatly helped to ensure that this new field remained closely connected with the rest of medical genetics, not just in the UK but across the rest of Europe through the European Society of Human Genetics.

Figure 3.13 Andrew Read (born 1939). Recorded interview 6/02/2007 [64]. (Courtesy of Andrew Read and Genetics and Medicine Historical Network.)

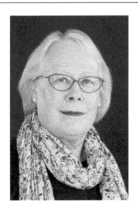

Dian Donnai is one of the significant number of medical geneticists in what has now become a predominantly female specialty, who have had their career progression delayed by family commitments and by the need to follow a husband's career geographically. Qualifying in medicine in 1968, she initially trained in paediatrics, moving first to Sheffield and then to Manchester. Here she joined Rodney Harris's department, initially as one of the first group of UK clinical genetics trainees, then as NHS consultant from 1986, and succeeding Rodney Harris as Professor and head of department in 2001. She likewise became Department of Health advisor for medical genetics.

She had already developed a special interest in congenital malformations before arriving in Manchester and became one of the founder

Figure 3.14 Dian Donnai (born 1945). (Courtesy of Dian Donnai. Recorded interview 6/02/2007 [63].)

clinical dysmorphologists (see Chapter 4), collaborating in the forming of the Dysmorphology Club with Robin Winter and other colleagues, and starting her own successful series of international dysmorphology conferences in Manchester. She has also pioneered studies in clinical dysmorphology across continental Europe, especially Scandinavia, establishing a collaborative approach in several countries where this had previously not been usual.

has been based at Manchester Children's Hospital, where for some years a separate medical genetics group also existed under Maurice Super (1936–2006), which subsequently merged with the main department.

Manchester's Christie Hospital, a major centre for cancer research, has also had a strong genetics component and between 1983 and 1997 was led by David Harnden, previously at Birmingham and originally at Edinburgh, whose early contributions to human chromosome research have been described in Chapter 1. From the 1990s the rapid development of clinical cancer genetics research and services (see Chapter 4) has seen Manchester play a leading role in this too, led by clinical geneticist Gareth Evans.

YORKSHIRE, SHEFFIELD AND THE TRENT REGION

Leeds has an interesting early background to genetics related to its longstanding involvement in the textile industry, in that William Astbury (1898–1961), pioneer in x-ray diffraction crystallography, took the first crystallographic images of DNA in Leeds in 1938. Promising contributions to medical genetics, though, by Robert Mueller, on familial deafness and on gene mapping by autozygosity analysis were cut short by his serious illness, while several other able colleagues moved elsewhere. Leeds and neighbouring Bradford have, however, played an important role in the development of genetic services for thalassaemias among its Asian minorities by Aamra Darr and her colleagues, especially through collaborations with Bernadette Modell in London (see Chapter 5).

The creation of new medical schools in the cities of *Nottingham* and *Leicester*, part of the same Trent health region of the NHS, geographically close to each other, and to the longer established medical school in *Sheffield*, has caused a number of problems for the development of medical genetics in all three centres; notably how to achieve a critical mass of workers and how to avoid duplication, especially of laboratory services. This is a situation that is now being played out on a larger scale across England with the advent of genomics, and it is not unique to medical genetics. Here I shall simply mention a few of the principal people involved in developing medical genetics in these health regions.

Sheffield developed a small human genetics department early, when Eric Blank (see Figure 3.15) was appointed in 1960 after training with Penrose.

Development of the Sheffield unit was hindered by initially being sited in a house unconnected to the main hospital. Blank was joined first by Dhavendra Kumar, later in Cardiff and author of a notable book on genetic disorders of the Indian subcontinent (Kumar 2004) and then by Oliver Quarrell (Figure 3.16a) as NHS consultant, who had developed a research interest in Huntington's disease while training in Cardiff and continued this work in Sheffield.

Both *Nottingham* and *Leicester* universities had flourishing basic genetics departments before their medical schools were opened, under Bryan Clarke and Robert Pritchard, respectively; Nottingham has continued this with important medically orientated molecular genetics research on myotonic dystrophy and other genetic disorders under David Brook. But the person whose work has been

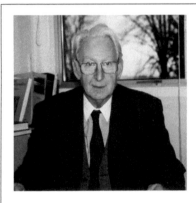

Figure 3.15 Eric Blank (1930–2007). Founder of medical genetics in Sheffield. (Photo courtesy of Catrin Blank. Interview with the author (not recorded but details available), 2004.)

Born in Brecon, South Wales, and trained in medicine in Cardiff, Eric Blank had originally planned a career in music (like several other geneticists in my interview series) and this remained a lifelong interest. The offer of an MRC research studentship took him to the Galton Laboratory under Penrose, where he undertook a major study of the disorder Apert syndrome (Blank 1960), which confirmed a paternal age effect for isolated cases (the majority) of this autosomal dominant disorder, an important finding in relation to genetic effects of radiation on mutation. More than 30 years later, the mechanism underlying this would be elucidated by Andrew Wilkie and colleagues (Goriely and Wilkie, 2012).

Blank's practice of combining business with pleasure led him to map out nearby golf courses while on Apert family visits around the country, something that apparently met with Penrose's disapproval until he was shown the successfully completed study, which was duly published in *Annals of Human Genetics*. Blank would have liked to stay on another year at the Galton, but Penrose firmly told him that 'it was time to go out into the real world'! He helpfully suggested several possibilities, among which was Sheffield, where Blank was to spend the rest of his career.

highly relevant, albeit indirectly, for medical genetics and many wider areas is Alec Jeffreys, discoverer of DNA fingerprinting (see Chapter 11). Based in Leicester throughout his career, he is a prime example of how an outstanding scientist can achieve worldwide success and renown from outside a large and well recognised centre.

It is perhaps understandable that, with the success of basic genetics so clearly displayed in Leicester through Alec Jeffreys' work, a more clinically orientated academic approach might not have been adequately supported to develop into a full academic department; this was sadly the case after Ian Young (Figure 3.16b), an outstanding clinical geneticist, was appointed primarily to develop NHS services there. Nor did the later creation of a Chair (without any support staff) help either him or Alexander Raeburn, from Edinburgh, in developing the field in nearby Nottingham, where a clinical genetics service had originally been started by paediatrician John Fitzsimmons. Changes in health region boundaries and the presence of three centres in a relatively small area were additional factors making it difficult to develop the necessary 'critical mass' in all these centres.

(a) (b)

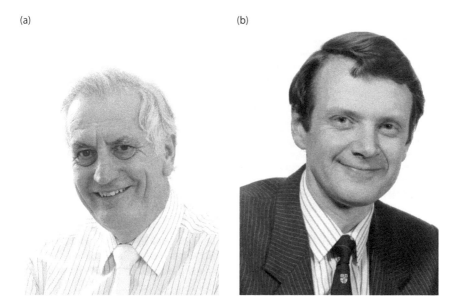

Figure 3.16 Medical geneticists across the east midlands and north of England. **(a)** Oliver Quarrell, Sheffield. (See text; photo courtesy of Oliver Quarrell.) **(b)** Ian Young, Leicester and Nottingham, who made major contributions to our understanding of mucopolysaccharidoses and other inherited bone dysplasias. (Courtesy of Ian Young.)

BIRMINGHAM

Birmingham has made major, though disjointed contributions to medical genetics over the years. Lancelot Hogben created a small research group there after his traumatic wartime experiences (see Chapter 1), but was limited by serious health problems. The university also had a small basic genetics department under Kenneth Mather and John Jinks, focused on Drosophila quantitative genetics, but though adjacent to the medical school these scientists seem to have had minimal contact with Hogben or others involved in human genetics there. As John Edwards notes in his recorded interview [14]:

> There was a little canal going through the middle of the campus and it could have been the Pacific from the amount of communication there was between the genetics department, Jinks and Mather, and the more direct approach of the human group.

John Edwards was the first person to develop medical genetics in Birmingham and his records are archived there, as are those of Hogben (Figure 3.17).

John Edwards' interests ranged widely over the field of medical and general genetics. His discovery of trisomy 18 (Edwards et al. 1960) has already been mentioned in Chapter 2, but his recognition of X-linked hydrocephalus (Edwards 1961) was another important clinical genetic study, while his paper 'the simulation

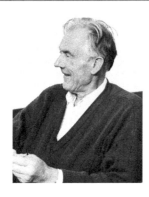

John Edwards had two main places of work, Birmingham and Oxford, but his major original contributions were mainly Birmingham based. He went there in 1956 after medical training and hospital clinical experience in London, in addition to a year as medical officer with the British Antarctic Survey. He worked with Lancelot Hogben (see Chapter 1), who was by then in poor health, and Thomas McKeown, epidemiologist, on seasonal variation in neural tube defects, but when the opportunity arose of joining the new MRC Clinical and Population Genetics Research Unit headed by Alan Stevenson (see Chapter 3), he moved to Oxford, only to find that numerous unforeseen problems existed (see the interview transcript), in particular the unit's isolation on a temporary site away from other academic departments. He returned to Birmingham where he was given a personal chair, but plans for a new institute there never materialised and after 20 years in Birmingham he again moved to Oxford, where he was appointed Professor of Genetics (but not human or medical genetics) in succession to Walter Bodmer.

Figure 3.17 John H Edwards (1928–2007). Recorded interview 23/08/2004 [14]. (Photo courtesy of Ross Shipman and Anthony Edwards.)

of Mendelism' (Edwards 1960) shows his ability to resolve what initially appeared to be complex mathematical situations. He later made close links with the Harwell geneticists, such as Anthony Searle [19] and Mary Lyon [18], in developing comparative gene mapping. Perhaps his biggest influence on medical genetics was through the series of small and informal meetings he organised during his Oxford years, which almost always resulted in new ideas, as did his own lectures, even though these were often difficult to follow!

Edwards was fortunate to have Sarah Bundey (Figure 3.18a) join him in Birmingham; she was an experienced clinical geneticist, a former colleague of Cedric Carter in London, with special expertise in neurogenetics. She also had good organisational skills, not John Edwards' strongest characteristic.

After Edwards had left for Oxford, his Birmingham chair was allowed to lapse for several years, only being revived by NHS funding, allowing Eamon Maher (Figure 3.18b) to be appointed, with a special interest in cancer genetics. He subsequently moved to Cambridge and the Birmingham University Chair again lapsed, the university having never been enthusiastic, or even supportive of it.

The NHS genetics service was robust, however, with the large West Midlands population allowing a considerable number of senior clinical and laboratory staff to be appointed, including Peter Farndon (see Figure 3.19, Box) who, after Sarah Bundey's early death, took on a lead role, not just for Birmingham but for medical genetics education overall in the UK, for training through the Royal Colleges and in building up and bringing together the professional UK genetics societies.

(a)

(b)

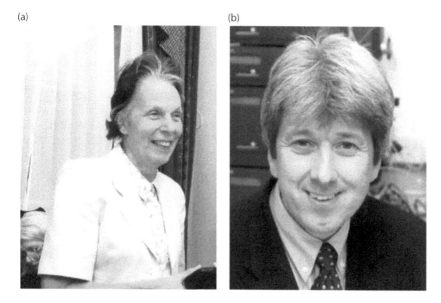

Figure 3.18 **(a)** Sarah Bundey (1936–1998), a key figure in Birmingham medical genetics. (Courtesy of Peter Farndon.) **(b)** Eamonn Maher, Professor of Medical Genetics in Birmingham and later in Cambridge. (Courtesy of Eamonn Maher.)

(a)

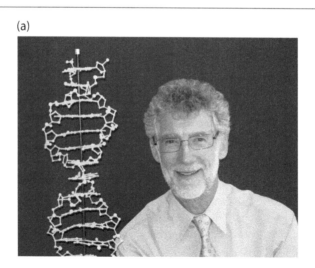

Figure 3.19 **(a)** Peter Farndon Born 1950. (Photo courtesy of Peter Farndon.) Recorded interview 7/11/2013 [97].

Peter Farndon trained in medicine in London and did an intercalated BSc degree at the Galton Laboratory, which convinced him to pursue a career in medical genetics. After a series of general clinical posts in paediatrics and adult medicine, he held one of the first medical genetics training posts in Manchester, finally taking up a permanent NHS-based consultant post in Birmingham. After mapping the gene for the familial tumour disorder Gorlin syndrome, he concentrated on service and education development in medical genetics, playing key roles in the formation of the British Society of Human Genetics from its components and the formation of the Joint Medical Genetics Service Committee of the Royal Colleges of Physicians and Pathologists. In 2005 he became Director of the new Genetics Education Centre, based in Birmingham, which formed part of the series of initiatives arising from the 2003 'Genetics White Paper' (see Chapter 8).

(b)

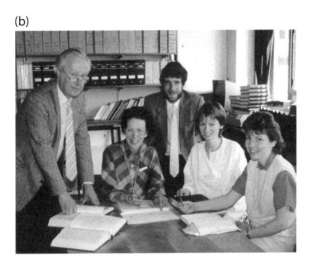

Figure 3.19 **(b)** The Birmingham clinical genetics team 1986, including Jack Insley (paediatrician), Sarah Bundey and Peter Farndon, with genetic nurses Jo Affleck and Barbara Gibbons. (Courtesy of Peter Farndon.)

LIVERPOOL

We have seen in Chapter 2 how Liverpool, under Cyril Clarke's leadership, had pioneered genetics in medicine in the 1960s; apart from Clarke's own contribution in the prevention of rhesus haemolytic disease of the newborn, his colleagues (all practising clinicians in adult medicine) included Richard McConnell (gastroenterology and genetics), seen in Figure 1.10, David Price Evans (pharmacogenetics), John Woodrow (rheumatology and immunogenetics) and David Weatherall (thalassaemias). But after Clarke's retirement and move to London in 1973 as President of the Royal College of Physicians, and David Weatherall's move to Oxford in 1974 (see below), the Liverpool interest in genetics faded, the only group remaining being the cytogenetics laboratory of Stanley Walker (a botanist by background), which became an NHS cytogenetics unit.

Thus the spirit of Liverpool medical genetics was very largely carried on at a distance, by people who had worked with and been influenced by Cyril Clarke but who ended up in other places, including David Weatherall in Oxford, Rodney

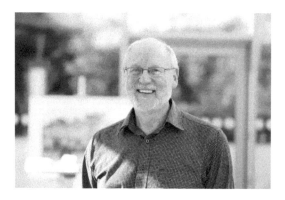

Figure 3.20 Alan Fryer, Liverpool.

Harris in Manchester, Marcus Pembrey and Michael Pope in London and myself in Cardiff.

When medical genetics was finally reborn in Liverpool, with the appointment of Alan Fryer (Figure 3.20) in 1990 as NHS clinical geneticist, it was at Alder Hey Children's Hospital.

Despite being at that time the largest children's hospital in Britain, this had previously had no significant genetics interest (apart from inherited metabolic disease) and no links with Cyril Clarke's era apart from some genetic counselling clinics done over many years by paediatrician David Fielding from neighbouring Chester.

OXFORD

Deciphering the history of medical genetics in Oxford is far from easy and not at all typical of the rest of Britain; the story could be written from several viewpoints – basic science, clinical medicine or medical genetics itself – and I shall here only try to mention some of the main components.

After the early MRC unit under Alan Stevenson had been closed on his retirement (see Chapter 2), most of the remaining members, notably Martin Bobrow, Peter Pearson and Clare Davison, found homes elsewhere; Peter Pearson moving to the Chair of human genetics in Leiden, Martin Bobrow (Figure 3.21a) to the basic genetics unit of Walter Bodmer, which formed part of the broader biochemistry department of the university, before also moving to a Chair in the Netherlands (Amsterdam). Clare Davison, co-author of Stevenson's genetic counselling book, moved to a clinical genetics post in Cambridge. Richard Lindenbaum (Figure 3.21b) remained on the site of the previous MRC unit as NHS consultant until his early death in 1991, and was joined by John Edwards part-time from his basic genetics university chair, as well as by George Fraser [32] who founded a familial cancer clinic.

Dick Lindenbaum deserves a special note here; he has been well described in the obituary by his colleague John Edwards (with an addendum by Lindenbaum's close childhood friend Oliver Sacks), as 'one of the last of the general clinical geneticists whose knowledge covered almost the whole field of genetic disease'.

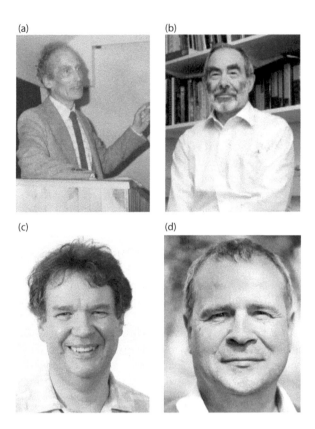

Figure 3.21 Some of the numerous contributors to Oxford medical genetics (see Chapter 2 for Alan Stevenson). **(a)** Richard Lindenbaum (see text). (Photo courtesy of Andrew Wilkie.) **(b)** Martin Bobrow (born 1938), subsequently Chair of medical genetics in Cambridge. (Photo courtesy of Martin Bobrow and the Genetics and Medicine Historical Network.) **(c)** Andrew Wilkie, worker at the Weatherall Institute for Molecular Medicine on the molecular basis of the craniosynostoses and on paternal age effects. (Photo courtesy of Andrew Wilkie.) **(d)** Richard Gibbons, whose work at Institute of Molecular Medicine on genes involved with brain development originated from early studies with David Weatherall on the thalassaemias. (Photo courtesy of Richard Gibbons.)

Born into a London medical family and educated there and at Oxford, he trained in paediatrics and joined the Stevenson MRC Oxford unit, collaborating closely there with both Martin Bobrow and Peter Pearson before transferring to the NHS.

Lindenbaum's personality reflects the remarkable breadth and depth of many of the early medical geneticists. A true polymath, he particularly excelled in his fluency in numerous European languages. Especially in his case, contributions cannot be measured solely in terms of his published work, though his recognition of the key importance to isolating the Duchenne muscular dystrophy gene of a girl with the disorder having a translocation involving the X chromosome, was a landmark advance (Lindenbaum et al. 1979). Perhaps his best memorial is his correspondence with physicians and patients, often exceptionally detailed, which gives an indication of the value of a talented, insightful and humane medical geneticist, albeit too much of a perfectionist to be able to function optimally in a busy service setting. It is a pity from a historical perspective that such patient-related (and hence confidential) records are rarely formally archived.

Looking outside the medical genetics unit itself, which remained (and still remains) largely unrecognised by the main Oxford academic structures, the principal development in the field over the past 30 years has undoubtedly been

Born in Liverpool and trained in medicine at Liverpool Medical School, David Weatherall first did clinical posts and then undertook his compulsory military service as a medical officer based in Singapore, where he encountered his first case of thalassaemia. A local pathologist helped him to do some simple haemoglobin studies, and interest in and publication of the case in 1960 resulted in a link with Herman Lehmann, in London, who had previously been the key clinical colleague for Max Perutz in his Nobel Prize-winning work on haemoglobin structure. Weatherall had already been greatly influenced by Cyril Clarke, who arranged a research fellowship for him in Baltimore with Victor McKusick between 1960 and 1962 soon after he had returned to Liverpool from the army.

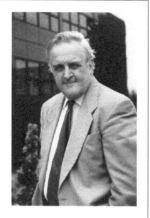

Figure 3.22 David Weatherall (1933–2018). Recorded interview 16/12/2004 [30] (See also Chapter 10).

The research was mainly on studies of the frequency of haemoglobin disorders in the Baltimore area but progressively moved towards studies of the mechanism of pathology in the thalassaemias with Johns Hopkins haematologist Lockhart Conley. Soon after returning to Liverpool after the end of the Fellowship, David Weatherall was invited to take up a staff position in Conley's unit, which met with disapproval from most of the Liverpool physicians who felt that he should complete his clinical training in the traditional manner. However, Cyril Clarke had a different, though possibly ambiguous view when Weatherall asked his opinion:

I had only just got back, about four months into a locum senior registrar post, when I got this letter from Hopkins inviting me back for a faculty post with Conley. I knew what I wanted to do, it would be very difficult to do at Liverpool at the time because there was no lab, there was no equipment. The Nuffield Institute had not been built then, so that's when I got my bit of career advice from Cyril. I just went and asked him whether I could go back to the States for a couple of years, because everybody told me it would wreck my career.......He didn't even look up from what he was doing and he said 'What do you want to do?' and I said 'I would like to go back at least for a year or two'. 'Well bugger off then' and that was it, so I buggered off and went back to try to develop some way of measuring haemoglobin synthesis in the test tube, which would start an interesting two or three years' work.

Returning again to Liverpool in 1965, with his research path now clearly established, and with facilities now available in Clarke's new Nuffield Institute of Medical Genetics, Weatherall was joined by John Clegg, a Cambridge-trained molecular geneticist who he had first met while in America. This paved the way for the thalassaemia work to move into molecular studies from 1974 onwards, which are described further in Chapter 10, and which set the scene for comparable work on the molecular pathology of other mendelian disorders. After 10 years in Liverpool both Weatherall and Clegg moved to Oxford in 1974 and persuaded MRC to create a molecular haematology unit, which proved to be the predecessor of the wider Institute of Molecular Medicine.

David Weatherall continued his thalassaemia work up to and beyond his retirement, when his colleague Douglas Higgs became head of the Institute. He has also had an immense wider influence, especially in taking the new molecular approaches to other countries, particularly in the tropics, and to fields such as malaria and other infectious diseases, along with colleagues; at the same time he remained close to his clinical roots through his position as Oxford's Regius Professor of Medicine.

the Institute of Molecular Medicine, pioneered by (and now named after) David Weatherall (Figure 3.22 [30]) and opened in 1989.

More than anyone else, David Weatherall was able to develop Cyril Clarke's vision of genetics being 'part of all medicine', something that never happened in Liverpool itself, and indeed could only really come to fruition somewhere with the abundant resources and range of talent possessed by Oxford. Weatherall managed to gather together a remarkable series of groups from different areas of medicine in the new institute, including, among others, children's infections (Richard Moxon), malaria research (Adrian Hill), neuromuscular disorders (Kay Davies, see Chapter 12) and his own field of thalassaemias.

But sadly medical genetics as such was not represented in its initial leadership, largely because there was no medical geneticist at the time in Oxford who could both lead molecular research and effectively represent the developing clinical speciality of medical genetics, while it would have been difficult to recruit someone from outside with John Edwards already present in a senior position. Weatherall's successor as Regius Professor of Medicine, John Bell, focused on common disease genetics, especially diabetes, through the study of association and linkage with genome wide molecular markers; more recently whole genome analysis, involving the Wellcome Trust Centre for Human Genetics, initially led by Peter Donnelly, has undertaken one of the first major applications of this to undiagnosed disorders (see Chapter 12). This unit, along with Walter Bodmer, has recently also made major contributions to the genetic origins of the British population; again, though, there has been little involvement with medical geneticists.

Turning to Oxford University itself, genetics has been fragmented among various departments from an early stage. In Zoology, EB Ford had pioneered the concept of genetic polymorphism in the immediate post war years, while Cyril Darlington developed cytogenetics in Botany, but any connections with human genetics were tenuous. The appointment of Walter Bodmer (see Chapter 4) to the genetics Chair (its location moved to Biochemistry) brought expertise in population and molecular genetics, and HLA research, but the only link with medical genetics was through Martin Bobrow after closure of the Stevenson MRC unit. The university may have felt that appointing John Edwards after Bodmer moved to London would have created such a link, but this in fact increased the fragmentation of medical genetics and Edwards' successor was entirely non-medical.

Even in more recent years those seeking to develop academic medical genetics in Oxford, such as Andrew Wilkie (Figure 3.21c) and Richard Gibbons (Figure 3.21d), both of whom have created outstanding research groups within the Institute of Molecular Medicine, have had to do so from a base other than medical genetics itself. Wilkie's work on the molecular basis of the craniosynostoses is a prime example of how work on a group of rare disorders can uncover important general molecular mechanisms (Wilkie et al. 1995, Wilkie 1997), in this case the basis of the relationship between mutation rate and paternal age (first identified by Eric Blank, as already noted); the same is true for Gibbons' research on key genes in human brain development arising from recognition of the alpha thalassaemia-mental retardation (ATRX) syndrome.

Thus despite its abundant available talent and very real achievements, an 'outsider' is left with the feeling that Oxford has missed successive opportunities for uniting the two complementary strands of 'medical genetics' and 'genetics in medicine' that could have gained much more by their closer integration.

CAMBRIDGE

Like Oxford, Cambridge has had an abundance of talent at its disposal but has often not used it well. Over a century ago William Bateson was forced to leave Cambridge on account of lack of funding support, while in the 1950s Max Perutz and his molecular biology colleagues had to be rescued by the MRC after the University refused to back a new centre for them. The experience of Peter Goodfellow (see interview [98] and Chapter 11), eventual successor in RA Fisher's university genetics chair, shows that little had changed even in the 1990s, with the prevailing attitude remaining that one should feel honoured to be there and not expect to be given much. Malcolm Ferguson-Smith (see section on Glasgow) seems to have been a fortunate exception.

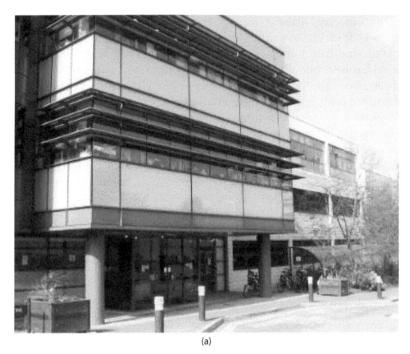

(a)

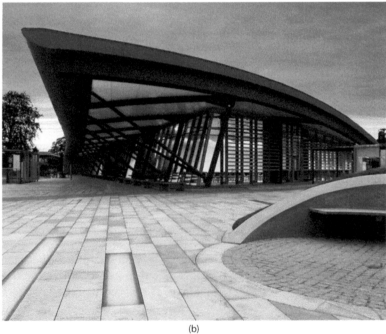

(b)

Figure 3.23 Two genetics research centres making a major impact on medical genetics. **(a)** The Weatherall Institute for Molecular Medicine, Oxford, opened in 1989. **(b)** The Wellcome Trust Sanger Institute at Hinxton, Cambridge.

Unsurprisingly, not much attention had been paid to medical genetics, whether service or academic aspects, until Ferguson-Smith's arrival from Glasgow with his clinical geneticist colleague John Yates, though Clare Davison, previously with Stevenson's Oxford unit, had already developed genetic counselling clinics. Then the later appointment of Martin Bobrow to a specific chair in medical genetics allowed consolidation of genetic services and research after Ferguson-Smith had retired from his broad Pathology Chair and moved to the Veterinary School. But even then, academic medical genetics remained insecure, with the chair left unfilled after Martin Bobrow's retirement until Eamon Maher's appointment to it in 2012, since when it has re-established its strength, in particular by linking closely with the Sanger Institute, as indicated below.

The biggest impact on Cambridge genetics from the late 1990s has come from the development by the Wellcome Trust of its genome campus at Hinxton on the edge of Cambridge, in the form of the Sanger Institute (Figure 3.23b), which ensured that the UK played a major role first in the Human Genome Project itself (Chapter 12) and then in the range of successor downstream projects. Although primarily focused on new technology and informatics, the clear and increasing applications in medical genetics research and diagnosis (see Chapter 12) have allowed valuable, even if somewhat belated clinical links to be built, as well acting as a major training centre in these areas for both clinical and laboratory geneticists. It has also attracted a number of outstanding scientists from abroad, including Leena Peltonen-Palotie (1957–2010) from 2007 until her untimely death. It must be said though that, as in Oxford, there was relatively little interaction between these research scientists and the wider British medical genetics community until very recently.

LONDON

We have seen in Chapter 2 that the earliest medical genetics centres (apart from the MRC units) were mostly London based, so it might have been expected that with the growth of university and NHS funding in the 1960s they would have become even more dominant. This did not prove to be the case, however, with the exception of Paul Polani's Paediatric Research Unit at Guy's Hospital Medical School, and it is worth looking at some of the reasons why.

Taking the exception first, there is no doubt that Paul Polani's own ability and foresight were a major factor. Having been fortunate to become well established thanks to generous charities' funding, he realised that this would not last indefinitely, but he was able to transfer much of his increasing diagnostic cytogenetics work, by now under John Hamerton (see Chapter 2), to NHS funding, while more basic research attracted mainstream research grant funds. He also realised early the need for more service-related clinical input and genetic counselling, especially with the advent of prenatal diagnosis, attracting John Fraser Roberts after his retirement from the MRC, and Caroline Berry (Figure 3.24a; [20]), who became one of the first formally trained clinical geneticists. She in turn provided the basis for regional development of clinics and laboratory referrals across the South-East Thames health region, bringing in other clinical

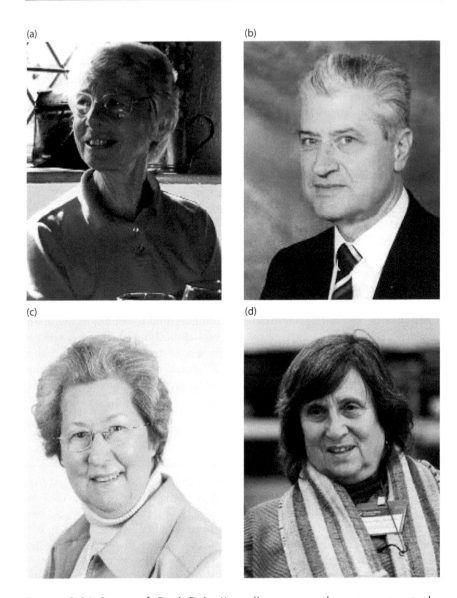

Figure 3.24 Some of Paul Polani's colleagues and successors at the Paediatric Research Unit, Guy's Hospital. See Chapter 2 for Paul Polani himself. **(a)** Caroline Berry (born 1937). Recorded interview 14/102004 [20]. Developer and leader of clinical genetics services for the South-East Thames region, based at the Paediatric Research Unit. (Photo courtesy of Caroline Berry.) **(b)** Francesco Giannelli (born 1936), the first worker at the Paediatric Research Unit to introduce molecular techniques, with special contributions to haemophilia. (Photo courtesy of Francesco Giannelli.) **(c)** Mary Seller, major contributor to experimental neural tube defect research. (Photo courtesy of Mary Seller.) **(d)** Ellen Solomon, successor to Paul Polani and Martin Bobrow as head of the Paediatric Research Unit, with her research mainly in cancer genetics. (Photo courtesy of Ellen Solomon and the Genetics and Medicine Historical Network.)

geneticists such as Frances Flinter, and leaving Polani himself and his able and innovative research groups to flourish largely unencumbered by service commitments. Notable workers over the early years have included Francesco Giannelli (molecular genetics and haemophilia, Figure 3.24b), Mary Seller (neural tube defects, Figure 3.24c) and Phillip Benson (lysosomal disorders). More recent contributors include Ellen Solomon (cancer genetics, Figure 3.24c), Richard Trembath and Chris Mathew (clinical molecular genetics) and Gillian Bates (Huntington's disease; see Chapter 11).

Polani's immediate successor, Martin Bobrow, inherited a healthy situation and as he succinctly put it in his recorded interview [24]:

> Paul had a natural flair for organisation, so he produced a structure that ...... was a sort of pyramid, it had individual divisions that had their own functions and some grew and some grew a little bit less. It had a reasonable substructure. He had a proper secretariat. He had proper books, it was financially sound and it really was just a going concern. If you go back to that department now, with the benefit of my having left it, it's an absolutely stunning place. Doubled in size. Doubled in space. So everywhere I leave does well! Mostly after I leave!

Interview with Martin Bobrow

Other London centres found it less easy to develop. Cedric Carter's MRC Clinical Genetics Research Unit remained small and almost entirely clinical and epidemiological, with no significant laboratory component; it was closed as an MRC unit on Carter's retirement, but just before this was able to act as the focus for the development of dysmorphology as part of medical genetics, thanks to the presence there of a group of young enthusiasts, in particular Robin Winter, Michael Baraitser, John Burn and Marcus Pembrey (see Chapter 4). Fortunately, charities' funding was able to produce a permanent post to succeed Carter, that would allow Pembrey (Figure 3.25) to develop his work and introduce molecular techniques; it could not hope to match the balanced all-round structure achieved by Polani's unit, though it has continued to flourish as a clinically orientated unit.

In terms of NHS health regions, the Galton Laboratory, for many years the centre of UK human genetics, found itself in the same health region as the unit at the Institute of Child Health, but its medical aspects had already declined since Penrose had retired, to be succeeded first by Harry Harris, then by Elizabeth (Bette) Robson, and finally David Hopkinson, all of whom focused on basic research, particularly enzyme polymorphisms. The highly respected Gerald Corney continued to run a genetic counselling clinic there, while its basic enzyme and gene mapping research continued to be prominent, with Sue Povey in particular making clinically orientated contributions, but there was little scope for clinical service activities. Likewise, neither North-West nor South-West London health regions were able to develop medical genetics centres comparable to that at Guy's Hospital or those of the larger UK regions.

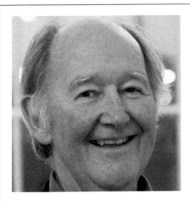

Figure 3.25 Marcus Pembrey (born 1943). Recorded interview 19/09/2006 [62]. (Photo courtesy Marcus Pembrey.)

Marcus Pembrey can claim the distinction of being the only British clinical geneticist to have worked with all the key founders of the specialty. Coming from a medical academic family and having trained in medicine in London, where he first had contacts with Cedric Carter and John Fraser Roberts, he also met Cyril Clarke, who (as others including myself also experienced) told Pembrey to go away and contact him again after passing his MRCP exam, but then offered him a research fellowship in Liverpool. Here he met and worked with David Weatherall, and continued research on mild variants of haemoglobinopathy in the Middle East after his return to London, being by then based with Paul Polani at Guy's Hospital, where he also again linked with John Fraser Roberts, taking over the authorship of his textbook. He took a permanent post, later a Chair, at the Institute of Child Health, soon before Cedric Carter retired, with a view to succeeding him, and was able to attract substantial funding to develop molecular genetics there.

Among his particular contributions have been his proposal (with Robin Winter) that Fragile X syndrome might involve a pre-mutational event (Pembrey et al, 1985), and the possibility of genetic imprinting as the basis for Angelman syndrome (Malcolm et al, (1991). He has also played major roles in the European Society of Human Genetics (ESHG) and in the European School of Medical Genetics. His continuing involvement with the Bristol-based 'ALSPAC' epidemiological study of children (see Chapter 10) has helped to maximise the genetic aspects of this.

This was in no way the fault of the able people involved, who made valuable specific contributions, including Michael Patton (Noonan syndrome) and Shirley Hodgson (cancer genetics, see Chapter 4), but rather part of a wider London problem affecting many specialist medical services. Put simply, London's traditional medical centres were mostly in the centre of the city, whose population had migrated outwards during the second half of the twentieth century, leaving too many services, too close together and often duplicating each other. This had been recognised long ago, but resistance from entrenched interests meant that plans for change were blocked until funds for logical redevelopment were no longer available, with smaller services such as medical genetics not able to influence the situation much. The academic situation was somewhat comparable, so it can readily be seen how regional centres, with genetic services and research departments, often integrated 'under one roof' (to use a phrase of Rodney Harris), and with well-defined and stable populations to serve and study, had the advantage over the more fragmented London groups.

Of course, this picture of the London medical genetics centres omits the important research role of the considerable number of major research units not specifically designated as genetic, but where genetic research of a variety of types has become increasingly prominent, especially after the spread of molecular techniques. The Institute of Neurology, the National Heart and Lung Institute and the Institute of Cancer Research are a few of the larger examples; more circumscribed units are provided by St Mark's Hospital (familial polyposis of the colon) and the Institute of Ophthalmology (the base for the pioneer ophthalmologist and medical geneticist Arnold Sorsby [Chapter 9]). This can be seen as an indication of how 'genetics in medicine' has finally, for clinically orientated research at least, become a reality for most fields of medicine.

WESSEX AND THE WEST OF ENGLAND

Southampton and its surrounding 'Wessex' area were too close to London to allow development of a separate medical school until 1971, but a small clinical genetics unit was developed by first David Siggers, trained by Victor McKusick in Baltimore, and then Nick Dennis (a trainee of Cedric Carter), in conjunction with the paediatric department. Unusually, a flourishing NHS cytogenetics laboratory

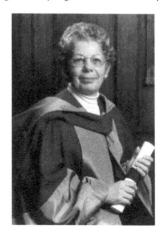

had already been developed in the non-teaching hospital at nearby Salisbury by Marina Seabright (Figure 3.26), who had been in the forefront of introducing chromosome banding techniques (see Chapter 10); when she retired in 1987 she was able to attract Patricia Jacobs, originally in Edinburgh (see Chapter 2) but then for many years in America, to succeed her, accompanied by her husband Newton Morton, renowned population and mathematical geneticist, who formed an MRC group in Southampton.

Patricia Jacobs not only transformed the Salisbury lab into an outstanding research as well as service unit, but quickly introduced molecular techniques so that the unit became one of the two English NHS genetics reference labs, revitalising the UK cytogenetics scene which had been becoming somewhat static. Even more importantly, she was able to develop laboratory medical genetics as a scientist while at the same time strengthening links with clinical geneticists, serving as President of the UK Clinical Genetics Society even though not medically trained.

Figure 3.26 Marina Seabright (1922–2007), Patricia Jacobs' predecessor at the Wessex cytogenetics laboratory, Salisbury; she was responsible for discovery of the trypsin-Giemsa chromosome banding technique. (Courtesy of John Barber and European Society of Human Genetics.)

(a) (b) (c)

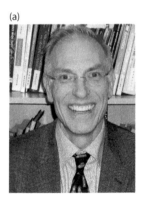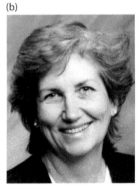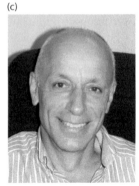

Figure 3.27 Pioneer workers in the late-to-develop South-West of England.
(a) Peter Lunt, Bristol. (Courtesy of Peter Lunt.) **(b)** Christine Garrett, Exeter.
(Courtesy of Christine Garrett.) **(c)** Peter Turnpenny, Exeter.

Moving further west to our final English health region, South-West England had been persistently backward from the beginning in any medical genetics developments, despite John Fraser Roberts having been based in Bristol when he wrote his landmark book in 1940. Even when the health authorities belatedly funded a clinical geneticist post (single handed and without any academic component) they refused to allow it to cover Devon and Cornwall, which had to wait for another decade. It is remarkable that those initially involved, Peter Lunt in Bristol, Christine Garrett and Peter Turnpenny in Exeter (see Figure 3.27) should eventually have been able to achieve so much with such minimal support, but also sad to think of the opportunities lost, especially for academic activities.

As in Salisbury, the laboratory components of medical genetics helped to rescue the situation; in Bristol, Linda Tyfield was able to develop molecular techniques from a base in medical biochemistry (cytogenetics under Alan McDermott had remained relatively isolated), while in Exeter molecular genetics under Sian Ellard, supported by clinician Andrew Hattersley, was finally able to ensure that the far South-West was on the map when the peninsula achieved its own medical school, giving much needed backing to Peter Turnpenny's longstanding efforts. Now the South-West as a whole is relatively well staffed, following the frequently seen pattern across the country that it is the initial steps that are the hardest to achieve.

WALES

Coming now to the author's own territory, I must first apologise to readers for writing a somewhat personal account; to do otherwise would be artificial, though I have tried to make it as objective as possible.

Wales can claim no longstanding tradition in genetics, apart from in the 1930s Aberystwyth being the headquarters of the Agricultural Research Council, leading to some early botanical cytogenetic studies there. I myself arrived in Cardiff from

Johns Hopkins in September 1971, just as it was undergoing a major expansion from having been a small provincial medical school to becoming a major medical teaching and research centre with a new integrated building at University Hospital of Wales. My remit was to develop medical genetics from within the Department of Medicine, and I had essentially a free hand as to how I should do it, with strong support from the clinical academic departments, in particular Medicine and Paediatrics, and as it proved later from clinicians generally across Wales. I was asked on arrival whether I wished to continue practicing general adult medicine (in which I had been trained, mainly in Liverpool) in terms of clinic referrals and acute medical intakes; somewhat rashly I said yes, it being far from clear at that point whether clinical genetics would prove to be a viable specialty in itself, but I did not expect that this aspect of my work would continue for more than 25 years! (Figure 3.28.)

Although I was appointed, like most others at the time, with no support staff, I was in fact not entirely alone, since the head of medicine, Robert Mahler, whose background was metabolic medicine, had just established PKU screening, while on the other side of the city paediatric pathologist Michael Laurence (see Figure 3.29), whose principal interest was spina bifida, had started a small chromosome laboratory in his unit, which later moved to the University Hospital site and finally came together with my own unit in 1985 in a new Institute of Medical Genetics. There was also an outstanding haemophilia unit under Arthur Bloom.

Peter Harper was born in Devon to a strongly medical family, and from an early stage tried to combine biology and medicine, medical genetics seeming a possible solution. After Oxford University and medical school in London, qualifying in 1964, he sought advice from Cyril Clarke, to be told (as were several others) to go away and come back after passing the MRCP exam. Two years later he duly went to Liverpool, his research there being on inherited oesophageal cancer, followed by a Fellowship with Victor McKusick at Johns Hopkins Hospital, Baltimore, where his MD thesis was on myotonic dystrophy.

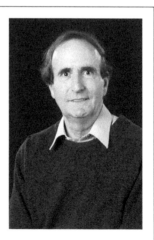

On return to Britain in 1971 he was appointed at University of Wales College of Medicine, Cardiff, where he developed medical genetics research and services, as described in the text , his own special field being the clinical and molecular genetics of myotonic and other muscular dystrophies and Huntington's disease. Since retiring from clinical work in 2004 he has focused on preserving and documenting the worldwide history of medical genetics.

Figure 3.28. Peter Harper (born 1939). Recorded interview 03/09/2004 [16] by Angus Clarke.

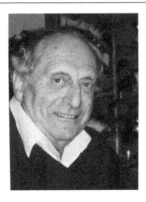

Michael Laurence was born in Berlin, coming to Britain as a refugee from Nazi Germany aged 11; he studied medicine at Cambridge and Liverpool universities, qualifying in 1949. After deciding to make a career in pathology, a post at Great Ormond Street Children's Hospital initiated his lifelong interest in neural tube defects; he also met Cedric Carter there and collaborated on his family study of spina bifida. After moving to South Wales as paediatric pathologist in 1960 he initiated further studies of neural tube defects in the South Wales valleys, documenting the geographical variation and correlation with social deprivation, leading to the strong suspicion of a nutritional cause, probably deficiency of folic acid, though his results fell just short of statistical significance to prove this. The development of prenatal diagnosis and screening techniques for neural tube defects encouraged his involvement with wider prenatal diagnosis, while his links with Cedric Carter made him one of the group involved in founding the Clinical Genetics Society. After joining Peter Harper in setting up the new Wales Institute for Medical Genetics, he retired in 1989 to live in Bern, Switzerland.

Figure 3.29 K Michael Laurence (1924–2018). Interview 23/07/2004 [13].

Starting medical genetics clinics in Cardiff, and soon in the other main hospitals across Wales, principally with the local paediatricians, I found to my surprise that in addition to families referred for genetic counselling, there were at least as many where the primary need was for an accurate diagnosis, which I was often able to provide thanks to my broad experience in rare disorders, paediatric and adult, acquired with Victor McKusick during my years at Johns Hopkins. This was not only good for relations with clinicians across Wales, but made me realise that Wales, with a stable population of 3 million, was an ideal base for the study of uncommon, mainly mendelian disorders, which formed, then as now, the bedrock of medical genetics practice.

A series of family- and population-based studies, mainly on neurogenetic disorders such as Duchenne and myotonic dystrophies, Huntington's disease and others, with registers for some of them, also gave the foundations for genetic linkage and gene mapping research, which I had already been involved with for myotonic dystrophy in America, and which evolved a decade later into DNA-based mapping and positional cloning.

After 10 years as the sole clinical geneticist, it was a great relief when it became possible to appoint Helen Hughes from Toronto (Figure 3.30a) to develop North Wales services, for which she was ideally suited from her long running experience in running the Ontario outreach clinics. Her dysmorphology skills also made a major contribution in this field, not just in Wales but across the UK. She was

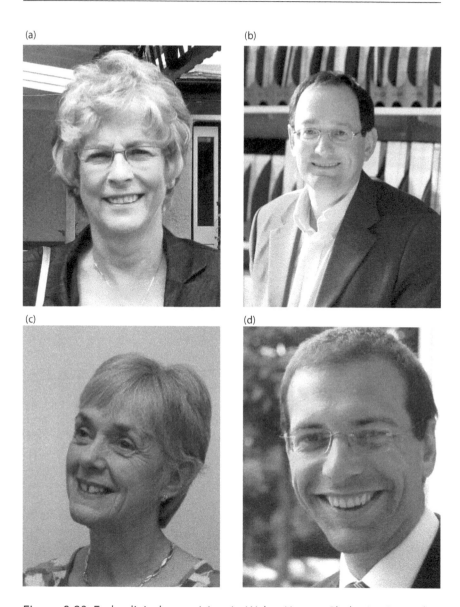

(a) (b)

(c) (d)

Figure 3.30 Early clinical geneticists in Wales (Angus Clarke is pictured in Chapter 7). **(a)** Helen Hughes, dysmorphologist and pioneer of 'outreach' genetics services for remote rural areas. (Courtesy of Helen Hughes.) **(b)** Julian Sampson, successor to Peter Harper as Head of the Wales Institute of Medical Genetics; leader of the international collaboration to isolate the tuberous sclerosis (*TSC2*) gene and discoverer of the recessively inherited form of colorectal cancer with polyposis. (Courtesy of Julian Sampson.) **(c)** Sally Davies, clinical geneticist responsible for genetic and other services for Marfan syndrome. (Courtesy of Sally Davies.) **(d)** Jonathon Gray, leader of the All-Wales Medical Genetics Service and developer of cancer genetics services for Wales. (Courtesy of Jonathon Gray.)

followed by Angus Clarke [96] (see Chapter 7), Julian Sampson (Figure 3.30b [91]), now head of the Institute, who led the international consortium that isolated the tuberous sclerosis (*TSC2*) gene, and Sally Davies (Figure 3.30c), to make up a balanced and harmonious clinical team, greatly helped by a succession of outstanding NHS and research trainees, many of whom went on to lead units elsewhere in Britain and abroad and are mentioned elsewhere in this book.

Turning to the laboratory research aspects, we were very fortunate in Cardiff to make a close and fruitful collaboration with Bob Williamson [61], Kay Davies [80] and colleagues at St Mary's Hospital London, just at the time, 1981, when the first DNA polymorphisms (RFLPs) were appearing (see Chapter 12). This allowed mapping of the Duchenne locus on the short arm of the X chromosome (Murray et al. 1982) and, after we had set up a molecular genetics lab in Cardiff, led initially by Duncan Shaw and Linda Meredith (see Chapter 10), for the Becker type to be shown as allelic to it by clinical genetics trainee Helen Kingston. Wider mapping projects allowed similar DNA-based linkage studies to be launched for myotonic dystrophy (building on my early work in America), and also for Huntington's disease, leading to our joining the successful international collaboration for isolation of the HD gene in 1993. Our family resource and all-round experience of medical genetics were essential factors in making Cardiff one of the first centres nationally and internationally to use molecular genetics not only for research but for services such as carrier detection and prenatal diagnosis.

Space does not allow description of what seems (with hindsight!) to have been a 'golden age' for positional cloning of a series of genes for mendelian disorders that had previously been little understood, but mention must be made of tuberous sclerosis (Julian Sampson) and neurofibromatosis (Meena Upadhyaya, Susan Huson) as well as the *Human Gene Mutation Database* pioneered by David Cooper and Michael Krawczak. A final very special Cardiff contribution has been the development of a series of collaborative studies of social and ethical aspects of medical genetics, especially genetic testing, by Angus Clarke, an aspect discussed further in Chapter 7.

It is also worth mentioning that Cardiff has proved to be a fruitful place for the writing of books on genetic topics, with no fewer than 55 over the last 40 years contributed by various members of the Department. It has also produced a large number of workers who have gone on to hold Chairs across Britain and in other European countries.

The issues posed for medical genetics in Wales by devolution and by overall changes in the NHS are considered in Chapter 8, but readers outside Wales may be feeling that I have already allowed it an over-generous ration of space (a separate small book is being prepared to celebrate 50 years of medical genetics in Wales), so we must conclude this account of the development of medical genetics across Britain by briefly considering Ireland.

IRELAND

Although not strictly part of 'Britain', it would be wrong to omit Ireland from this account, since the links for medical genetics have always been very close.

Northern Ireland, with its compact and stable population of around 1.5 million, for many years provided a service for families from the Republic of Ireland, where medical genetics was notable by its absence until recently and prenatal diagnosis lacking on account of an absolute ban on termination of pregnancy.

Most regions of the UK have seen the development of medical genetics occur initially around a single key individual, and this was certainly the case for Northern Ireland, where it was founded and for many years shaped by one individual, Norman Nevin (see Figure 3.31, Box).

While development of medical genetics in Northern Ireland has been influenced extensively by political and social factors, this is even more the case for the Republic of Ireland. Here its perceived associations with termination of pregnancy (still illegal though this seems likely to change) effectively prevented any genetic services, including genetic counselling, being established up to the 1980s; families needing them were forced to go to Belfast or to the British mainland. The absence of a comprehensive national health service and dependence on private practice are further factors that have hindered the progressive developments seen elsewhere in Britain and the rest of Europe. Even now, despite there being no lack of able Irish workers to develop the field (see

Born, educated and medically trained in Belfast, Norman Nevin was attracted to medical genetics by the lectures of Alan Stevenson (see Chapter 2) who was at the time Professor of Social Medicine and Epidemiology in Belfast, and with whom he did an intercalated degree. He qualified in medicine in 1960 and initially went into Pathology, but in 1965 went for two years to Cedric Carter's London unit on an MRC Fellowship, where he received a thorough grounding in medical genetics. On return to Belfast in 1967 as lecturer in human genetics, based at first in medical statistics with Eric Cheeseman, a former colleague of Stevenson, he progressively built up an all-round medical genetics department. Initially he focused on mendelian disorders, for which Stevenson's early epidemiological

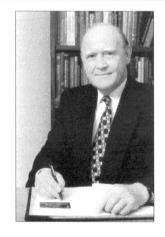

Figure 3.31 Norman C Nevin, Belfast (1935–2014). Recorded interview 4/11/2004 [26]. (Photo courtesy of Alun Evans and Patrick Morrison.)

studies had provided foundations, but his biggest contribution was his leading role in the multicentre trial of vitamin supplements for the prevention of neural tube defects, described in Chapter 11, for which Northern Ireland had the extraordinarily high frequency of 1 in 100 births. He was also much involved in the early development of the Clinical Genetics Society.

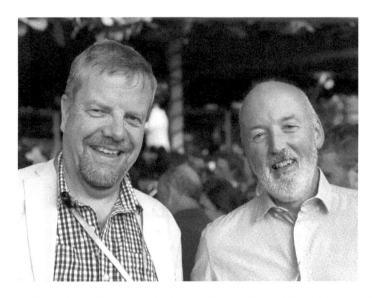

Figure 3.32 Andrew Green, clinical geneticist (left) and David Barton, head of genetics laboratories, Dublin. Pioneers of medical genetics in difficult circumstances in the Irish Republic. (Photo courtesy of Simon Patton.)

Figure 3.32), and the existence of close European links, it still proves difficult for them to overcome the combination of under-resourcing, political inertia and religious conservatism that have held things back.

CONCLUSION

This survey of the development of medical genetics across Britain has proved to be longer than I had anticipated, but it is important to recognise the diversity both of its origins and of its spread across the country. Unlike some other European countries it cannot be traced to a single founding source, while the key players have also been a diverse mixture in terms of their backgrounds and interests; for the most part they have been medically trained and have indeed remained clinically orientated, in contrast to most of their counterparts in continental Europe, who have frequently been scientists who have needed and obtained a medical qualification, rather than true clinicians. The founders were also almost exclusively male, despite there being a number of talented and prominent women undertaking research in the field, even from the early years. This is likely to have been due to multiple causes, not just to prejudice and the discouragement of women in medicine generally; the long and often antisocial hours to build a successful unit from the ground up, with little consideration for family commitments, did not help, while many of the most able female workers preferred to devote their time to their own research or clinical work rather than to undertake the extensive administrative duties necessitated by a large department in a rapidly expanding field.

British medical genetics has now moved into a different era, with its laboratory base increasingly centralised and genomic in nature, while for clinical geneticists and genetic counsellors the psychological aspects now receive much greater recognition. Together with this has come a marked gender shift in the specialty, with women now the majority among both clinical and laboratory staff. This is not unique to medical genetics, being seen in many fields of medicine, nor is it confined to Britain. It will probably take some years for a new equilibrium to become established, but meanwhile this and other beneficial changes have come about as a natural progression.

How the structure of medical genetics services across Britain will progress over the coming years is very much an open question and is discussed briefly in the final chapter of this book. The changes may well depend not just on scientific and technological advances, but also on wider medical and political issues, notably the overall future structure of the National Health Service.

REFERENCES

Blank E. 1960. Apert's syndrome (a type of acrocephaly-syndactyly): Observations on a British series of thirty-nine cases. *Ann Hum Genet.* 24:151–164.

Brock DJ, Bolton AE, Scrimgeour JB. 1974. Prenatal diagnosis of spina bifida and anencephaly through maternal plasma-alpha-fetoprotein measurement. *Lancet.* 1(7861):767–769.

Brock DJ, Sutcliffe RG. 1972. Alpha-fetoprotein in the antenatal diagnosis of anencephaly and spina bifida. *Lancet.* 2(7770):197–199.

Edwards JH. 1960. The simulation of mendelism. *Acta Genet Stat Med.* 10:63–70.

Edwards JH. 1961. The syndrome of sex-linked hydrocephalus. *Arch Dis Child.* 36:486–493.

Edwards JH, Harnden DG, Cameron AH, Crosse VM, Wolff OH. 1960. A new trisomic syndrome. *Lancet.* 1(7128):787–790.

Emery AE, Dreifuss FE. 1966. Unusual type of benign x-linked muscular dystrophy. *J Neurol Neurosurg Psychiatry.* 29:338–342.

Goriely A, Wilkie AOM. 2012. Paternal age effect mutations and selfish spermatogonial selection: Causes and consequences for human disease. *Am J Hum Genet.* 90:175–200.

Hogben A, Hogben A. (eds.). 1998. *Lancelot Hogben, Scientific Humanist: An Unauthorised Autobiography.* Woodbridge, Suffolk, UK: Merlin Press.

Johnston AW, Warland BJ, Weller SD. 1966. Genetic aspects of angiokeratoma corporis diffusum. *Ann Hum Genet.* 30:25–41.

Kumar D (ed.). 2004. *Genetic Disorders of the Indian Sub-continent.* New York: Springer.

Lindenbaum RH. Clarke G, Patel C, Moncrieff M, Hughes JT. 1979. Muscular dystrophy in an X; 1 translocation female suggests that Duchenne locus is on X chromosome short arm. *J Med Genet.* 16:389–392.

Malcolm S, Clayton-Smith J, Nichols M, Robb S, Webb T, Armour JA, Jeffreys AJ, Pembrey ME. 1991. Uniparental paternal disomy in Angelman's syndrome. *Lancet.* 337:694–697.

Moorhead P, Nowell P, Mellman W, Battips D, Hungerford D. 1960. Chromosome preparations of leukocytes cultured from human peripheral blood. *Exp Cell Res.* 20:613–636.

Murray JM, Davies KE, Harper PS, Meredith L, Mueller CR, Williamson R. 1982. Linkage relationship of a cloned DNA sequence on the short arm of the X chromosome to Duchenne muscular dystrophy. *Nature*. 300:69–71.

Pembrey ME, Winter RM, Davies KE. 1985. A premutation that generates a defect at crossing over explains the inheritance of fragile X mental retardation. *Am J Med Genet*. 21(4):709–717.

Wilkie AO. 1997. Craniosynostosis: Genes and mechanisms. *Hum Mol Genet*. 6:1647–1656.

Wilkie AO, Slaney SF, Oldridge M. et al. 1995. Apert syndrome results from localised mutations of *FGFR2* and is allelic to Crouzon syndrome. *Nature Genetics*. 9:165–172.

4

Branching out: Specialties and subspecialties in medical genetics

ABSTRACT

As medical genetics has grown, with increasing applications to different areas of medicine, so it has also differentiated. The degree of involvement of medical geneticists in different fields and the nature of the links with the various specialties involved have varied considerably, though none of the different areas have become completely separate from medical genetics as a whole. The longest established subspecialty has been clinical dysmorphology, the study of congenital malformations, largely developed in Britain by medical geneticists rather than by general paediatricians. Its combination of clinical pattern recognition, creation and use of clinical databases and links with work on developmental defects in experimental species have made it a valuable area of basic research as well as of clinical diagnosis, especially with increasing recognition of the underlying molecular and genomic defects. Clinical cancer genetics has likewise become an important field, now closely linked with cancer diagnosis and basic cancer research, largely through the recognition of single gene subsets of common cancers.

The natural tendency for any new topic in medicine or science is to start as part of an already existing speciality or scientific field and then, once it has grown to a certain point, to evolve into a specialty, or at least subspecialty, in its own right. Medical genetics is no exception to this general rule, but is more complex than most.

To begin with, medical genetics is a 'hybrid' discipline, which has both clinical and laboratory elements, joined more recently by genetic counsellors strongly linked to psychology and the social sciences. Clinical genetics, at least in most countries, including Britain, cannot trace its origins to a single parent medical specialty, but has roots in both adult internal medicine and in paediatrics, and to some extent other specialties. The mixture varies between countries, but in Britain the contributions of adult medicine and paediatrics have been close to equal, most of the founders coming from adult medicine, with a swing towards paediatrics in the 1970s and 1980s, and to some extent back again in more recent years. The number from obstetrics has been few throughout, despite the prominence of prenatal diagnosis.

Likewise the laboratory aspects of medical genetics have been derived from a wide range of scientific technologies, including basic genetics and other areas of biology, notably cytology, as well as serology, biochemistry and molecular biology, while there has been a close connection from the start with mathematics and statistics, which has again become more prominent recently with the importance of this in genomic analysis.

As this already complex mixture crystallised during the second half of the twentieth century into a distinct field of 'medical genetics', some areas within this began to become especially prominent, and to a varying degree became separate from medical genetics generally; I shall try to trace a few of these strands in this chapter for clinical genetics, while the development of laboratory-based medical genetics is covered, though less fully, in Chapter 10.

A further complexity is that during the past half century other medical specialties have themselves been evolving and their relationship with medical genetics has also changed, with marked differences in this between different specialties. As a field that inevitably crosses age and specialty boundaries, the development of medical genetics needs to be considered in the light of these changes in other specialties. Thus, in the 1960s 'general internal medicine' covered a number of fields that have since become individual and largely separate specialties, such as cardiology, endocrinology and renal medicine, with the role of the general physician diminishing accordingly. The role of the hospital and acute inpatient medical care has also declined by comparison with outpatient and community-based medicine. Overall one might consider that Cyril Clarke's vision of medical genetics becoming part of the whole of medicine has been fulfilled, but in very different ways to what he envisaged 50 years ago.

BIRTH DEFECTS AND DYSMORPHOLOGY

Chapter 2 has described how in Britain the first workers in medical genetics were from a wide range of mainly adult specialties, but with a major swing towards paediatrics when the availability of chromosome analysis made it possible to identify a specific cause for an increasing range of congenital malformations. This resulted in a considerable number of paediatricians coming to work in, and in some cases founding, genetics centres across the country, partly to provide genetic counselling, but also to diagnose and delineate previously unrecognised syndromes. While in America and in some other countries such as France, the lead role in this was taken by paediatricians themselves, such as David Smith of Seattle, most general paediatricians in Britain did not show a major interest in this area of dysmorphology, leaving it largely to the growing number of paediatrically trained clinical geneticists. It is of interest that no attempt was made in Britain by paediatricians as a whole to 'claim' medical genetics as a subspecialty of paediatrics, as occurred for a time in France, or at least in Paris (Harper 2018). Chapter 9 shows how when the new Royal College of Paediatrics and Child Health was formed (as late as 1996), medical geneticists were definite that they preferred to remain with the broader Royal College of Physicians.

The rapid and highly successful development of clinical dysmorphology as part of British medical genetics, principally during the 1980s and 1990s, can be attributed to a number of causes, but notable among these has been the high calibre of the founding workers, both in terms of their clinical diagnostic skills and their academic achievements. Added to this should be the strong tradition of collaboration between individuals and different centres around the country, leading to the delineation of new disorders which would have been difficult or impossible without the sharing of information on puzzling or apparently unique cases. Many of those involved also had a highly developed skill of pattern recognition that allowed the identification of new specific syndromes. The population base for medical geneticists was a further important factor for these mostly rare or very rare disorders. Whereas an individual paediatrician might serve a defined population of 100,000, a medical geneticist would commonly cover a population of 1,000,000 or even more.

The collaborative nature of this field can be well seen in the development of such regular meetings as the Dysmorphology Club, where individuals, often trainees, could present specific cases that would often form the basis for the recognition of new disorders, and where this would probably have not occurred unless the population base was essentially that of the entire UK. This in turn led to the development of computerised databases that could extend the process further and more internationally and could lead to definitive publications based on a series of patients.

The key people involved in these developments were young (at the time!) and often in relatively junior positions, working mostly 'out of hours' with a high degree of single-mindedness and devotion to their research – something that it should be said has characterised the field of medical genetics in all areas throughout its formative years. It is difficult to single out key individuals, but among those deserving special mention are Robin Winter (Figure 4.1a), sadly lost far too young, and Michael Baraitser (Figure 4.1b; [33]), both of the Institute of Child Health, London; Dian Donnai [63] (see also Chapter 3), who initiated the regular Manchester Dysmorphology Conference; and Helen Hughes (Toronto and Cardiff [90]).

From these cooperative activities, and also from a patient and systematic searching of the international literature, evolved the *London Dysmorphology Database*, curated by Winter and Baraitser, which became one of the main tools for the medical genetics community internationally in the delineation of new syndromes, together with the newly founded journal *Clinical Dysmorphology*, whose youthful editorial board is shown in Figure 4.2.

(a) (b)

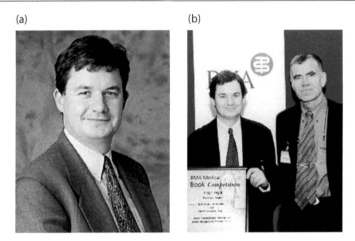

Figure 4.1 UK pioneers of clinical dysmorphology.

(a) Robin Winter (1950–2004). Based initially at Northwick Park Hospital and then at Institute of Child Health, London, Robin Winter combined a remarkable ability for recognising the features of rare or undelineated dysmorphic syndromes with an extensive knowledge of basic and statistical genetics, and of the applications of computers. His longstanding collaboration with Michael Baraitser, and with others at the Institute of Child Health, with its unrivalled clinical opportunities from tertiary and international referrals, resulted in the new field of clinical dysmorphology becoming a recognised scientific as well as clinical research field within medical genetics. His early death was a major loss to medical genetics as a whole. (Photo from Witness Seminar, Clinical Geneticsin Britain, Harper et al. (2010); Courtesy of Tilli Tansey.) **(b)** Robin Winter and Michael Baraitser, creators of the *London Dysmorphology Database*.

Michael Baraitser describes the beginnings of the database:

…both Robin and I knew that it was an absolutely ridiculous waste of time for one to turn pages of a book, to find the right diagnosis. …And then he, being so very bright with computers, probably said to me, let's start computerising this. And that's how we started it. There was a main frame computer based at Northwick Park and you had to throw punched cards into the computer. We basically sat down with early volumes of all the genetics journals, mostly from volume 1 and we paged through these and put the data into the computer. We concocted our list of features and it took off from there.

Interview with Michael Baraitser

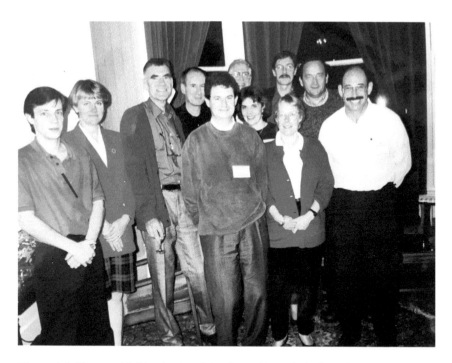

Figure 4.2 The youthful (and colourful) editorial board of *Clinical Dysmorphology*, 1990. (Courtesy of Dian Donnai.)

John Burn gives an idea of the intensity of the work involved in his description of Robin Winter:

> …immensely talented, hardworking – too hardworking I think – and he developed the database and was really at the front edge of the mouse models and of the dysmorphology database with Michael. And so, again, he had an encyclopaedic knowledge. A rather quiet-spoken, thoughtful chap but with a great sense of humour as well. I mean we got on extremely well and his loss was devastating to the community. But I'm not that surprised, in the sense that his lifestyle became very monk-like. You know, it was almost as if he was writing the Lindisfarne Bible when he was doing his databases. He would just get up early in the morning and sit and plough through photocopies of papers and get them onto the database. He was completely obsessed with getting that database comprehensive. And he did become completely encyclopaedic in his knowledge because of that, in the same way that Victor [McKusick] did with his Mendelian Inheritance in Man.

Andrew Wilkie and Dian Donnai have written a valuable obituary of Robin Winter, which can be read on the Academy of Medical Sciences (https://acmedsci. ac.uk). His contribution was especially unique because he combined his great clinical skills with mathematical approaches to genetic risk analysis and to

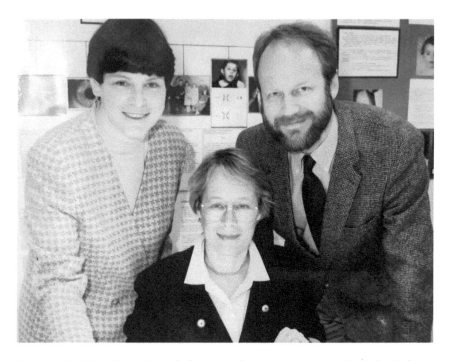

Figure 4.3 Dian Donnai and the Manchester International Birth Defects Conference (1994). Left to right: Jill Clayton-Smith, Dian Donnai, founder of the meeting, with Max Muenke. (Courtesy of Dian Donnai.)

recognition that human malformations could be the key to uncovering the basic molecular defects, not just for the human disorders but for experimental species also; in other words, that clinical dysmorphology was a two-way process in which it could not only learn from basic developmental processes but also contribute importantly to their understanding.

Clinical dysmorphology in the UK was not confined to London (Figure 4.3). Dian Donnai describes the origin of the Manchester Birth Defects meeting:

PSH: When was the first year you held your Manchester dysmorphology meeting?

DD: That was 1984, and do you want to know how that started?

PSH: Yes.

DD: Well it was all Peter Farndon's fault and two gins and tonics. After I was appointed as a consultant in 1980, Peter Farndon was the next senior registrar here and we used to go down to the CGS meetings and to the dysmorphology club meeting in London..., we were staying in London overnight in the Railway Hotel near St Pancras and we were waiting to go out and meet some people for dinner, so we had a gin and tonic in the bar and so I said, I'm fed up with staying in London and I was tired because I had got up early that morning etc etc and Peter said 'Well why don't you organise a meeting in Manchester?' and I said I don't suppose anybody would come you know. They just assume that they are always going to be in London. 'Go on' he said, 'Go on'. Anyway he bought me another drink and well, I have always thought, I had this slight resentment because people in London by then had been referring to the dysmorphology meeting as 'colleagues from all over the country come to London to ask our advice.' It was like a red rag to a provincial bull, that. And so I thought oh damn it. I will try to organise an international meeting, because I think I had just been that year, or I was just about to go to my first David Smith meeting in the US, so I thought, let's have a meeting. Instead of people just having a few slides in their pockets and describing their cases, let's have people actually present work at a formal meeting. So we had the first Manchester birth defects meeting in 1984 and I have had one every two years since then and I don't know how many people we had at the first one. Probably about thirty, and now people fight to have a place to come and we have to limit membership.

Interview with Dian Donnai [63]

Most of these early dysmorphologists were strongly clinical in their approach, but they were keenly aware that a detailed knowledge of embryology and teratology was essential for the understanding of congenital malformations and that the disorders resulting from environmental factors were intimately related to those caused by genetic defects. They also recognised the value of studying malformations in other species, which could provide homologues for human malformations and were more amenable to experimental approaches. In this they were greatly helped by experimental studies, largely on mice, notably the early work of Hans Grüneberg, based at University College London, part of the constellation of talent in genetics there represented by Penrose, RA Fisher, JBS Haldane and others (see Chapters 1 and 2). Grüneberg, like his American counterpart Josef Warkany, was a refugee from Nazi-controlled Europe, and his book *Animal Genetics in Medicine* (Grüneberg 1947) gave a firm foundation on which later more clinical workers could build. A number of these early workers, especially in America, were primarily pathologists and regarded themselves as 'teratologists', focusing more on the developmental basis of malformations than on their diagnosis during life.

At a more specifically genetic level workers such as Mary Lyon [18] and colleagues at Harwell delineated a series of mendelian mutants, again mainly in mice, which could be used to study their human counterparts, while the basic developmental genetics studies of Conrad Hal Waddington in Edinburgh, followed by Anne McLaren in London, were also highly relevant.

During the first post-war decades there had thus developed an extensive body of basic research, strongly supported by the Medical Research Council, on which clinical dysmorphologists could build; furthermore, a number of the basic scientists involved were themselves interested in the human applications and happy to collaborate with clinical workers, most of whom were clinical geneticists. It may well be asked why more general paediatricians outside medical genetics did not become involved in the field when it represented an increasingly important cause of childhood death and morbidity. The UK pattern forms a contrast to the United States, where paediatrician David Smith had a considerable influence in developing dysmorphology across paediatrics generally. The first medical genetics developments in France were also stimulated by the recognition of paediatrician Robert Debré in Paris that malformations were the new challenge for reducing infant mortality (Harper 2018). Perhaps the field of premature birth and neonatal care offered more scope for therapeutic skills, but the fact that clinical geneticists usually serve a population of more than a million, as noted above, and also have been keen to share their experience across the country, has undoubtedly been a factor, as have their close links with more basic scientists in the field.

When molecular genetics became applicable to normal developmental processes and to congenital malformations from the late 1990s, it soon became clear that many showed underlying gene mutations that had not been detectable by previous chromosome studies. This applied equally to many birth defects that had not previously been considered as genetic due to lack of any obvious familial clustering and which were now often revealed to be the result of new dominant mutations. The clinical delineation based on dysmorphic features could now be refined by molecular analysis, allowing a combined clinical-molecular classification that was both of practical use in diagnosis and genetic counselling, and which has contributed to a greater understanding of the developmental basis of the conditions.

Many of the molecular defects in human malformations proved to be the counterparts of those already recognised in other organisms, not just mammals but distantly related, though well-studied organisms such as Drosophila, yeast and bacteria. This widened the concept of 'model organisms' still further, and strengthened the scientific basis of clinical dysmorphology to the extent that human and especially medical data are now often the 'model' on which research in other species can be based. The field has now matured to the extent that individual disorders can be attributed to defects in specific developmental pathways, giving a network of 'inborn errors of development' akin to the 'inborn errors of metabolism' foreseen by Garrod at the beginning of the twentieth century. In the same way that inherited metabolic disease was accompanied by a landmark handbook, *The Inherited Basis of Metabolic Disease* (Stanbury et al. 1960), so the molecular basis of congenital malformations now has its own comparable volume, Charles Epstein and colleagues' *Inborn Errors of Development*, first published in 2004.

Despite this progress, it has to be said that clinical data in relation to dysmorphic syndromes (and other genetic disorders) often remain undervalued by comparison with laboratory information, even in situations where these details are of key importance. This especially applies to publications in high profile journals, in which clinical details are usually relegated to 'supplementary material' or sometimes omitted altogether. Perhaps this reflects the still widespread lack of respect in which clinical research is held by some basic scientists involved in the reviewing of papers and editing of journals?

It might be considered that the recent advent of whole genome analysis as a first-line approach to genetic diagnosis would remove the need for a detailed clinical assessment, but this is most unlikely. Previous experience with the use of chromosome analysis in the 1960s and with fragile X testing for mental handicap in the 1990s, to name but two, has shown that a 'blunderbuss' approach can be inefficient in comparison with use together with a skilled clinical and general genetic assessment. The Deciphering Developmental Disorders (DDD) study (2015), described in more detail in Chapter 11, shows how effective a combined genomics and clinical genetics approach can be in this respect, also permitting an 'iterative' approach that allows the phenotypic characteristics to become better defined. This improved definition will undoubtedly be increased as whole genome sequencing is increasingly applied to critically ill newborns without obvious syndromic features.

An important British contribution to note here is the international role across continental Europe in encouraging collaboration between different workers and centres in sharing data on malformations, something not widespread in most of these countries, even though most have had individuals interested and experienced in the field. The willingness of such people as Dian Donnai to encourage collaborative initiatives on the ground in different countries is an example of the value of such 'networking' activities.

As noted at the beginning of this section, dysmorphology, despite its rapid development, has not become separated from medical genetics overall, and this has quite possibly contributed to its continued vitality by allowing cross-fertilisation with human molecular genetics and with new genomic developments, quite apart from a shared need for genetic counselling and other core components of medical genetics. The fact that most regional medical genetics centres now contain at least four or five senior medical staff, together with the need to provide an all-round training for those entering the field, means that one or more individuals with particular expertise in clinical dysmorphology are now available in all centres to provide a service and to draw on the wide range of patients who can contribute to the still-growing understanding of this field.

When we come to look at the various adult medical (and surgical) specialties, we find that there are marked variations in the extent and the way in which medical genetics interacts with them. In some cases most of this interaction and the resulting developments have been initiated by medical geneticists, in others by the specialty itself; in some fields the interaction remains slight. It is well worth examining the specific situations. In historical terms, Rushton (2009) has documented in detail the early descriptions of genetic disorders according to clinical speciality; it is interesting to see how numerous and often how early these descriptions were. As noted in Chapter 1, they provided strong support for the establishing of mendelian inheritance as a general principle, while in recent years they and later clinical reports have at times proved valuable for isolation of the underlying specific genes, through permitting the tracing of the original families.

CANCER GENETICS

The development of cancer genetics has been the most striking area of expansion in terms of medical genetics services over the past 40 years, as well as illustrating the fruitful interplay of basic scientific research with clinical genetics. Not only have British workers made numerous and major research contributions to this field (see Chapter 11), but a co-ordinated policy approach to cancer genetics services across the country has allowed an efficient, yet economical delivery of these services that has been a model for other countries and contrasts with the more fragmented approach seen in some (e.g. the USA).

Genetics has been a prominent aspect of basic cancer research for a century or more – in fact ever since Theodor Boveri's recognition of cancer as a 'genetic disorder' of the cell (Boveri 1914). The chromosomes of tumours were a subject of active research by the 1950s and it was the need to have a clear normal reference point that led to the discovery of the normal human chromosome number by Tjio and Levan in Lund, Sweden, in 1956. A number of early American workers, notably Madge Macklin, Eldon Gardner and Henry Lynch, took an interest in large 'cancer families' apparently following mendelian dominant inheritance, but there was little connection between cancer research and medical genetics in Britain until around 1980, when Walter Bodmer, previously Professor of Genetics in Oxford (Figure 4.4; [68]),

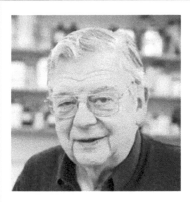

Figure 4.4 Walter F Bodmer (born 1936). Recorded interview 12/06/2017 [68]. (Photo from Clinical Cancer Genetics, Jones and Tansey (2013), courtesy of Tilli Tansey.)

Walter Bodmer has been a pivotal figure in UK and worldwide human and medical genetics for the past 50 years. Born in Germany but brought up from an early age in Manchester, he originally studied genetics with RA Fisher in Cambridge, before moving to America in 1961 to work on microbial genetics with Joshua Lederberg at Stanford University; here he was also involved in early research on the HLA system, together with his wife Julia, and began population genetics collaborations with Luca Cavalli-Sforza. Returning to Britain in 1970 as Professor of Genetics in Oxford, he built a team that made major discoveries in human molecular genetics before moving to London as Director of the Imperial Cancer Research Fund in 1979, where his main contributions were on familial colorectal cancer and polyposis. He was also much involved in the human gene mapping workshops and the Human Genome Project. Since his return to Oxford he has studied the genetic origins of the British people, as well as being involved with many wider science policy areas.

became director of the then Imperial Cancer Research Fund (ICRF) and linked with workers at St Mark's Hospital, located nearby in London, which had a longstanding interest in familial polyposis coli, including a register of families.

The recognition that this and other rare inherited cancer syndromes following mendelian inheritance, the only cancer patients regularly seen until then by medical geneticists, might be relevant to the basic understanding of common cancers, led to the formation of the Cancer Families Study Group (now the Cancer Genetics Group), for which ICRF funded workers, mainly genetic nurses or counsellors, across the country. This led for the first time to regional medical genetics centres developing clinical cancer genetics as a specific interest, something which increased dramatically a decade later when the molecular basis of these familial cancers began to be discovered and especially after it was found that a subset of 5%–10% of common cancers, such as colorectal and breast cancer, also showed germline mutations, giving high risks to family members.

While this might only form a small proportion of these common cancers, it greatly exceeded the overall number of the previously recognised mendelian tumour syndromes and presented a major organisational challenge to existing genetic services in terms of capacity for the provision of molecular diagnosis, genetic counselling and predictive genetic testing. In addition, widespread media publicity, especially regarding breast cancer, resulted in the referral of a large number of 'worried well' family members whose genetic risks were in fact low, necessitating some form of prioritisation or 'triage'. Around half of all referrals to genetics clinics are now related to cancer.

It is of interest that in the UK, in contrast to America, most of the necessary service development to handle the situation efficiently was undertaken by medical geneticists, oncologists and specialist surgeons working closely together, and that in fact most of the expanded workload and workforce, both clinical and laboratory, was based in medical genetics centres, whose cancer-related work rose to equal or even exceed all other referrals over the next decades. Far from feeling threatened by this, as might perhaps have been expected, surgeons and oncologists were in fact relieved by it, realising that the process of identifying high-risk groups and the considerable time involved in genetic counselling and prediction for healthy relatives was increasingly distracting them from their core activities of diagnosing and treating affected patients. This approach was brought together in a 1996 report, *Genetics and Cancer Services*, endorsed by the Department of Health and a good example of the Department's valuable approach at that time of responding to advice based on expert professional opinion (Department of Health, 1996).

An important factor in the successful development of clinical cancer genetics within the overall framework of UK medical genetics and cancer services has been the availability of clinical geneticists with a broad background in adult medicine, already noted and contrasting with the situation in many other countries, notably Australia and France, where the almost exclusive origin of medical genetics from paediatrics has made it less easy for clinical geneticists to relate to and be accepted by mainly adult specialties such as oncology and surgery.

The evolution of clinical cancer genetics has also given scope for an increased and more independent role of the non-medical specialist genetic counsellor (see

(a)　　　　　　　　　　　　　　(b)

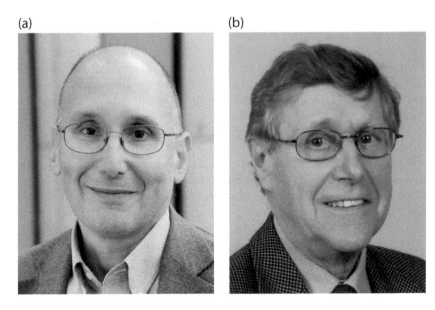

Figure 4.5 Medical genetics research and the major cancer research institutes. **(a)** Michael Stratton (born 1957), head of the Cambridge Sanger Institute since 2010 and former director of the Cancer Research Campaign Laboratories, where he was involved with isolation of the *BRCA2* and other cancer-related genes. (See also Chapter 11). (Photo courtesy of Wellcome Trust Sanger Institute.) **(b)** David Harnden (born 1932), early human cytogeneticist, who developed the Christie Institute, Manchester, into a major centre for genetic aspects of cancer research. Recorded interview 18/03/2004 [08]. (Photo courtesy David Harnden.)

Chapter 6), since the need for clinical and diagnostic skills is usually much less for the common cancers than in more general genetic counselling for rare disorders, while the psychological aspects are correspondingly greater.

Key people in the development of clinical cancer genetics include former directors of the major cancer research units, notably Walter Bodmer (already mentioned), Michael Stratton (Figure 4.5a) in London (now head of the Sanger Institute, Cambridge), and David Harnden (Figure 4.5b; [08]) at the Christie Hospital, Manchester, who were able to bring clinical geneticists into their units, as well as to link with those in other regional medical genetics centres. Among the numerous clinical geneticists making major contributions to developing the field have been Gareth Evans (Manchester), John Burn (Newcastle [100]; see Chapter 3), George Fraser (Oxford [32]), and in London Victoria Murday, Rosalind Eeles and Shirley Hodgson, some of whom are shown in Figure 4.6.

Interestingly, and probably appropriately, clinical cancer genetics in Britain, despite its rapid and continuing growth over the past 30 years, has not become a formally recognised separate specialty, remaining as a subspecialty and special interest area, predominantly but not exclusively based within medical genetics, though also closely linked with oncology. Its connections with multiple specialties

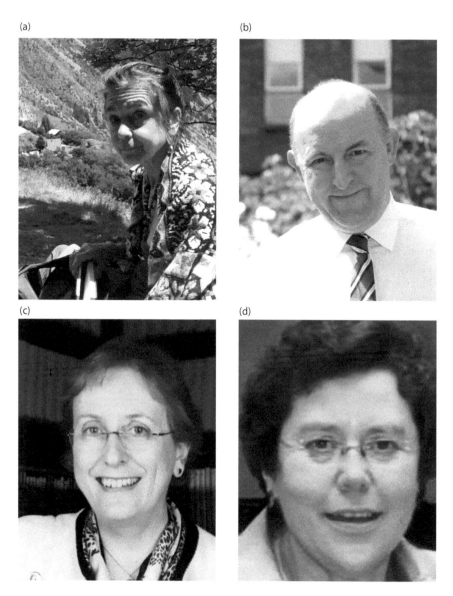

Figure 4.6 Some of the key workers in different areas of UK clinical cancer genetics. **(a)** Shirley Hodgson; Cambridge, London. (Familial colorectal cancer). **(b)** Gareth Evans; Manchester. (Familial breast cancer). **(c)** Rosalind Eeles; London. (Familial prostate cancer). **(d)** Susan Huson; Oxford, Manchester. (Neurofibromatosis).

may well be one reason, as with dysmorphology, for its continuing vitality at a point where many specialties plateau and become more rigid.

Alongside the increased demand for cancer genetics services, and to a considerable extent responsible for it, has been a major change in the public and professional perception of the nature of cancer generally. Although a genetic predisposition was widely recognised in the nineteenth and the first part of the twentieth century, cancer later became generally considered by the population at large to be largely environmental in its causes, with factors such as diet and viruses the main focus. Now, however, with the publicity given to gene discoveries, the main basis is felt to be 'genetic', despite the fact that specific genes in the germ line giving a high risk to relatives are only involved in a small minority of cases, most mutations being purely somatic. It is interesting to contrast this change in perception with some other disorders such as peptic ulcer, formerly considered mainly genetic and the subject of long chapters in genetics textbooks, where the genetic aspects have become of less interest now that specific external factors have been recognised.

NEUROGENETICS

It is now well over a century since the London Neurological Society (soon to become part of the Royal Society of Medicine), invited William Bateson to speak to them in 1906 on the topic of mendelian heredity (Bateson 1906; see also Harper 2005). Bateson had been assiduous in collecting evidence for the universal operation of mendelian inheritance and had found a rich source among specialist clinicians in London, including neurologists (Figure 4.7a). In his published text Bateson showed a strikingly modern approach by combining a range of mendelian situations from

(a)   (b)

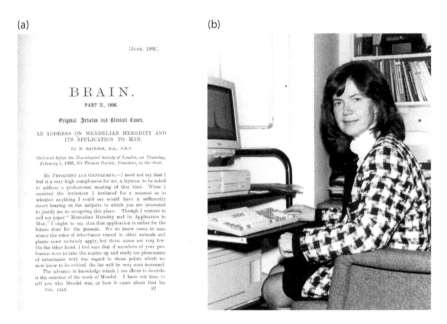

Figure 4.7 Genetics and neurology. **(a)** Title page from William Bateson's 1906 lecture to the London Neurological Society. **(b)** Anita Harding (1952–1995) One of the first modern neurologists to develop neurogenetics in a molecular context. (Courtesy of Sarah Tabrizi; See also Sarah Bundey (1936–1998), Figure 3.18, and Kay Davies, Figure 11.4b, the first molecular geneticist to study the basis of neuromuscular disorders.)

widely differing species in a single image. Sharp-eyed readers will notice that Bateson begins his lecture 'Mr President and gentlemen' and uses a deferential approach; the London neurologists were clearly perceived then as an elite and seemingly exclusively male group, something that took a long time to change!

Bateson gave his audience clear practical advice on how they should go about studying the families that they encountered – advice as valuable now as then:

> Finally, I would say something as to the way in which evidence must be collected if it is to be used in the study of heredity. First, the facts must be so reported as to be capable of analysis. It is for want of such analysis that all examination of the facts by pre-Mendelian methods failed. The tabulations must present each family separately. Miscellaneous statistics are of little use. Secondly, it is absolutely necessary that the normal or unaffected members should be recorded, together, if possible, with information as to their offspring. In the records hitherto published these essentials have too often been omitted, the doctor's attention having been more or less exclusively directed to the individuals manifesting the disease. Next, if similar families are to be added together, it is scarcely necessary to insist that the cases added must be in reality similar. For instance, there are abundant genealogies of deaf mutism, but the various families present such inconsistencies in the heredity rules which they follow that there can be no doubt that not one, but many, pathological states are concerned. Accurate diagnosis is the first preliminary in dealing with these phenomena.

The field of neurology indeed proved to contain a remarkably high proportion of mendelian disorders, involving not only the brain but the neuromuscular system; after the promising start made by Bateson's lecture, though, most British neurologists showed little interest in the genetic aspects, especially since chemical or other investigations showed few abnormalities that might lead to understanding or treatment. One exception was Julia Bell's *Treasury of Human Inheritance* (see Chapter 1) which over the period 1930–1950 produced a series of key studies on neurological conditions, including Huntington's disease (Bell 1934), myotonic dystrophy (Bell 1947), Leber's optic atrophy (Bell 1931) and Charcot-Marie-Tooth disease. These monographs combined an assiduous collection of all reported families worldwide with a detailed quantitative analysis of the genetic aspects (Harper 2006).

The abundance of large, multi-generation families with clear mendelian patterns gave special opportunities for gene mapping once DNA markers became available, but again few British neurologists were interested initially in undertaking this, while the laboratory basis for molecular genetic analysis was at first limited to genetics centres, so it fell largely to medical geneticists to map (beginning in the 1980s) and then to isolate (from the 1990s) the genes for a key series of neuromuscular and central nervous system (CNS) disorders. British groups were prominently involved in these discoveries and, while the general topic of gene mapping is considered later (Chapter 12), it must be stressed that collaboration was the key to success, involving neurologists (adult and paediatric), medical geneticists, and basic molecular research laboratories.

Only when gene mapping studies had led to the identification of specific genes and mutations did neurologists in general begin to take a lead role in using molecular approaches for diagnosis. This change, when it did happen, occurred very rapidly, so that medical geneticists and molecular genetics laboratories found that their role was changing to one that principally involved the extended family and such areas as genetic counselling in relation to carrier detection and predictive testing. It is of interest, though, that the difficult and time-consuming field of presymptomatic (predictive) testing for such late onset disorders as Huntington's disease, for which careful protocols have been worked out, has largely remained with clinical geneticists and specialist genetic counsellors (Harper et al. 2000). As with cancer genetics, most clinical neurologists understandably prefer to devote their time to affected patients rather than to healthy individuals at risk, particularly when, as in the UK, there is a comprehensive network of colleagues with the relevant genetic and psychological skills.

Who were the principal individuals responsible for the development of neurological genetics? In fact, despite Bateson's early encouragement, very few names stand out in the first half of the twentieth century. Julia Bell has already been mentioned, though she was not herself a neurologist, working closely with several of the London neurologists based at the National Hospital for Nervous Diseases. Only in the 1980s, when molecular genetics began to revolutionise the field, do we find key individuals involved from genetics, notably Anita Harding (Figure 4.7b) and Sarah Bundey (see Chapter 3), both linked to the London institutes of Child Health and of Neurology. As a practicing neurologist based at the Institute of Neurology, London, Anita Harding was especially well placed to modify the rigid clinical and social traditions of British neurology; both were also strongly influenced by Cedric Carter in their basic medical genetics training. It is sad that both died relatively young, with much more still to be contributed. A sensitive obituary for 'Munk's roll' (lives of Fellows of the Royal College of Physicians, volume 11) has been written on Sarah Bundey by Peter Farndon. Another major London contributor has been Michael Baraitser (see above and Chapter 3), who pioneered the use of computerised databases for neurogenetic conditions, together with Robin Winter. Neurogenetics has also been my own main area of research in the areas of Huntington's disease and myotonic and other muscular dystrophies.

At a research level, much neurogenetics has now become fused with wider neuroscience, but in terms of clinical practice, it remains largely as a subspecialty, with some workers based in neurology, others in medical genetics. Huntington's disease provides a good example of the longstanding, close and fruitful links between the two specialties: the World Federation of Neurology Research Group on Huntington's Disease (with a strong British representation) has had a powerful influence on genetic research for this disorder for over 50 years, while the UK Huntington's Prediction Consortium, involving all UK centres undertaking this difficult area of medicine, has also been a major factor in helping both specialties to develop high standards of practice in presymptomatic testing, which have proved a paradigm for other late-onset genetic disorders.

Neuromuscular disorders, just as much as those of the CNS, are an area where UK medical geneticists, both laboratory based and clinical, have made major discoveries, especially during the 1980s and 1990s when positional cloning identified most of the key genes involved (see Chapter 12). The group of Bob Williamson [61] and Kay Davies [80] at St Mary's Hospital, London, working closely with the Cardiff medical genetics unit, began this process with the mapping of the Duchenne muscular dystrophy gene (Murray et al. 1982), and this and subsequent mapping discoveries also made accurate carrier detection and prenatal diagnosis possible for a series of neuromuscular disorders for which there had previously been almost no previous understanding of the basic defect. Clinical geneticists also took a lead role in the organising of specialist clinics, notably in Newcastle and Glasgow, working closely with the few paediatric neurologists at the time interested in muscle disorders. An important role was also played by Alan Emery (see interview [48]) in coordinating the series of international workshops run by the European Neuromuscular Centre (ENMC) from 1992, which has now held over 250 meetings, mostly on rare inherited neuromuscular disorders.

OPHTHALMIC GENETICS

The eye has been fertile territory for the involvement of medical geneticists ever since the earliest years of genetics. As with neurological disorders, the abundance of non-lethal, multigeneration and clearly mendelian families made it relatively easy to identify patterns of inheritance, while 50 years or more later these same families and others were suitable for gene mapping studies. William Bateson found enthusiastic collaborators in such ophthalmologists as Edward Nettleship (Figure 4.8a) who actually gave up his London practice to allow more time for studying inherited eye disorders; he is commemorated in Julia Bell's extensive 'Nettleship Volume' of her *Treasury of Human Inheritance*, published in several parts from 1922 onwards.

Close and active collaborations at a clinical level were essential, since few general medical geneticists, then or now, had the skills for an accurate diagnosis. Even so, it is remarkable how many important basic contributions to wider genetics were made by ophthalmologists, such as Arnold Sorsby (Figure 4.8b), who produced the early book *Clinical Genetics* (Sorsby 1953), and was also founding editor of the *Journal of Medical Genetics* in 1964. His research fellow, George Fraser [32],(born 1932), produced an important book, *The Causes of Blindness in Childhood* (Fraser 1967), among many wider contributions. A similar broad interest was present across continental Europe, with ophthalmologists such as Petrus Waardenburg (1886–1979) in the Netherlands), Jules François (1907–1984) in Belgium and Adolphe Franceschetti (1896–1968) in Switzerland, all making contributions to genetics well outside their own specialty.

In Britain at least, the interest of ophthalmologists in genetics declined over subsequent decades outside a few centres (it should be said that the earlier

(a)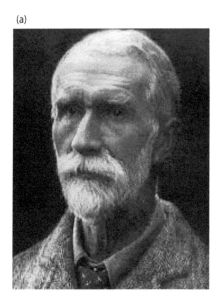

(b)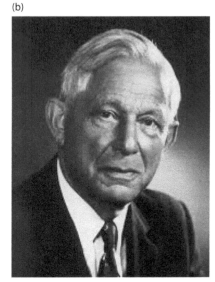

Figure 4.8 Two UK pioneers of ophthalmological genetics. **(a)** Edward Nettleship (1845–1913). **(b)** Arnold Sorsby (1900–1980). First editor of *Journal of Medical Genetics* (see Chapter 9).

contributions were also only from a very small minority of clinical workers). Molecular developments and the possibility of localised gene-based therapies have now, though, again become an important part of eye research, while collaborative clinics between ophthalmologists and medical geneticists provide a basis for genetic counselling and testing.

DERMATOLOGY AND GENETICS

Inherited skin disorders, like those of the eye, lend themselves to the identification of clear mendelian patterns, though this has included some false trails, notably in the claims for Y chromosomal inheritance of the disorder ichthyosis hystrix, which took a painstaking restudy by Penrose and Stern (1958) to show that the apparent confinement to and transmission by males was the result of selective reporting and inadequate study of female relatives. A notable British contributor was Edward Cockayne, children's physician at Great Ormond Street Hospital, London and author of the classic book *Genetic Disorders of the Skin and its Appendages* (Cockayne 1933). More recent workers such as Michael Pope and Celia Moss have continued the dermatological genetics tradition.

The skin has also been important in the identification of mosaicism, notably the phenomenon of X-inactivation, though Mary Lyon's original discovery of this (see Chapter 10) was made on mouse rather than human observations. Mosaicism at the chromosomal level in a number of malformation syndromes has also had important theoretical consequences for human genetics generally.

CARDIAC GENETICS

The genetic aspects of heart disease, both in adults and in children, have attracted the attention of those working in medical genetics from early times. It was Paul Polani's studies on congenital heart disease in the mid 1950s that led to the recognition of a high frequency of aortic coarctation in Turner syndrome (Polani et al. 1954), and in turn to the finding that these phenotypic females showed an XO chromosome constitution (Ford et al. 1959). It should not be forgotten that in America Victor McKusick was originally a cardiologist, coming to medical genetics via his studies on Marfan syndrome.

Coronary heart disease also received some early attention in Britain from the work of Joan Slack at the Institute of Child Health; her family studies of coronary heart disease (Slack and Evans 1966) and of familial hypercholesterolaemia (Slack and Nevin 1968) at Cedric Carter's London unit (see Chapter 2) led to the gradual appreciation that the latter was a specific mendelian disorder, unlike most coronary heart disease. But it took a long time before people realised how common and under-diagnosed it was (and indeed still is). Even slower was any attempt to do something about this, despite it being one of the few major treatable genetic disorders, UK medical geneticists being largely responsible for highlighting this neglect as little short of a disgrace. It would be worth a detailed study of why this should have been so, and what we can learn from it.

Several reasons stand out: first, the disorder does not fall under a single clinical discipline. Some cases are seen by cardiologists, but rarely stand out from the overall body of coronary heart disease; others are seen by metabolic physicians dealing with lipid disorders. Neither group has been trained to deal with (or even think about) the tracing of extended families. Nor have there been until recently specific biochemical or molecular tests to provide confirmation that a genetic rather than a secondary cause is operating. Direct referrals to medical genetics services have been rare, perhaps because coronary heart disease is so common in the general population.

Recently, collaborative efforts involving all these three groups are beginning to emerge, perhaps stimulated by what has happened for the mendelian subset of common cancers and by recognition of the benefits that early detection and preventive therapy can offer.

Another area of adult heart disease that is belatedly receiving attention from the genetic viewpoint is that of the arrhythmias. Here the problem has been that the familial nature of these has often been concealed by the high proportion of undiagnosed and asymptomatic cases, many of whom may never develop problems. As widespread cardiac screening and, more recently, molecular tests have increased, this has brought cardiologists face to face with unfamiliar situations such as how to handle (and hopefully to avoid) the undesirable consequences of incidental discovery of an abnormal result, something that medical geneticists have already become familiar with in the context of genetic testing for late-onset disorders generally.

A third important disorder prominently involving medical geneticists (most notably, in historical importance, Victor McKusick in America) has been Marfan syndrome, where early detection of aortic problems now gives major possibilities for reduction in mortality.

All these areas of cardiology have created the need for collaborative initiatives between cardiologists and medical geneticists to ensure that services are introduced carefully and equitably, rather than based on enthusiasm and on what is technically possible. On the whole these new developments, in genetic heart disease as in most other fields, are progressing in a responsible manner in the UK, helped in part by most of them being delivered through the NHS rather than as the result of commercially driven pressures, and also helped by the generally close links between clinical geneticists and other clinical specialties.

GASTROINTESTINAL GENETICS

Richard McConnell's 1966 book, *The Genetics of Gastrointestinal Disorders*, was the first volume in the series of Oxford University Press 'Monographs on Medical Genetics' (see Chapter 9) and written, as stated in its preface, 'to provide the clinician with information about the influence of heredity in the gastro-enterological conditions which he meets in practice'. McConnell (see Figure 2.10b) was a practicing physician and gastroenterologist in Liverpool, a close colleague of Cyril Clarke; he also handled the relatively few genetic counselling requests in Liverpool at this time. It is of interest how much space in McConnell's book is devoted to the genetics of peptic ulcer, in which the genetic aspects were already well recognised, especially associations with the ABO blood groups, but where the environmental factors (apart from gastric acid itself) were as yet unknown. As with other common conditions, such as cancer and tuberculosis, the perception of a disorder being genetic or environmental changes according to the extent to which environmental factors can be identified or treated.

Also in McConnell and Clarke's minds were the remarkable and perhaps unique Liverpool families with dominantly inherited oesophageal cancer (Howel-Evans et al. 1958), and their contrast with most oesophageal cancer which shows little familial aggregation in the British population.

The gastrointestinal system, especially the liver, shows numerous relatively rare adult and childhood genetic conditions, but not so prominent as to give the need or demand for specific 'gastroenterological geneticists'. Cystic fibrosis provides an interesting example: in the author's experience at least, genetic counselling referrals were rare before the molecular defect was discovered; then they become abundant for a few years, after which paediatricians became comfortable with interpreting the results of DNA testing and incorporated these into their own practice.

The iron storage disorder haemochromatosis provides a more recent object lesson in how *not* to interpret and apply genetic advances. This had long been known to be an uncommon (at least in Britain) disorder, with a frequency of around 1 in 8000, but following identification of the main predisposing gene in the HLA region (Feder et al. 1996), enthusiasts claimed it as 'the commonest adult genetic disorder' by confusing the genotype frequency of homozygotes (at least 50 times greater) with the frequency of the clinical disorder; then by insisting that population screening was needed to find the 'missing' patients and even treating these healthy individuals unnecessarily by venesection with, needless to say, excellent results! This example shows the continuing need for training in simple but basic genetic principles for all those involved with inherited disorders.

BLOOD DISEASES: HAEMOPHILIA AND HAEMOGLOBIN DISORDERS

Blood disorders have figured strongly in the history of genetics in medicine for many years. Haemophilia, in particular, played a major role, though the first well documented families were from America (Otto 1803, Hay 1813). The fact that Queen Victoria was a carrier, with disastrous consequences for the royal families of Europe, gave it much publicity (see Rushton 2009); the disorder was largely responsible for the firm establishment of X-linked inheritance, while the work of Julia Bell and JBS Haldane established both the first human genetic linkage (Bell and Haldane 1937) and estimates for mutation rate (Haldane 1935).

Haemophilia services in the UK have had a long tradition of forming self-contained regionally based centres for management and therapy, something that has undoubtedly raised standards. In terms of carrier testing and genetic counselling, the degree of involvement with wider medical genetics has been variable; in my own experience these links have been mutually beneficial and have helped to ensure that extended family members are appropriately counselled and tested. Before accurate molecular testing was possible, X chromosome inactivation caused problems comparable to those encountered with other X-linked disorders, and haemophilia centres were among the first to use the Bayesian approaches to risk estimation pioneered by medical geneticists for Duchenne muscular dystrophy.

The other large group of blood disorders where both research advances and service applications have come mainly from outside medical genetics is the group of haemoglobin disorders, a recurring theme throughout this book. In Britain the thalassaemias have played a leading role in our understanding of the molecular pathology of genetic disorders generally, thanks to the work of David Weatherall [30] and others (see Chapter 10), while the applications of the advances in prenatal diagnosis, pioneered by Bernadette Modell [70] are described in Chapter 5.

For sickle cell disease, even though largely affecting different ethnic minority communities to the thalassaemias, a community-based approach to prevention and management has likewise proved the most fruitful one. For many years, services for the condition, both genetic and management, tended to fall in between haematology and medical genetics. It took a persistent and activist approach for this to change, pioneered notably by Elizabeth Anionwu (Figure 4.9) in London, whose recent autobiography (Anionwu 2016) gives a vivid account of both the successes and the difficulties she encountered in establishing services.

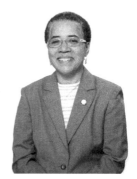

Figure 4.9 Elizabeth Anionwu. Pioneer of community-based services for sickle cell disease. (Courtesy of Elizabeth Anionwu.)

PSYCHIATRIC GENETICS

Mental illness has been closely connected to genetics from the earliest years of the field, with both Fraser Roberts and Penrose having a background in psychiatry, specifically in mental handicap. The principal area of both research and practice, though, for most psychiatrists in recent years has been that of the major psychoses, schizophrenia and depression, and this has originated from very different traditions. Its beginnings in this respect came largely from the German schools of psychiatry, which became progressively and inextricably involved with the Nazi eugenics and race hygiene policies, leading to the infamous 1933 'eugenics law' and to the atrocities carried out under the guise of research in the concentration camps.

The founder of modern psychiatric genetics in Britain, Eliot Slater (Figure 4.10), trained originally in Munich in 1934 with Ernst Rüdin, despite Rudin's Nazi links and his close involvement with the recently enacted 1933 law enforcing sterilisation of those with serious mental illness and other major genetic disorders. It seems impossible that Slater was unaware of this, especially since his senior colleague at the Maudsley Hospital, London, Aubrey Lewis, wrote a highly critical *Lancet* editorial on the subject (Anon 1933). In the discussion following Penrose's 1949 address to the Eugenics Society (see Chapter 2), both Lewis and Slater are noted as supporting Penrose's criticisms of the Society; it would have been interesting to have had an eyewitness account of this meeting.

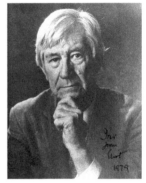

Figure 4.10 Eliot Slater (1904–1983), pioneer of modern psychiatric genetics. (Courtesy of Peter McGuffin.)

On his return to Britain Slater initiated a series of extensive family studies of major psychoses at the Maudsley Hospital, including twin studies, which later formed the basis for an MRC unit and attracted talented colleagues including James Shields, Valerie Cowie and Irving Gottesmann. Slater shared Penrose's insistence on publishing all raw data, something that would prove valuable in the face of the various and often conflicting theories surrounding genetics and schizophrenia, as well as the persistent, though totally unfounded view among some schools of psychiatry (principally in America), that mental illness had no genetic component whatever.

With the advent of molecular genetic analysis it was hoped that this might soon help to unravel the genetic basis of schizophrenia and depression, but despite much effort and very large samples this has proved to be extremely difficult, though the studies have shown that dependence on one or just a few specific major genes is improbable. Despite the difficulties though, the goals remain extremely worthwhile in the light of the immense burden of morbidity from these common mental illnesses, especially if the studies identify genes that may contribute to new therapies. Continuing work based largely in Cardiff by Peter McGuffin, Michael Owen and colleagues has led a major MRC supported initiative to tackle this difficult area.

While on the subject of controversies, mention must be made of research on the genetics of intelligence. This highly important area has long been in the minds of medical geneticists, psychiatrists and psychologists since the time of Penrose and even before (e.g. Francis Galton), and early studies on mental handicap established that severe cases were likely to have a specific cause, often mendelian or chromosomal, whereas milder cases were likely to represent one end of a 'normal' distribution. The progressive identification of the specific genes involved in severe mental handicap has continued the line of work initiated by Penrose in his 1938 Colchester study, to the extent that what used to be thought of as a single category is now recognised as a large series (several hundred) of specific but individually rare disorders, including many due to new dominant mutations, which usually show no familial aggregation. Analysis of whole genomes, most notably of the X chromosome as studied by workers at the Cambridge Sanger Institute and elsewhere, has revealed the extent of this situation (see Chapter 11). To a considerable extent this work has also linked with the identification of dysmorphic syndromes mentioned earlier.

A natural hope has been that understanding these conditions might lead to determination of the main genetic factors involved in intelligence generally, but so far this seems a long way away, not surprising given the extreme complexity of the pathways involved. Studies of genetic variation in normal groups with high and low IQ have, as with major mental illness, largely excluded the action of a few genes with major effect. A disturbing aspect of such research has been the manner in which some investigators, especially behavioural scientists, have embarked on such studies seemingly unaware of the inherent sensitivity of the topic, the near impossibility of eliminating confounding biases, and the likelihood that politicians and the media will almost certainly distort and misuse any findings that might occur.

Turning to the service aspects of psychiatric genetics, these are at present minimal for the major common mental disorders, making a striking contrast to cancer genetics, as described earlier. This is largely because no significant subsets following mendelian inheritance have so far been identified, so that there is no possibility of excluding risk for members of a family with multiple cases. Add to this the fact that the population risk is high for everyone, regardless of family history, and it can be seen that the scope for genetic counselling is limited, with just the well-established 'empiric risks', as established by Slater and his colleagues over 50 years ago, to fall back on (Slater and Cowie 1971).

The author found this clearly shown when he and his colleague Peter McGuffin, head of Psychological Medicine in Cardiff and an expert in psychiatric genetics, set up a joint genetic counselling clinic, in anticipation of a possible surge in demand as had recently happened for cancer genetics. In fact, demand proved minimal, with only a very few families (mostly with a family history of dementia) showing any added value of such specialist input. This reinforces what has been learned from other adult specialties, that genetic counselling for common non-mendelian conditions can mostly be handled by those in the specialty, provided (and it is a big proviso) that any mendelian subset has been carefully excluded.

If we attempt to put together the information in the different sections of this chapter, can we learn any overall lessons from what may seem a series of very different situations? I think that we can, and that some at least are important for the future as well as for the past.

The first is that medical genetics itself has broadened and branched, and that this has usually involved the formation of close links with colleagues in a variety of medical specialties, as well as networks with other medical geneticists across Britain and internationally. And second, awareness and skills related to genetic problems have indeed spread out to other clinical specialties; not just diffused, but actively encouraged by medical geneticists. Third, the ways in which clinical specialities interact with and utilise medical genetics services is highly variable, depending on the nature and inheritance patterns of the particular conditions, as well as on the local situation. Finally, all of these very positive developments happened as the result of professional links and discussions, usually involving lay societies and backed up by guidelines involving professional societies, and with a virtual absence of 'top down' directives from health departments or other comparable bodies, a strong contrast with the situation over the past few years, at least in England (see Chapter 8). Policy makers planning to encourage the future development of genetic (including genomic) services across medicine as a whole will be wise to learn from what has happened over the past 60 years, and to listen to the workers directly involved on the ground before issuing directives.

REFERENCES

Anionwu EN. 2016. *Mixed Blessings from a Cambridge Union*. London: ELIZAN.

Anonymous. 1933. Eugenics in Germany. *Lancet*. 2:297–298.

Bateson W. 1906. An address on mendelian heredity and its application to man. *Brain*. 29:157–179.

Bell J. 1931. *Hereditary optic atrophy (Leber's disease)*. In: Pearson K (ed.). *Treasury of Human Inheritance*, vol. 2, part 4. London: Cambridge University Press, pp. 325–423.

Bell J. 1934. *Huntington's chorea*. In: Fisher RA (ed.). *Treasury of Human Inheritance*, vol. 4, part 1. London: Cambridge University Press, pp. 1–67.

Bell J. 1947. *Dystrophia myotonica and allied diseases*. In: Penrose LS (ed.). *Treasury of Human Inheritance*, vol. 4, part 5. London: Cambridge University Press, pp. 343–410.

Bell J, Haldane JBS. 1937. The linkage between the genes for colour-blindness and haemophilia in man. *Proc R Soc Lond B*. 123:119–150.

Boveri T. 1914. *Zur Frage der Entstehung Maligner Tumoren [On the problem of the origin of malignant tumors]*. Translated by Marcella Boveri. Jena: Fischer.

Cockayne EA. 1933. *Inherited Abnormalities of the Skin and its Appendages*. London: Oxford University Press.

Department of Health. 1996. *Genetics and Cancer Services*. London: HMSO.

Epstein CJ, Erickson RP, Wynshaw-Boris A (eds.) 2004. *Inborn Errors of Development: The Molecular Basis of Clinical Disorders of Morphogenesis*, 2nd edn 2008. New York: Oxford University Press.

Feder JN, Gnirke A, Thomas W. et al. 1996. A novel MHC class I-like gene is mutated in patients with hereditary haemochromatosis. *Nat Genet.* 13:399–408.

Ford CE, Jones KW, Polani PE, De Almeida JC, Briggs JH. 1959. A sex-chromosome anomaly in a case of gonadal dysgenesis (Turner's syndrome). *Lancet.* 1(7075):711–713.

Fraser GR. 1967. *The Causes of Blindness in Childhood.* Baltimore: Johns Hopkins University Press.

Grüneberg H. 1947. *Animal Genetics and Medicine.* London: Hamish Hamilton Medical Books.

Haldane JBS. 1935. The rate of spontaneous mutation of a human gene. *J Genet.* 31:317–26.

Harper PS. 2005. William Bateson, human genetics and medicine. *Hum Genet.* 118:141–51.

Harper PS. 2006. Julia Bell and the *Treasury of Human Inheritance. Hum Genet.* 116:422–432.

Harper PS. 2018. Conversations with French medical geneticists. A personal perspective on the origins and early years of medical genetics in France. *Clin Genet.* 94:115–124.

Harper PS, Lim C, Craufurd D. Ten years of presymptomatic testing for Huntington's disease: The experience of the UK Huntington's Disease Prediction Consortium. *J Med Genet.* 2000;37(8):567–571.

Harper PS, Reynolds LA, Tansey EM (Eds). 2010. *Clinical Genetics in Britain: Origins and Development.* London: Wellcome Trust Centre for the History of Medicine at UCL.

Hay J. 1813. Account of a remarkable haemorrhagic disposition, existing in many individuals of the same family. *N Engl J Med.* 2:221–225.

Howel-Evans W, McConnell RB, Clarke CA, Sheppard PM. 1958. Carcinoma of the oesophagus with keratosis palmaris et plantaris (tylosis): A study of two families. *Q J Med.* 27(107):413–429.

McConnell RB. 1966. *The Genetics of Gastrointestinal Disorders.* Oxford: Oxford University Press.

Murray JM, Davies KE, Harper PS, Meredith L, Mueller CR, Williamson R. 1982. Linkage relationship of a cloned DNA sequence on the short arm of the X chromosome to Duchenne muscular dystrophy. *Nature.* 300:69–71.

Otto JC. 1803. An account of an haemorrhagic disposition existing in certain families. *Medical Repository.* 6:1–4.

Penrose LS. 1938. *A Clinical and Genetic Study of 1280 Cases of Mental Defect.* Medical Research Council. London: His Majesty's Stationery Office.

Penrose LS, Stern C. 1958. Reconsideration of the Lambert pedigree (ichthyosis hystrix gravior). *Ann Hum Genet.* 22:258–283.

Polani PE, Hunter JF, Lennox B. 1954. Chromosomal sex in Turner's syndrome with coarctation of the aorta. *Lancet.* 2:120–121.

Rushton AR. 2009. *Genetics and Medicine in Great Britain, 1600–1939.* Bloomington, IN: Trafford Publishing.

Slack J, Evans KA. 1966. The increased risk of death from ischaemic heart disease in first degree relatives of 121 men and 96 women with ischaemic heart disease. *J Med Genet*. 3(4):239–257.

Slack J, Nevin NC. 1968 March. Hyperlipidaemic xanthomatosis. I. Increased risk of death from ischaemic heart disease in first degree relatives of 53 patients with essential hyperlipidaemia and xanthomatosis. *J Med Genet*. 5(1):4–8.

Slater E, Cowie V. 1971. *The Genetics of Mental Disorders*. Oxford: Oxford University Press.

Sorsby A. 1953. *Clinical Genetics*. London: Butterworth.

Stanbury JB, Wyngaarden JB, Frederickson DS (eds.) 1960. *The Metabolic Basis of Inherited Disease*. New York: McGraw-Hill.

The Deciphering Developmental Disorders Study. 2015. Large-scale discovery of novel genetic causes of developmental disorders. *Nature*. 519:223–228.

Tjio J-H, Levan A. 1956. The chromosome number of man. *Hereditas*. 42:1–6.

5

Prenatal diagnosis and reproductive genetics

ABSTRACT

The possibility of diagnosing serious genetic disorders prenatally by amniocentesis coincided closely with the legalisation of termination of pregnancy in Britain and other countries during the 1960s and 1970s. Initially applied to Down syndrome and other chromosome disorders, then to neural tube defects, prenatal diagnosis gave parents the option of avoiding genetic risk and achieving a healthy family, but at psychological cost. Ethical issues were increased as more general prenatal screening was introduced, often without adequate information for the women involved or full consideration of their wishes. Medical geneticists have taken a cautious and at times critical approach to these developments but have been closely involved with studies of safety, early approaches such as chorion villus sampling, and noninvasive prenatal testing by analysis of fetal DNA in maternal blood. They have also worked for the provision of molecular prenatal diagnosis of disorders, such as the thalassaemias, in specific ethnic groups. New developments, such as preimplantation genetic diagnosis and gene editing technology, continue to give both ethical and practical challenges in reproductive genetics.

It is now 60 years since the advent of techniques allowing the prenatal detection of genetic disorders in early pregnancy, something that has radically changed the face of medical genetics and linked it inevitably, regardless of the views of those in the field, to the topic of abortion. Prior to this, the main link between genetics and reproductive issues had been through infertility, male and female, where analysis of first the sex chromatin and then of the sex chromosomes themselves, had been a useful, if restricted, diagnostic aid. Thus the first generation of medical geneticists grew up with little contact with obstetrician-gynaecologists, and the converse was also true. An exception in the UK was the Liverpool research on the prevention of rhesus haemolytic disease, described in Chapters 2 and 11.

Table 5.1 Successive new technologies in applied reproductive genetics

Amniocentesis
Prenatal chromosome analysis
Amniotic fluid enzymes and other proteins
Ultrasound obstetric imaging
Maternal serum alphafetoprotein
Fetoscopy and fetal blood sampling
Chorionic villus sampling (CVS)
Molecular analysis of CVS samples
Preimplantation genetic diagnosis
Free fetal DNA in maternal serum (NIPT)
Gene editing

AMNIOCENTESIS

Amniocentesis, the first in a series of techniques in prenatal diagnosis (Table 5.1) was until recently the most widely used (apart from fetal ultrasound). It had already been in use for some years during late pregnancy, again mainly for the detection of rhesus haemolytic disease, in Britain and elsewhere, but there was no indication for exploring its application to early pregnancy until termination of pregnancy became legal, something that occurred at different times in different countries.

Not surprisingly, the first use of amniocentesis in the early prenatal diagnosis of genetic disorders occurred in Scandinavia (Fuchs and Riis 1956, Riis 2006), where termination of pregnancy for fetal abnormality was already legal, rather than in Britain or America. This was initially in relation to fetal sexing for haemophilia using the sex chromatin body, and it was almost a decade later that full chromosome analysis was shown to be feasible on cultured amniotic fluid cells in USA. The first systematic UK study came from Scotland (Ferguson-Smith ME et al. 1971), benefiting from the application of ultrasound to placental localisation and other obstetric uses from 1957 by Ian Donald (1910–1987), Professor of Obstetrics at University of Glasgow, though it should be noted that Donald was strongly opposed to its use in connection with prenatal diagnosis and pregnancy termination.

This early UK experience of prenatal diagnosis is of interest and importance in setting the tone for a long-lasting caution and at times ambivalence of medical geneticists in relation to prenatal diagnosis and reproductive genetics generally. Apart from Ian Donald, an obstetrician and a devout Catholic, several medical geneticists early in the field had strong religious affiliations that must have generated feelings against prenatal diagnosis, but they were also faced in their regular genetic counselling practice by the tragedies associated with inherited disorders in high-risk families and the dilemmas posed for these families when the possibility of achieving healthy children through prenatal diagnosis finally became a reality – though at the possible cost of terminating a much-wanted pregnancy. Most medical geneticists were or soon became aware of these keenly felt issues and adopted the view that, where couples wished for prenatal diagnosis in such situations, it was right to offer it, to give support and to work towards making it safer and more widely feasible.

An example of this situation is provided by Northern Ireland, where Norman Nevin [26] had early on developed a medical genetics service (see Chapter 3), but where termination of pregnancy was allowable only in exceptional situations, and which received genetic referrals from the neighbouring Irish Republic, where termination for any reason was totally illegal. As a strict Protestant Christian himself, his position was a difficult one, but he managed to retain the respect of the highly traditional community and to provide a valued medical genetics service. It also helped that UK centres documented their experience in detail, for example on safety aspects of amniocentesis, which helped to ensure that both the obstetricians and laboratories involved maintained high standards of practice. Indeed, a specific journal on the topic, *Prenatal Diagnosis*, was founded in 1980, edited for many years by Malcolm Ferguson-Smith. A historical article (Ferguson-Smith and Bianchi 2010) charts its development over the following 30 years. It gives an indication of the succession of new techniques that have advanced the field, as well as of the very extensive studies on their applications in practice, many of these published in the journal.

The thoughtful and responsible attitude to prenatal diagnosis taken by the British medical genetics community generally in these early years can be seen in its submissions through the Clinical Genetics Society to government bills relating to abortion during the 1980s, and may have contributed to a much less polarised position on the topic by comparison with, for example, the USA. Likewise, in countries such as Norway, Belgium and France, leading medical geneticists frequently had close links with government and were influential in the introduction of prenatal diagnosis. Examples can be seen in my recorded interviews with such workers as Kåre Berg [49], Herman Vanden Berghe [66], Joelle and André Boué [43] and Jean-François Mattei [94], all accessible at (www.genmedhist.org/interviews). International collaborations across Europe on the safety of amniocentesis and on the efficiency of cell culture techniques were also carried out.

Initially the principal indication for amniocentesis was for high risk of Down syndrome or other chromosome disorder, most commonly due to advanced maternal age, but a major advance was the finding by David Brock and colleagues in Edinburgh that a high proportion of fetuses with open neural tube defects showed a raised level of alphafetoprotein (AFP) in amniotic fluid (Brock and Sutcliffe 1972), (see also Chapters 3 and 10 for details of Brock's life and work).

It is easy to forget now how common these malformations were (1% of all births in parts of Wales, Western Scotland and Ireland) and how great the morbidity and mortality was that they caused. I myself remember on first coming to Cardiff finding a complete hospital ward devoted to spina bifida patients and their complications. The situation changed further when it was found that maternal serum AFP could be used to detect the defects (Brock et al. 1974), opening the way, along with increasingly sensitive fetal ultrasound, to prenatal screening for neural tube defects.

The ethical aspects of these developments were in part defused by the discovery (again UK work in multicentre collaborations), that preconceptional dietary supplementation by folic acid could provide a large measure of prevention against neural tube defects (Smithells et al. 1981; Medical Research Council (MRC) Vitamin Study Research Group 1991), particularly in high-risk areas, so that now they are relatively uncommon in early pregnancy as well as in live births.

More serious ethical dilemmas have resulted from early screening approaches to Down syndrome, initially the use of a combination of biochemical and ultrasound measures, while more recently the detection in maternal blood of free fetal DNA of placental origin during early pregnancy (see below). Much of the Down's screening development, in the UK and elsewhere, has been led by obstetricians, some of whom have tended to promote it as a part of routine antenatal care, giving rise to concerns that women were being pressured into having tests or, at the least, were being given inadequate information on the limitations and consequences of testing. For medical geneticists, with a long tradition of 'non-directive' genetic counselling, this has given rise to considerable criticism of prenatal screening programmes, especially where, as in Down syndrome screening, a 'public health' approach, based primarily on cost saving, has been a prominent, even if usually unspoken factor in promoting them.

For some years the psychological effects of prenatal Down's screening on pregnant women were largely ignored, the focus being more on technical aspects, on safety, and on factors such as efficiency in detection of abnormality and false positive rate. Medical geneticists and other genetic counselling staff, though, became increasingly concerned by the numbers of women referred, often in a distressed state, who had been given little or no information on the consequences of Down's screening, on the nature of the disorder itself, and on the possibility of false positive or false negative results. These women (and their partners) were a very different group to those originally seen for amniocentesis, who were mostly already aware of their increased risk and were prepared to accept the consequences of prenatal testing and potential abortion.

These concerns led to the first systematic psychological studies of prenatal screening, which were initially carried out mainly in Britain, helped by the fact that the NHS base for most testing allowed a relatively unbiased sample. Theresa Marteau (Figure 5.1), psychologist at Guy's Hospital Medical School, London, and working closely with the clinical genetics service there, was a leader in the initial studies (Marteau et al. 1993), which were followed by numerous other series in the UK and around the world, all showing a significant level of adverse psychological effects and a lack of communication that can only be considered as failure of good medical practice.

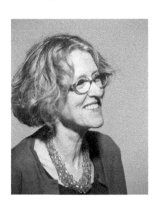

Figure 5.1 Theresa Marteau. (Courtesy Theresa Marteau.)

The recognition of these problems led to the gradual improvement of the screening system, notably the recognition that screening is not simply a laboratory process but also needs full communication and consent to be built in (and funded). It also resulted in increased communication between obstetric and medical genetics services, and increasingly to the involvement of non-medical genetic counsellors who, along with clinical geneticists, often found themselves acting as advocates for women and as critics of potentially harmful screening programmes generally. Even so, the experience resulting from prenatal screening has created an attitude of reserve among the medical genetics community towards new reproductive developments and technologies generally.

FIRST TRIMESTER PRENATAL DIAGNOSIS AND CHORIONIC VILLUS SAMPLING

One of the inevitable drawbacks of amniocentesis, especially when involving cultured cells, was the late diagnosis and correspondingly late termination of pregnancy involved. The possibility of first trimester prenatal diagnosis based on chorionic villus sampling (CVS), with a diagnosis possible by the 10–12th week of pregnancy, was thus a major advance in terms of acceptability, particularly for members of religions where later termination is forbidden but early termination before 'ensoulment' has occurred may be acceptable, as in Islam. Britain cannot claim to be an innovator of this technique, which was established by obstetrician Bruno Brambati and his scientist colleague Giuseppi Simoni in Italy (Brambati et al. 1986); an even earlier (and undoubtedly premature) attempt had been made in China (Anon 1975). Over the following years a major international initiative was coordinated by Laird Jackson (Philadelphia) through the *CVS Newsletter*, which provided worldwide data on safety and accuracy.

Whereas CVS has been used in many countries for chromosomal prenatal diagnosis, often in pregnancies at low genetic risk, this was much less the case in Britain, partly due to the occurrence of false positive abnormal findings due to placental mosaicism, but also by the widespread experience and relative safety of amniocentesis. Where it rapidly proved to be of great value was for the less frequent but much higher-risk situations in recessively inherited conditions, such as inherited enzyme disorders and haemoglobinopathies. UK obstetricians especially involved with the early development of CVS include Humphrey Ward and Charles Rodeck, both based in London.

A particularly valuable contribution made by British workers in this area was in relation to molecular prenatal diagnosis, initially of the thalassaemias, then later of a wide range of disorders where a molecular defect or linked DNA marker had been identified. The key people involved initially for beta thalassaemia were Bernadette Modell in London and Bob Williamson, molecular geneticist at nearby St Mary's Hospital [61], who together pioneered the use of CVS for the first trimester prenatal diagnosis in the Greek Cypriot and Pakistani communities in London and the North of England. Later John Old, working in Oxford with David Weatherall, provided a more systematic prenatal diagnosis laboratory service for the haemoglobinopathies. The recorded interview with Bernadette Modell [70] (see Figure 5.2, Box) describes graphically the benefits that affected families gained from this, as well as the traumas and disappointments that they were prepared to accept along the way. In particular, it became clear that most families who previously had an affected child had already decided against risking a further recurrence (1 chance in 4) unless some form of prenatal diagnosis could be offered, a point of general relevance to genetic counselling taken up in the next chapter, where the somewhat different situation for sickle cell disease is also described.

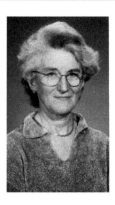

Figure 5.2 Bernadette Modell (born 1935). Recorded interview 14/12/2007 [70]. (Courtesy Bernadette Modell and the Genetics and Medicine Historical Network).

Bernadette Modell initially studied Zoology and undertook laboratory research at both Oxford and Cambridge Universities, before deciding to train in Medicine. During clinical paediatric work at University College Hospital, London, she encountered patients with beta thalassaemia, mainly of Cypriot origin, and built up a clinic for specialised treatment. This led to the introduction of carrier screening and prenatal diagnosis which was extended in collaboration with Dr Aamra Darr to the Pakistani community in the north of England as first trimester prenatal diagnosis became feasible. Her work became the basis for international programmes of thalassaemia prevention through the World Health Organisation, and for wider approaches to genetic screening.

Initially the only possible approach to prenatal diagnosis of thalassaemia involved fetal blood sampling from the umbilical cord by direct fetal visualisation (fetoscopy), with a high risk of miscarriage and a late termination in the event of an abnormal result. Even so, families were often prepared to accept this traumatic procedure, that had been pioneered by John Scrimgeour in Edinburgh (Scrimgeour 1973) and Charles Rodeck in London. But matters changed when molecular diagnosis became possible and Modell set up a collaboration with Bob Williamson, then in Glasgow (see Chapter 10); the following passage from the interview shows how important are the mundane aspects of obtaining material before work in the lab can even start:

BM. It must have been 1974, when Bob was still using the biochemical methods. They were still using biochemical methods to try to sort out the messenger and the binding of DNA and so on, and Bob was still working in Glasgow, but I thought this was extremely interesting …I said 'Well, I've got loads of patients and you need material to try and get your message out for alpha and beta thalassaemia and so forth, so what can I do to help?' So he said 'If there are any splenectomies we could do with a spleen'. So I said fine. The operations then were done at … St Pancras Hospital, paediatric operations were done there, at that time. And so I had a sit-up-and-beg bicycle and I went on this bicycle with a container of liquid nitrogen in front of me, would go into the operating theatre, we had a lovely surgeon and he would say 'Oh yes, Dr Modell's come', and get me to explain what it was all about, and as soon as the spleen was out, it was straight into the liquid nitrogen and then it went on the night train up to Glasgow, packed in dry ice. And …. in other ways I did everything I could to provide Bob with his stuff and I didn't realise at the time that this was going to be what we really needed. It took quite a while for the penny to drop once he was successful, that the one thing that really mattered was to move prenatal diagnosis into the first trimester and this was going to be the way to do it; and once the penny dropped of course we started working together.

A further collaboration with obstetrician Humphrey Ward resulted in a catheter that could be used safely to obtain chorionic villus material, and first trimester molecular prenatal diagnosis for thalassaemia became a reality. By this time Modell was working with the Pakistani community in Bradford and Leeds, along with locally based social scientist Aamra Darr; they found that the potential demand for prenatal diagnosis from thalassaemia families was as high as it had proved to be with those from the London Cypriot community, and that the difference between first and second trimester prenatal diagnosis was striking.

So now among these families, there was one, and actually he was an Imam, a Mullah, and they had a child with thalassaemia. They were one of these families that came down to London for prenatal diagnosis, mid trimester prenatal diagnosis and they came and the fetus was affected and they had a mid trimester abortion and they felt obviously terrible, as one does. And she got pregnant again. Aamra had told them about our efforts for first trimester diagnosis, so they came down to London to see us, and said they wanted us to try and I said to him, I asked him whether he felt that by doing this they would be contributing to developing techniques that were acceptable to their community and he said yes, they also thought that. So that was our first real case and we did it here at the Temperance Hospital, in the same operating theatre where we had been doing the research. This was interesting because sometimes you are so focused on what you are doing that you don't realise what's going on around you. The theatre sister burst into tears. She said, it was wonderful seeing something good come out of all of this. There are so many good people and they become so involved in the objective that you are trying to reach and sometimes you don't see them because they are behind you, not in front. Now that fetus was affected too and she had an early abortion. And when Aamra went to see the family later in Bradford, she said 'It's wonderful. I can't tell you the difference'. And they got pregnant again and it was alright the next time. When we finally published on the first series, in the acknowledgements, I felt I had to acknowledge the 22 brave ladies who had made all these decisions which led us on and on to getting something which was better.

As in many other areas of genetics and medicine, haemoglobin and its disorders proved a paradigm for genetic disorders more widely; molecular genetics progressed, with the identification first of linked DNA markers and then of specific mutations for an increasing number of genetic disorders, such as Duchenne muscular dystrophy and cystic fibrosis, CVS gave the possibility of early prenatal diagnosis for essentially any mendelian disorder with a known molecular basis, greatly helping numerous affected families, though also raising difficult issues as to where the limits should lie in terms of clinical severity, variability and age at onset.

CVS proved to be not without its pitfalls, though the sharing of information through the CVS newsletter and other channels reduced the impact of these. For chromosome disorders the finding that placental mosaicism was relatively frequent, and that a CVS result might not always reflect an abnormality in the fetus, was a reason for caution in interpreting results.

In part because of these concerns, and because its safety in terms of pregnancy loss was consistently slightly greater than that of amniocentesis, CVS never replaced amniocentesis as the main test for low-risk pregnancies, at least in the UK, but has proved of the greatest value for molecular and biochemical diagnosis, where the recurrence risks are high (usually 1 in 4), as seen with the thalassaemias.

ULTRASOUND AND PRENATAL DIAGNOSIS

Ultrasound has already been mentioned in connection with placental localisation during amniocentesis, and it has likewise proved a valuable aid for CVS, but as its resolution developed it became an increasingly powerful prenatal diagnostic tool in its own right. Initially the relatively crude images could only detect such major conditions as twinning and anencephaly, but the detection of progressively smaller abnormalities became feasible, with major consequences, some intended, others not.

Neural tube defects provide a good example of how ultrasound has changed prenatal diagnostic practice. In high incidence areas, it was at first mainly used in conjunction with amniotic fluid AFP analysis after a raised maternal serum AFP had been found, but as ultrasound was developed, this increasingly allowed amniocentesis to be avoided. In low-risk regions or countries it frequently led to population maternal AFP screening being avoided altogether, especially as ultrasound became used for all pregnancies. High resolution ultrasound has increasingly been used for the detection of limb, cardiac and other structural defects.

These developments have not always proved to be true advances in medical practice and, as they were pioneered primarily by radiologists and obstetricians, and often explained to pregnant women as forming part of 'routine antenatal care', a number of unintended consequences arose which might have been avoided if medical geneticists had been more fully involved from the outset. Patterns of practice varied greatly across Britain, but now most have a designated fetal medicine multidisciplinary team, containing an expert ultrasound radiologist, an obstetrician/gynaecologist, and a medical geneticist, who can discuss problem situations.

Among the commoner problematic issues arising from the increased use and resolution of ultrasound have been the following. First, the experience of those using and interpreting ultrasound in the early years frequently lagged behind the technology, something that has improved over the years with training courses and defined standards of practice. In particular, satisfactory normal ranges for measurements such as limb length were initially inadequate or even absent. A second deficiency, which medical geneticists could have readily identified from their experience of Bayesian approaches in other fields, was the lack of consideration of context. Thus, an ultrasound finding or measurement that might strongly indicate fetal abnormality in a situation of high prior genetic (or other) risk would more often simply reflect variability within the normal range if the prior risk were low or if the finding had resulted from a general 'screening' situation. Radiology and its related imaging techniques are particularly prone to such 'incidentaloma' generating situations generally.

An example (many years ago) from my own experience remains in my mind of a healthy couple whose first child had achondroplasia being told that their second pregnancy would probably also be affected since the ultrasound limb length appeared to be 'slightly short', though at that time there was no clearly defined normal range established. After examining the affected child and confirming the diagnosis of classical achondroplasia, it was clear that the prior genetic risk to the second pregnancy was minimal, the affected individual representing a new dominant mutation; the pregnancy continued and a normal child was duly born.

A final issue in the use of ultrasound generally in pregnancy is that it has often been unclear, in overall policy as well as individual situations, what is the primary aim. Is it to help with monitoring the general growth and development of the fetus? Or is it to identify and eliminate any 'abnormality' that may be incidentally discovered? Most pregnant women are told only the former, leading inevitably to distress and confusion if an apparent abnormality, or finding of uncertain significance, is detected by ultrasound. This is just one aspect of a general situation in the use of 'screening' procedures throughout medicine, which fortunately is more tightly regulated in Britain (at least in NHS practice) than in many other countries. Medical geneticists can and do play a valuable part in minimising problems of this nature, both in their own areas of work and in helping other specialities to become aware of them.

PREIMPLANTATION GENETIC DIAGNOSIS

The research and service applications described briefly above for the prenatal diagnosis of genetic disorders, extensively involving both clinical and laboratory medical genetics across Britain, have shown how an inevitably sensitive and at times controversial field could be developed and introduced into medical practice, for the most part, in a responsible way and with a high degree of consensus among all involved. Sadly, this was not always the case for preimplantation genetic diagnosis (PGD) based on in vitro fertilisation (IVF).

IVF itself was very much a British development, due to the efforts and collaboration of Cambridge basic geneticist and embryologist Robert Edwards and NHS- employed obstetrician Patrick Steptoe, based in Oldham, not an academic centre (Figure 5.3).

After the birth of the first IVF baby, Louise Brown, in 1978, it rapidly became clear that this would become a major advance in the management of infertility; plans were put forward to the MRC for a major research and NHS centre in Cambridge but unfortunately were rejected, forcing Edwards and Steptoe to seek funding from private sources and reducing the research aspects. The pattern thus became set for IVF to be developed mostly in the private sector, while research in the field largely moved abroad, despite the presence of expert scientists in developmental genetics, such as Anne McLaren (see Figure 5.4), in Britain. Edwards (1925–2013) belatedly received a Nobel award in 2010 for his work, but Patrick Steptoe (1913–1988) had sadly already died by then, as had their nurse-embryologist colleague Jean Purdy, who Edwards considered had received insufficient recognition.

When molecular and chromosomal techniques for PGD based on single cell analysis became possible a few years later, they mostly became an appendage

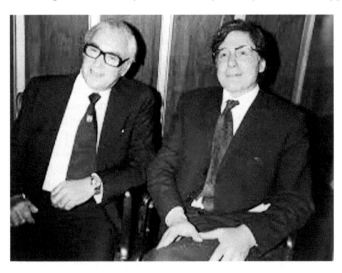

Figure 5.3 Patrick Steptoe (Oldham) and Robert Edwards (Cambridge), the first workers to apply in vitro fertilisation resulting in a human birth.

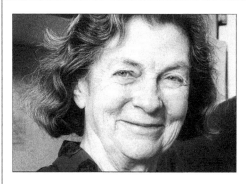

Anne McLaren initially studied biology at Oxford and London universities, developing research in mammalian early embryonic development. After some years in Edinburgh she returned to London to lead the MRC Mammalian Development Unit, continuing her research after retirement at Cambridge up to her death at age 80 in a car accident. While her research used mostly mice, she linked closely with workers on human development and was involved, together with Mary Warnock, in developing ethical guidelines for research and practice of IVF and related areas that led to the 1978 Warnock Report and the establishment of the Human Fertilisation and Embryology Authority (HFEA).

Figure 5.4 Anne McLaren (1927–2007). (Photo Courtesy Wikipedia.)

of IVF services, again largely involving the private sector and often lacking the standards of accuracy that had evolved for prenatal diagnosis, and also initially lacking significant contact or collaboration with medical genetics services. The result was that patients were often unprepared, without prior genetic counselling or even at times a secure diagnosis; medical genetics centres were correspondingly reluctant to refer patients or to recommend this new approach when those involved could provide few or no data on experience, accuracy or safety. While most of these problems were eventually resolved, and while most PGD centres now link closely with medical genetics services, it was unfortunate and largely unnecessary that these poor standards of practice should ever have occurred in the first place. In most other countries, including the USA, the same problems have occurred, with a few notable exceptions (e.g.: the comprehensive centre in Brussels).

This is perhaps an appropriate place to mention the role of the Human Fertilisation and Embryology Authority (HFEA), now responsible legally for licensing any research or service applications involving the creation or use of human embryos and one of the few UK bodies involved in genetics whose recommendations carry the weight of law. Initially it was concerned mainly with the regulation of IVF itself and did not examine the genetic diagnostic aspects in detail, but this has now been corrected. The existence of the HFEA has largely ensured that medical practice and research in this area has become responsible both ethically and scientifically, something that would almost certainly not have happened otherwise, given the early problems of the commercial involvement with IVF and the uncertain quality of PGD mentioned above.

Recently the unit at University College London has coordinated worldwide data on PGD, and a book edited by Joyce Harper gives a valuable account of the field (Harper 2009). It is interesting that, contrary to some early views that PGD might largely replace early prenatal diagnosis through avoiding early pregnancy termination, it remains relatively infrequently used at present, perhaps owing to the hormonal side effects and other technological aspects of IVF.

NONINVASIVE DNA-BASED PRENATAL TESTING (NIPT)

The most recent approach to early prenatal diagnosis, particularly for Down syndrome, has been the recognition that cell-free DNA, of placental origin, can be detected in the maternal circulation during early pregnancy. While this might be considered to be an extension of the other screening techniques described above, it has the difference that it has proved sufficiently accurate and specific to be used as a primary diagnostic test, not just for preliminary screening, though confirmation by other tests is still usually recommended in many circumstances, especially when it is used as a population screening test.

The original discovery that fetal DNA was present in the maternal circulation was a largely British one, made by Dennis Lo and colleagues, working at first in Cambridge and later in Hong Kong. The work was then developed further in America by Diana Bianchi and co-workers. The initial focus was on the analysis of fetal cells present in maternal blood, but despite much effort this did not provide a sufficiently accurate prediction for widespread use.

The realisation that free fetal DNA, of placental origin, existed in maternal plasma, and that it was present in the first trimester, changed the situation radically, especially in combination with improved genomic techniques. Rapid application, driven largely by commercial involvement, has led to its use as a screening tool for diagnosing Down syndrome and other autosomal trisomies with a quantitative imbalance of fetal DNA. While it has shown a high specificity for these, wider use to detect microdeletions is still much less certain in its benefits, though this has not stopped the use and active promotion of NIPT for this in the private sector internationally and in the UK.

The unbiased evaluation of NIPT as a population screening service has been made difficult by these largely commercial settings, and it has been systematic studies, undertaken largely in Britain, that have been especially helpful, thanks to the existence of comprehensive NHS-based services that can provide the basis for extensive and largely unbiased studies. (For medical genetics developments these have proved even more important in evaluating new services than they have in medicine generally.) The last decade of evaluation of NIPT has not only allowed detailed analysis of accuracy but has also given a greater opportunity for the public to make decisions on the way this should be offered, something that was largely absent when earlier Down's screening programmes were being introduced.

The use of NIPT in a low-risk screening situation has been analysed in a clear and at times critical recent report from Nuffield Council on Bioethics (2017). To what extent this approach will prove feasible and acceptable for the use of whole genome screening remains to be seen. A current research study on how whole genome sequencing may be able to identify abnormalities in pregnancies found to be at risk from ultrasound and other tests should provide information on this.

OTHER REPRODUCTIVE ADVANCES AND MEDICAL GENETICS

Among the other advances in reproductive technology that are especially relevant to genetic disorders, mitochondrial replacement deserves a mention, not just because the main initial research advances and applications have come from Britain, but also because the disorders involved, while rare, are often extremely severe and also intractable in genetic terms, with no possibility of definitive prenatal diagnosis, and with especially high risks to offspring in the maternal line. The possibility of transferring the nucleus of a fertilised egg where the mitochondria are likely to be abnormal into a donated egg with normal mitochondria is now allowing these disorders to be avoided, while retaining the full complement of nuclear genes from the parents. While the possible ethical aspects have received much publicity, they are much less significant in practice than for many other genetic situations. A level-headed report from Nuffield Council on Bioethics (2012) giving cautious approval shows how valuable it is to have such reports before the issues become sensationalised and potentially polarised.

A further development that needs careful consideration before it enters clinical practice is gene editing, which gives the possibility of repairing the mutational defect in a gamete resulting from a severe mendelian disorder. Here the ethical concerns focus mainly on the fact that this approach would also affect future generations; while this might be an advantage for a genetic disorder, it could be open to abuse if used for 'genetic enhancement'. Again, a Nuffield Council report (2018) has clearly set out the facts and issues involved.

One potential advance in reproductive genetics that has not so far happened (perhaps surprisingly), but which will undoubtedly have a major practical and ethical impact when it does, is the ability to separate X- and Y-bearing sperm and thus achieve pre-conceptional sex selection. This will be much more difficult to regulate than current approaches involving pre-implantation or prenatal diagnosis.

A final development that has repeatedly been claimed, without evidence, to have occurred over the past decade, is human reproductive cloning. Again, British technology, ('Dolly the sheep' at the Roslin Institute, Scotland), has made such a possibility potentially feasible, but social restrictions are likely to prevent it in humans, at least in Britain, though it is a topic that needs to be kept a close eye on. Medical geneticists have not been involved in this scientifically and ethically dubious field, whether in Britain or (to my knowledge) in other countries. Intermittent claims from occasional 'rogue operators' outside Britain in this and related areas have so far never been substantiated and have been widely condemned, most recently in the use of gene editing.

A final, not entirely anecdotal comment from a historian colleague, who had submitted a paper on British medical genetics services to a historical journal, may be relevant to quote here, if only to illustrate the lack of knowledge about medical genetics among historians until very recently. One reviewer of the paper commented that 'these medical geneticists seem to be very busy people. When do they find time to do their cloning?' (Leeming 2003). It is not entirely clear if molecular or human cloning was meant (probably the latter), but it shows the still widespread ignorance concerning what we actually do (and do not do) as medical geneticists!

REFERENCES

Anonymous. 1975. Fetal sex prediction by sex chromatin of chorionic villi cells during early pregnancy. *Chin Med J.* 1:117–126.

Brambati B, Simoni G, Fabro S (eds.) 1986. *Chorionic Villus Sampling.* New York: Marcel Dekker.

Brock DJ, Bolton AE, Scrimgeour JB. 1974. Prenatal diagnosis of spina bifida and anencephaly through maternal plasma-alpha-fetoprotein measurement. *Lancet.* 1:767–769.

Brock DJ, Sutcliffe RG. 1972. Alpha-fetoprotein in the antenatal diagnosis of anencephaly and spina bifida. *Lancet.* 2:197–199.

Ferguson-Smith MA, Bianchi DW. 2010. Prenatal diagnosis: Past, present and future. *Prenatal Diagnosis.* 30:601–604.

Ferguson-Smith ME, Ferguson-Smith MA, Nevin NC, Stone M. 1971. Chromosome analysis before birth and its value in genetic counselling. *Br Med J.* 4(5779):69–74.

Fuchs F, Freiesleben E, Knudsen EE, Riis P. 1956–1957. Antenatal detection of hereditary diseases. *Acta Genet Stat Med.* 6(2):261–263.

Fuchs F, Riis P. 1956. Antenatal sex determination. *Nature.* 177:330.

Harper J (ed.). 2009. *Preimplantation Genetic Diagnosis.* Cambridge: Cambridge University Press.

Leeming W. 2003. *Second International Workshop on Genetics, Medicine and History*, Brno. www.genmedhist.org/workshops

Marteau TM, Kidd J, Michie S, Cook R, Johnston M, Shaw RW. 1993. Anxiety, knowledge and satisfaction in women receiving false positive results on routine prenatal screening: A randomized controlled trial. *J Psychosom Obstet Gynaecol.* 14:185–196.

Medical Research Council (MRC) Vitamin Study Research Group. 1991. Prevention of neural tube defects: Results of the Medical Research Council Vitamin Study. *Lancet.* 338:131–137.

Nuffield Council on Bioethics. 2012. *Novel Techniques for the Prevention of Mitochondrial DNA Disorders: An Ethical Review.* London: Nuffield Council on Bioethics.

Nuffield Council on Bioethics. 2017. *Non-invasive Prenatal Testing: Ethical Issues.* London: Nuffield Council on Bioethics.

Nuffield Council on Bioethics. 2018. *Genome Editing and Human Reproduction.* London: Nuffield Council on Bioethics.

Riis P. 2006. First steps in antenatal diagnosis, 1956. *Hum Genet.* 118:772–773.

Scrimgeour JB. 1973. Other techniques for antenatal diagnosis. In: Emery AEH (ed.). *Antenatal Diagnosis of Genetic Disease.* New York: Churchill Livingstone, p. 49.

Smithells RW, Sheppard S, Schorah CJ et al. 1981. Apparent prevention of neural tube defects by preconceptional vitamin supplementation. *Arch Dis Child.* 56:911–918.

6

Genetic counselling

ABSTRACT

Genetic counselling, one of the key parts of medical genetics, was also one of the earliest, beginning in Britain almost immediately after the end of World War II, at Great Ormond Street Hospital, London. Over the following decades a comprehensive network of genetic counselling clinics developed across Britain, mainly based in regional medical genetics centres under NHS clinical geneticists and closely linked with other genetic services. Accurate genetic risk estimation and genetic diagnosis were initially the principal elements, but psychological aspects became progressively more recognised and important, especially as non-medical genetic counsellor posts were introduced and training programmes for them created. With increasing genetic and genomic applications and their use in wider medicine, the need for genetic counselling is greater than ever and its nature is continuing to evolve, as is its relationship with other aspects of medical genetics.

BACKGROUND

Genetic counselling forms one of the most important parts of medical genetics, and of genetics in medicine generally; it deserves much more than a single chapter of this book to be devoted to its history and development, but so far no satisfactory and comprehensive account has been written. I am also aware that, despite beginning to undertake genetic counselling myself over 50 years ago, and having written a book on the subject, *Practical Genetic Counselling* (Harper 1981–2010), which has proved useful, I have not done it justice in my own historical work, particularly in my interview series, mainly because I was focusing on capturing the memories of the oldest workers in the field, primarily clinicians and scientists. Thus I hope that the short account given here will be a stimulus to others to undertake the detailed historical studies needed, and I have been pleased to learn recently that such an initiative is under way for Britain.

Looking back to the earliest years of genetics, the pioneering book of Joseph Adams, published in 1814, has already been mentioned in Chapter 1. Not only did Adams recognise the types of heredity that would later become clearer as 'mendelian' and 'multifactorial', but he incorporated these concepts into his medical practice and his advice to patients and their families.

Yet, in the most serious of all hereditary peculiarities, the great susceptibility to madness, celibacy has been recommended as a duty. Before we venture to propose measures contrary to one of the strongest impulses of Nature, and to the first blessing which the Almighty Fiat bestowed on man, it becomes us seriously to weigh the consequences.

Were this opinion universal, it would probably produce its effects only on the most amiable and best disposed, whilst the profligate and unprincipled would indulge themselves, regardless of posterity: it is scarcely necessary to hint at the result. To interdict marriages with the healthy individuals of such families, might do much towards extinguishing that enthusiasm, which, when well directed, proves the source of those achievements which aggrandize families, which encrease the glory of nations, and improve the condition of mankind. Nor is this confined to heroes and statesmen, but extends to the effusions of genius, and to the cultivation of the softer virtues.

Adams, 1814
Accessible at www.genmedhist.org/digitisedresources

For the next century I can find almost nothing that might be considered relevant to modern genetic counselling, if one leaves aside the promotion of eugenics by Francis Galton and his colleagues in Britain and a range of workers in other countries, especially America. The eugenicists were concerned with the health and 'quality' of populations rather than with the wishes and concerns of individuals, whereas genetic counselling is now properly regarded as primarily a matter for individuals, or at least for individual families.

William Bateson, in the chapter on human inherited disorders of his 1909 book, *Principles of Mendelian Inheritance* (Bateson 1909), says almost nothing about advice to families, though Norwegian Otto Lous Mohr, in his book *Genetics and Medicine* (1934), cautiously advocated such advice from physicians, to whom his book was primarily addressed.

The individual medical practitioner is most frequently consulted as to the possible consequences of marriage in cases where one or even both partners belong to a family in which pathological hereditary traits occur. Provided he is really familiar with the mechanism of segregation of autosomal and sex-linked traits and has grasped the essentials of dominant and recessive inheritance he may, by aid of one of the now existing text-books on the known pathological hereditary traits in man, give valuable advice in quite a few cases. But his judgment should always be given with the reservation involved in the fact that genetics primarily deals with probabilities.

Mohr was writing in the 1930s, at the time when pressure was developing for basic geneticists to support proponents of eugenics, who existed in Norway as well as in Germany, but Mohr and his colleagues in the Norwegian genetics community were resolute in opposing this. As can be seen in Mohr's book he recognised that the individual and the population aspects of genetics might conflict:

As will be realized, most of the measures outlined tend to prevent hereditary pathological states from coming to the surface. This brings the physician into the conflicting situation that his advice in the interest of the individual very frequently runs counter to the interests of the population, since it favors the further transmission of undesirable genes through unaffected heterozygous carriers. The same is true of our therapeutic measures in trying to alleviate the symptoms in the affected individuals themselves. It is of no use to hide this paradoxical situation which will prevail until perhaps a method is found by which we are enabled also to identify the heterozygous, normal carriers of recessive genes. So far nothing indicates that we are even approaching this goal.

It is not surprising that Mohr was arrested and imprisoned following the 1940 Nazi invasion of Norway.

In Britain, John Fraser Roberts makes no mention of what might be interpreted as genetic counselling in the original edition of his *Introduction to Medical Genetics* (1940), despite the fact that he is credited with establishing the first genetic counselling clinic at Great Ormond Street Children's Hospital in 1946. France was virtually devoid of genetics until the end of the war, and genetic counselling was absent initially from the main Paris units, though in Lyon Jacques-Michel Robert was early in establishing it during the 1950s. Germany was neither physically nor psychologically prepared for any activities based on human genetics after what had happened during the Third Reich; Walter Fuhrmann, working with Friedrich Vogel in Heidelberg, was the first to develop genetic counselling systematically (Fuhrmann and Vogel 1969).

Thus we have to look to America for the origins of modern genetic counselling, specifically to the work of Sheldon Reed, whose book *Counseling in Medical Genetics* (1955) can fairly be considered as marking its starting point. Fortunately, Reed himself, in his book and in other publications, has written about his early work, and a good account of his life and career has been given recently by Stern (2012). Reed was a Drosophila geneticist by background, but in 1941 he accepted the post of director of the Dight Clinic, in Minneapolis, Minnesota, which had been endowed by Edward Dight for seeing families to discuss genetic risk as part of a eugenics programme. Reed made it clear from the outset that he had no intention for his role to be related to eugenics. When looking back over the more than 4000 families that he had seen during his career, he admitted that he had no idea as to whether the effects had been eugenic or dysgenic; it is fortunate that his sponsors left him alone to practice as he considered best.

Reed coined the term 'genetic counseling' (usually spelt 'counselling' outside America) in 1947, in the absence of any satisfactory previous term, defining it loosely as 'a kind of genetic social work without eugenic shackles'; he was adamant that if those he was seeing had considered it as forming part of eugenics, it would never have been acceptable. By the time he wrote his book in 1955, his experience had been extensive; he writes confidently, clearly and simply, so that we gain a clear impression of his wider views and his character, as well as of the range of genetic problems with which he was involved. He comes across as a warm and kindly person, well aware of his own limitations, not being medically trained, as well as those of the field overall.

In fact, several of these early non-medical geneticists involved in genetic counselling seem to have had similar qualities, which at times caused them considerable stress. Thus Arthur Steinberg, as quoted in the book of Kevles (1985), commented:

> They'd had a baby with some awful business, and all you could say was that they had a 25% risk of its recurring. Couldn't do much of anything for them. I'd come home after clinic and my wife would take a look at me and say, 'you had heredity clinic today'.

I suspect, though, that such families often gained much more benefit from genetic counselling than Steinberg, and many others after him, realised. Even just being able to listen can be strongly therapeutic.

Returning to the development of genetic counselling in Britain, the first genetic counselling clinic seems to have been set up in 1946 by John Fraser Roberts, at Great Ormond Street Children's Hospital, London. We have already encountered Roberts through his book, *An Introduction to Medical Genetics* (first edition 1940) and through his pre-war research (Chapter 1), which was later supported by the MRC in the form of a small unit at the Institute of Child Health (Chapter 2), adjacent to Great Ormond Street Children's Hospital, where he was joined and later succeeded by Cedric Carter.

It is not entirely clear though, what kind of clinic this was, since Roberts, unlike Sheldon Reed, did not write about it directly. It was not funded by or connected with any eugenics body, such as the Eugenics Society which still lingered in post-war Britain. As well as receiving referrals from Great Ormond Street and other hospitals it may have catered for families seen primarily as part of the numerous studies, principally on common malformations, mental handicap and other childhood disorders, that were the primary function of the unit. It did not at that time have a diagnostic function; Roberts is said by his later colleague Marcus Pembrey to have 'hung up his stethoscope' as soon as he had qualified in Medicine. Roberts' secretary, later his second wife, stated that she prepared a summary of each family to be seen before the clinic was held (Harper et al. 2010).

The problems involved seem to have been essentially medical, with an absence of the racially slanted referrals frequently encountered by Sheldon Reed in America.

In addition to his London-based clinic, Roberts maintained clinical links with the hospitals for the mentally handicapped in Bristol and Colchester, where he had worked previously following Penrose, this later becoming part of the North-East Thames regional genetics service.

Cedric Carter, Roberts' colleague and successor, did describe the nature of the Great Ormond Street clinic (Carter 1978), as did Alan Stevenson for his clinic at the Oxford MRC Clinical and Population Genetics Research Unit. From their papers it would seem that they received a wide range of referrals from clinicians, both hospital-based and general practitioners, together with some self-referrals, not unlike the situation today, covering both mendelian and multifactorial disorders, with chromosome abnormalities an increasing source after 1960.

By around 1950 there had thus become established, in both America and Britain, a small core of genetics clinics where families with or at risk of a genetic disorder could obtain advice and which contained at least some of the elements that we would today recognise as genetic counselling. At this point, we need to look in more detail at what these elements are and how they have evolved over the following 60 years.

SOME DEFINITIONS

A number of definitions of genetic counselling have been proposed over the years, attempting to combine its key elements in a single sentence or paragraph. Not surprisingly for such a complex process they have been somewhat cumbersome. Probably the earliest, and also perhaps still the best, is that suggested by a working group of *American Society of Human Genetics* led by Frank Clark Fraser of Montreal, one of the first and most inspirational leaders of medical genetics, in 1974:

> Genetic counseling is a communication process which deals with the human problems associated with the occurrence, or the risk of occurrence, of a genetic disorder in a family. The process involves an attempt by one or more appropriately trained persons to help the individual or family to (1) comprehend the medical facts, including the diagnosis, probable course of the disorder, and the available management; (2) appreciate the way heredity contributes to the disorder, and the risk of recurrence in specified relatives; (3) understand the alternatives for dealing with the risk of recurrence; (4) choose the course of action which seems to them appropriate in view of their risk, their family goals, and their ethical and religious standards, and to act in accordance with that decision; and (5) to make the best possible adjustment to the disorder in an affected family member and/or to the risk of recurrence of that disorder.

> *Fraser, 1974*

This represents a fair summary that includes the main elements of genetic counselling in the last quarter of the twentieth century, not just in America but across most of Europe also; it remains largely valid today, despite the major technological changes underpinning medical genetics.

Clinical geneticist Thaddeus Kelly (1980) gave a more succinct definition:

> An educational process that seeks to assist affected and/or at risk individuals to understand the nature of the genetic disorder, its transmission and the options open to them in management and family planning.

However, the emergence of the non-medical graduate genetic counsellor in the 1980s and 1990s, discussed below, and in particular the professional separation from medical genetics overall which resulted from this divergence in much of America, though not in the rest of the world, led to a change in what should be included in the meaning of genetic counselling – or perhaps more accurately in what should *not* be included.

The American National Society of Genetic Counselors (NSGC) proposed a different definition in 2005, which essentially reflects genetic counselling in the narrower sense of it being 'what genetic counsellors in America do' rather than a multi-faceted activity that may involve several professional groupings.

> Genetic counseling is the process of helping people understand and adapt to the medical, psychological and familial implications of genetic contributions to disease. This process integrates the following:
>
> Interpretation of family and medical histories to assess the chance of disease occurrence or recurrence.
> Education about inheritance, testing, management, prevention, resources and research.
> Counseling to promote informed choices and adaptation to the risk or condition.
>
> *Stern 2012, p.14*

It is probably better to leave these definitions, especially since Britain has been largely free from the divisions concerning who should do genetic counselling seen in America, and to look in more detail at the key elements that form genetic counselling, and how these have evolved.

THE KEY ELEMENTS OF GENETIC COUNSELLING

The 'key elements' given in Table 6.1, are taken from the 7th edition of my own book *Practical Genetic Counselling* (2010) and represent those which I have found most central to my own practice of genetic counselling over the past 40 years.

Table 6.1 Genetic counselling: The main elements

Diagnostic and clinical aspects
Documentation of family and pedigree information
Recognition of inheritance patterns and risk estimation
Communication and empathy with those seen
Information on available options and further measures
Support in decision-making and for decisions made

Note: Based on Harper PS. *Practical Genetic Counselling* (1981) 1st edn. Bristol: John Wright. 7th edn. 2010 London: Hodder Arnold. An 8th edition (2020) by Angus Clarke is imminent.

I make no claim for any authority or official standing for them – though over this long time nobody has written or spoken to me voicing their disagreement!

In an historical account such as this, Table 6.1 might also be arranged chronologically as in Figure 6.1, with risk estimation the earliest distinct element of genetic counselling, from the time of Sheldon Reed and John Fraser Roberts (the 1940s onwards), and refined by Bayesian approaches, as introduced by Edmond (Tony) Murphy and by Alan Stevenson in the late 1960s. Clinical and diagnostic aspects became increasingly important from the 1960s onwards with the recognition of extensive genetic heterogeneity and the detailed study by clinical geneticists of dysmorphic syndromes, with increasing laboratory support from chromosome analysis. The introduction of psychological aspects, at first informally and then more formally, by both clinical geneticists and genetic counsellors, dates from the mid 1970s.

None of these developments has superseded the earlier approaches, so that genetic counselling has increasingly become a composite and often multidisciplinary activity and it would be wrong to see the different elements as mutually exclusive, which is the impression given at times by Stern's account for America.

Alongside these trends must be seen the growth of essential laboratory aspects, initially cytogenetics and subsequently molecular and genomic analysis, which have radically altered the context of genetic counselling.

Readers may be surprised to see that in Table 6.1 I list *diagnostic and clinical aspects* first, but this reflects my firm view, unchanged after half a century, that these form the 'bedrock' for satisfactory genetic counselling. To me, and I think to

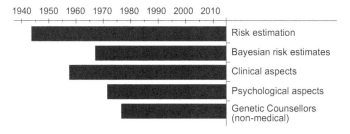

Figure 6.1 Genetic counselling: an approximate chronology for its different elements.

most people, it is self-evident that a firm and clearly established medical diagnosis is essential if one is to give secure genetic risk estimates, or other aspects of genetic counselling for relatives. Equally necessary is the clinical experience to know or to sense when the diagnosis is insecure or even completely wrong. Any differences of opinion on these points relate not so much on whether they are important, but whether they should be considered actually to form part of genetic counselling itself.

We have already seen that the earliest workers giving genetic counselling were non-medical, like Sheldon Reed, or if indeed medical, like John Fraser Roberts, would not attempt to challenge or revise a diagnosis themselves. But this predated the arrival of the medically trained and experienced clinical geneticists of the 1970s onwards who, in particular fields, were likely to be at least, and at times more experienced diagnosticians for rare disorders than the referring clinician. This period also saw the rapid development of recognition of specific syndromes and the heterogeneity of genetic disorders generally. Repeatedly I, like most other colleagues, have found that patients and families referred for genetic counselling really need a firm diagnosis first. The non-medical genetic counsellor is placed in a difficult position here, especially if not based in a general medical genetics unit, and is now often hindered more than helped by the multiplicity of tests, genetic or otherwise, that are available or may have already been done before a family is seen. It seems unlikely that whole genome sequencing, if used as a 'blanket' approach prior to genetic counselling, will alter the situation greatly (see Chapter 12). Most people involved in genetic counselling, whether or not medically trained, develop highly sensitive 'antennae' to the possibility of an incorrect diagnosis or early unnoticed features of a specific disorder (Huntington's disease is a good example), but it is much more difficult to question this if one is not medically trained and experienced oneself.

The obvious answer, which has developed almost universally across the UK, is for clinical geneticists and non-medical genetic counsellors to work closely together, giving the patients and families the benefit of the widest possible range of skills. For most UK regional centres, based in teaching hospitals, the 'under one roof' concept, allowing genetic counsellors, clinical geneticists and laboratories to work closely together, often with research groups nearby, has been a particularly productive one, allowing the different disciplines to learn from each other. In practice, this is also the situation found most often in America, where genetic counsellors and clinical geneticists also commonly, though not always, work as part of a team. I was saddened though, recently, to hear one experienced American genetic counsellor state that they had never throughout their long career worked with a clinical geneticist, and had not regretted this. It does not seem to me that the 'stand-alone' and isolated genetic counsellor is a satisfactory solution to the needs of most families.

Genetic risk

Most families seen for genetic counselling come because of actual or perceived risk of a genetic disorder to themselves or for family members. What they hope for is for this risk to be excluded, but from the earliest years of the field it has been recognised that it is uncommon to be able to tell someone that there is *no* risk; rather, risk may be reduced, often greatly, or alternatively it may be raised. The recognition, and at times acceptance, of uncertainty is something that is built into the fabric of medical genetics, including genetic counselling, and how to handle it is undoubtedly a key element.

This attitude to uncertainty is in strong contrast to that of most medical specialties, for whom risk is normally regarded as something to be got rid of if possible, and where it cannot, is regarded as a failure or, all too often, denied or at least not mentioned to those concerned. This attitude has been very slow to change in most fields of medicine and deserves a full historical study in its own right. Only recently have laboratory and clinical disciplines outside medical genetics begun to include approaches to risk estimation in their training, even though all areas of medicine actually carry considerable uncertainty in their practice.

How damaging the dogmatic pronouncement of an apparent certainty can be, especially when given by an 'expert', has been shown by a relatively recent UK legal case; it took the evidence of a determined medical geneticist, among other factors, to overturn the conviction of a mother accused of murdering her children on the grounds of the extreme unlikelihood of two successive cot deaths, using evidence from an eminent paediatric 'expert witness' whose ignorance of medical genetics, Bayesian risk estimates and elementary statistics resulted in a risk of 1 in 73,000,000 for the chance occurrence of two sudden deaths in sibs being given to the jury, giving the impression of certainty, whereas the true situation was that the evidence was much more evenly based.

It is thus not surprising that the first individuals involved in genetic counselling regarded accurate risk estimation as the central part of their work, particularly if they were non-medical scientists or, if medical, not experienced clinically. Apart from chromosome analysis from 1960, there were almost no laboratory tests at that time that might allow greater precision. But in fact there was considerable scope for helping families even in what might appear to be a very limited situation. First, most people seen for genetic counselling had been given little or no previous information on genetic risks or, worse still, had been given dogmatic statements that they should not have further children, or that recurrence was 'impossible'. Expectations were thus often low, and most families were appreciative of a careful family analysis and, most of all, for the time spent listening to their questions, even if the risk assessment might prove pessimistic. In addition, the majority of those seen for genetic counselling actually receive a low risk, something that those outside the field often do not recognise.

It was indeed fortunate that the early workers, such as Lionel Penrose and John Fraser Roberts in Britain, like Sheldon Reed and Arthur Steinberg in America, were in general sympathetic characters, often contrasting strongly with the eugenicists of a decade or two earlier (e.g.: Charles Davenport and Edward East in America), who seemed to regard families with a genetic disorder as a social 'problem' rather than as individuals. In Britain, this meant that when medically trained clinical geneticists became predominant in genetic counselling in the 1960s and 1970s, there was a firm human as well as scientific foundation for their work.

The recognition of mendelian inheritance for the disorder in a family gave, and still gives, greatly increased provision for a genetic risk estimate, allowing it to be reduced to minimal for offspring of those with rare recessively inherited disorders, or for male offspring of a man with an X-linked condition such as haemophilia. Where no mendelian inheritance was present, as for most common childhood and adult disorders, 'empiric risks' could be derived from the numerous meticulous studies pioneered especially by John Fraser Roberts and Cedric Carter. Fifty years on, many of these estimates have never been superseded.

A later, but extremely important approach to risk estimation was introduced in the 1970s, which was the Bayesian modification of primary risk in the light of additional or secondary (conditional) information, and its quantification in the setting of a specific family (see Chapter 1 for a note on Thomas Bayes). Thus, to take an example, such as a female sib of a male with an X-linked disorder such as haemophilia or Duchenne muscular dystrophy, one can intuitively see that if she has had a large number of healthy sons but none have been affected, then she is less likely to be a carrier herself, with her own daughters' risks correspondingly reduced. Likewise where a test exists with a substantial overlap between the normal and affected ranges, a greater resolution can be obtained by deriving a 'likelihood ratio' for normality than by simply using a single cut-off point attempting to divide 'normal' from 'abnormal'; a quantitative combination of this with the appropriate prior genetic risk and with other conditional family information, can give final risk estimates that are considerably more precise and accurate than those based just on the original mendelian pattern. The importance of recognising the limitations for screening of general populations, where the prior risks are very low by comparison for the risk within an affected family, is particularly relevant.

I have found it difficult to work out exactly when and how Bayesian risk estimations first entered genetic counselling. Karl Pearson and RA Fisher both mention Bayesian approaches as a theoretical mathematical problem and one might have expected workers such as Penrose and Haldane to have appreciated their practical use, but it does not feature in their writings; neither John Fraser Roberts nor Sheldon Reed mention it in their respective books. But it is the subject of several papers (Murphy and Mutalik 1969) and a subsequent book, *Principles of Genetic Counseling* (Murphy and Chase 1975) by Edmond (Tony) Murphy and colleagues working at Johns Hopkins Hospital in Victor McKusick's department in the late 1960s; it also features in Alan Stevenson and colleagues' book *Genetic Counselling* (1970). Was there a point of common origin? Both Murphy and Stevenson were from Ireland and both had a background in epidemiology. I had hoped to resolve this by interviewing Tony Murphy after his retirement from America to Europe, but sadly he suffered a major stroke the day before the interview was due, and never recovered from this.

Bayesian risks were first generally adopted into UK genetic counselling following a questionnaire sent to all UK clinical geneticists by Sarah Bundey in 1978, based on a series of pedigrees involving the X-linked disorder Duchenne muscular dystrophy; the results showed, to the embarrassment of all concerned, that only a minority was using them correctly. Apparently they were even unfamiliar to Cedric Carter, to the surprise of his colleagues and trainees. Marcus Pembrey [62] states:

> When pedigree calculations came up, ... I said, look, I don't know how to do this really. Michael [Baraitser] said, well I don't know how to do it, but there's a young chap who is working with me called Robin Winter who knows how to do it. And Joan [Slack] said, well I've had a go at it but I don't know. I said well, look, let's just make it a rule, from now on every pedigree we will do it, right there in front of everybody. We'll work it out. We've got to learn, we've got to get our heads around this. So it was completely open. It was the first change that happened. So when Cedric came in, it was the overlap period, we said "Cedric, can you help us on this? We've decided the three of us are going to really get this sorted." And we assumed that he could do this because he gave that indication. He said "oh no, this needs a wet towel round my head!"

> *Interview with Marcus Pembrey*

Following much discussion, Bayesian risk estimates were introduced generally into the training of UK clinical geneticists and, later, of non-medical genetic counsellors and molecular genetics laboratories. Full details can be found in the book on risk estimation by Ian Young (2000).

It is fair to say that, despite recognition of their importance, few people working in the genetic counselling field, apart from a few devotees, actually *liked* Bayesian calculations, so that one might have expected them to disappear from the scene when DNA-based genetic testing became widespread. Surprisingly, the reverse proved to be the case, since most early testing was based on linked markers, with a significant risk of errors from genetic recombination and other factors, so the result was a generation of molecular diagnostic laboratory workers who needed to learn Bayesian and similar probability calculations for constructing their reports. Andrew Read (Manchester) can take particular credit for this.

A Bayesian approach to risk estimation has gradually infiltrated other fields of medicine over recent decades, though with little credit given to medical genetics as the first specialty to introduce it systematically, and probably still the only one to think in a Bayesian way. A recent interesting general book on the topic (McGrayne 2012) also fails to mention the applications in medical genetics.

Pedigrees and family details

I shall confine myself to a very brief note here but would emphasise that these are an essential part of any genetic counselling interview, though some details are commonly collected in advance, either at a home visit or by telephone. I have found personally that the taking of family details gives a relatively 'neutral' introductory period during which the counsellor and the family can adjust to each other before more emotionally charged issues are raised. The symbols and other conventions used were actually standardised close to a century ago by fieldworkers in eugenics, and are valuable not only for a specific consultation but for identifying the extended family who may be at risk. They also form an important long-term record for future generations, as well as for research; thus the pedigree information collected in Julia Bell's *Treasury of Human Inheritance* has formed the starting point for a number of modern molecular genetic investigations. A variety of programmes to produce computer-generated pedigrees has been available for some years, but I have never personally found them particularly helpful.

Communication and empathy: Psychological aspects of genetic counselling

So far, the 'key elements' discussed have contained little in the way of 'counselling' in the psychological sense of the term, something that was not lost on American psychiatrist Seymour Kessler, who made a major contribution towards changing the balance for this. Kessler rightly stated that:

> How a field which deals intimately with so many emotionally charged issues could have evolved from biology and remained isolated from clinical psychology and psychiatry for so long a period of time is a matter on which students of the history of science need to ponder.

Kessler 1979

Kessler equally saw, unlike some of his American successors, that the medical and psychological approaches were not mutually exclusive, so it remains valid, 40 years later, to emphasise the value of the two remaining closely integrated.

The 'key element' that I have listed as *communication and empathy* in Table 6.1 is central to all aspects of genetic counselling, whoever undertakes it, and has been so since the beginning. It is abundantly shown in Sheldon Reed's book and in the passages that Stern (2012) gives from his papers, to the extent that she implies that the present-day American genetic counsellor is the direct lineal descendant of Reed, rather than passing through the generations of clinical geneticists in between. This view would do a grave injustice to this large and often eminent body of workers, including Clarke Fraser quoted above, who over the past half century or more have provided genetic counselling to the great majority of families seen worldwide, and who continue to do so, at least in most countries outside America.

In Britain it is certainly true that a few of the early clinical geneticists found communication with patients and families difficult – Cedric Carter was a notable instance, as described in Chapter 2. Some others have been too detailed or technical in their approach to be readily understood by those seen by them, or perhaps just rather difficult to understand – John Edwards (Chapter 3) might have been considered such an example. But most of those providing genetic counselling have been good communicators, partly because of their broad medical background but also on account of their empathic personality.

What one can certainly fault in the early years is the relative lack of time in medical genetics training programmes for the teaching of basic counselling skills and psychological principles, though many of these were absorbed subconsciously as the result of experience. In the case of our Cardiff unit we were fortunate to have had for some years the input of a highly experienced psychiatrist and psychotherapist, Christine Evans, from whom we learned an immense amount that was helpful in our regular genetic counselling practice. She in turn encouraged and surprised us by telling us that in many situations we were already following established psychological principles but that we were often unaware that we were doing so, and that these principles had names and a well-established theoretical basis. I strongly suspect that across the country many clinical geneticists giving genetic counselling have in the same way frequently been following these principles without realising it, but it is equally true that everyone could improve their communication and counselling skills by formal training.

Whatever one's approach to genetic counselling, an essential element is *time*, something particularly precious in most healthcare settings where there is continual pressure for greater 'efficiency' and where most medical specialties are forced to fit consultations into much less than the one hour normally considered essential for an adequate initial genetic counselling session. Yet one cannot fulfil the key aspects outlined above of listening, risk assessment and information giving without adequate time, and attempting to reduce this is no more logical or satisfactory than attempting to do the same for a complex surgical operation. How this was incorporated and to a large extent has been preserved (with a few regrettable exceptions) in an NHS system where time is one of the biggest factors in the cost of a service, is something that deserves a detailed study.

'Non-directiveness' in genetic counselling

The concept of 'non-directiveness' has been a fundamental tenet of genetic counselling over many years and it is difficult to pinpoint a precise origin. One factor was certainly a reaction to the prescriptive nature of eugenics, as can be seen in Sheldon Reed's statement, noted earlier, that genetic counselling would have never been acceptable to families had it been considered to be part of eugenics. It seems already to have been the norm by the 1950s in Britain too, since Cedric Carter notes that he changed his non-directive policy in some low-risk situations to encourage these families to have further children (Carter et al. 1971). An important factor reinforcing the non-directive approach by clinical geneticists and genetic counsellors was the dogmatic approach frequently taken by their clinical colleagues, notably in relation to the 'routinisation' of prenatal diagnostic tests discussed in Chapter 5. By the time that presymptomatic testing for Huntington's disease became feasible during the 1980s, a non-directive approach was firmly built into the testing protocols.

It has naturally been pointed out, by Kessler (1979), Clarke (1997) and others, that it is easy to be non-directive in a subliminal or even subconscious way through the language one uses or the way one describes the disorders involved, and this is another strong reason for all those involved in genetic counselling to have some formal training in general counselling skills. But it has also been questioned whether a non-directive approach is necessarily the best one, and whether it may leave families feeling unsupported. This lends further strength to the element of 'supportiveness' being a crucial and integral part of genetic counselling.

A further factor that is increasingly leading genetic counselling away from an entirely non-directive approach is the growing availability of effective therapies. Phenylketonuria has long been the classical example of this, as mentioned earlier, but the incentive of early detection and treatment for the familial cancers (Chapter 4) is another powerful example, and the number of treatable genetic disorders is increasing steadily. Nevertheless the principle of respect, with support, for the decisions of those seen remains the bedrock of genetic counselling. A valuable discussion of the overall topic is given by Clarke (1997) in his essay 'Beyond Non-directiveness'.

OUTCOMES OF GENETIC COUNSELLING

In all fields of medicine one is, rightly, increasingly asked to justify the efficacy and value of what one does; genetic counselling and other aspects of medical genetics are no exception, but the question arises, what does one mean by 'value' and 'success' and what outcome measures are appropriate? The eugenicists would have had no problem answering this, at least in theory, either in terms of increasing 'high quality' births in the population or reducing the frequency of abnormal ones. Medical geneticists have turned their backs on eugenics, so what outcome measures should be used? Population prevention of serious genetic problems may indeed be desirable, but only if this is in tune with the wishes of the individual patients and families involved – some prenatal screening programmes have come perilously close to the old eugenics.

As far as genetic counselling is concerned, the first attempt to examine outcomes was the study mentioned above of Cedric Carter and his colleagues in a retrospective comparison of births to couples given either a high or low risk (Carter et al. 1971). When they reviewed the reproductive outcomes for the families which Carter and John Fraser Roberts had seen over the years between 1952 and 1964, they found that the group given a risk of less than 10% for having an affected child (271 couples) had gone on to have 229 further children, 2% of which were affected, compared with 94 children (17 affected) for those (185 couples) given a 'high' risk of over 10%. Carter is definite that he did not attempt to 'deter' those in the high-risk category, but he does state, as noted above, that he changed his practice to give 'positive encouragement' to those at low risk. While few giving genetic counselling today would be so overtly directive, Carter's approach was probably not so different in practice to present day 'supportive' genetic counselling.

While producing data on factual outcome measures is relatively straightforward and has also been done for specific conditions such as thalassaemia (see Chapter 5) and for Duchenne muscular dystrophy, it is much more difficult to decide on what counts as 'success' when the only options are prenatal diagnosis or refraining from child-bearing. Attempts have been made to assess 'satisfaction' by those receiving genetic counselling, but the variability in both the nature and complexity of the situations encountered in genetic counselling referrals remains an issue. It is easier to decide on what criteria should *not* be used, such as number of affected births or pregnancy terminations.

OPTIONS FOR PREVENTION, THERAPY AND OTHER MEASURES

Genetic counselling does not happen in a vacuum and, quite apart from reproductive decisions and associated genetic tests, those seen will want to know what useful measures they can take, especially if they are actually affected with the particular disorder. A major and growing part of the work of clinical geneticists is now participation in management, usually as part of a team. Many genetic disorders are multisystemic and do not fall naturally under the work of a single specialty; it is often the medical geneticist who helps to link them and make sure that the patient does not 'fall between the cracks'. In Britain a number of such specialist multidisciplinary clinics have been established for such disorders as Marfan syndrome and neurofibromatosis, for example, though the organisation and NHS financial support for these clinics has been a challenge at times.

In my own experience these specialist clinics, however valuable, are not easily combined with genetic counselling; their ambience and organisation are very different, and they are too 'medical' for satisfactory counselling. They do however give scope for a different type of worker, the specialist nurse, whose role is complementary to the non-medical genetic counsellor, as discussed later in the chapter.

In terms of information on other aspects and options, lay societies and support groups now form perhaps the most valuable source (see Chapter 8); this is a major change since genetic counselling began when few such societies existed, and where lobbying and fund-raising for research was their primary purpose. The family with a genetic disorder is now much less isolated than was the case 50 years ago and the links between lay groups and genetics professionals much stronger.

Returning to more specifically genetic aspects of the 'options' related to and arising from genetic counselling, one that is often ignored, though arguably the most important, is the freedom to do nothing, that can be opened up by the exclusion, or at least sizeable reduction, of a potentially high risk. This was illustrated in the early study of Carter et al. (1971) mentioned above, and since at the time of this study prenatal diagnosis was not generally available, these results showed that many families were only prepared to have further children if they could be at least moderately confident of not having an affected child. The figure of 10% as a dividing line between 'high' and 'low' risk chosen by Carter et al. may seem a high one today, when we have a greater range of options to offer, but then it was a question of either taking or not taking the risk, and there is no doubt that for the families given a 'low' risk this gave the possibility of having a healthy child which previously they had felt was not open to them.

Once prenatal diagnosis – initially through amniocentesis, then in the first trimester by CVS – became feasible for some conditions, further options were created, especially for conditions such as Down syndrome and neural tube defects, as we saw in the previous chapter. This raised a number of troubling issues, though, both for families and for those involved in genetic counselling. Foremost among these was the fact that, at least in the early years of prenatal diagnosis, many women undergoing amniocentesis, usually at relatively low risk and with no family history of the disorder, were receiving little or no information about the risks and limitations of the procedure, or on the nature and severity of the condition, let alone wider genetic counselling. In many antenatal clinics prenatal tests became 'routinised', especially once blood and ultrasound tests permitted non-invasive screening before amniocentesis. Obstetric practice varied greatly, often without good reason, some obstetricians working closely with geneticists while others had little or even no contact. Lack of time, as well as of inclination, was a major factor in this unsatisfactory situation, especially as the increasing use of prenatal diagnostic testing in low-risk or 'screening' situations meant that many women had no personal experience of the genetic disorders concerned, in contrast to the situation for thalassaemia and other recessively inherited disorders, where those undergoing prenatal diagnosis were at high risk for a disorder already in the family.

These and other problems provided fertile ground for a series of studies during the 1980s and 1990s, primarily by psychologists, ethicists and others in the social sciences, encouraged by the funding that had become available and by their increasing awareness of genetics as relevant to their fields of work. Theresa Marteau (Chapter 5) and Martin Richards (Chapter 7) were among the first in Britain to document these issues from the psychological viewpoint.

Among the various ways of improving this largely unsatisfactory situation, one was to involve non-medical staff in providing information and genetic counselling. At this point in the UK there were relatively few formally trained genetic counsellors, so nursing staff were the ones primarily involved, some attached to medical genetics units, others part of the antenatal service. Few of these had any formal training in genetics, but it could be argued that this might not be needed in such a specific situation, provided that those involved had good links with medical geneticists if a complex situation were encountered. At the least this ensured that women undergoing prenatal diagnosis had the time and opportunity to have their questions answered and be given accurate information.

TIME AND TIMING

The essential factor of having adequate time in undertaking genetic counselling has already been highlighted in this chapter and elsewhere in the book, but the related topic of *timing* also needs emphasising. This arises in a variety of contexts, some of them of considerable practical significance. I have all too often during my career received a hospital ward referral shortly after the birth, or sometimes the death, of a child with serious abnormalities where it has been expected that I should give genetic counselling; it is usually clear in such situations that the parents are too distressed to take in any information other than that directly relevant to the outlook for or loss of their child, and where it is better to postpone any detailed discussion of genetic aspects to a later occasion. But on the other hand, too much delay can equally cause problems and I can recollect situations where I have given a high recurrence risk only to find that the mother was already pregnant again but had not previously mentioned it.

Since pregnancy is clearly not the best time for giving genetic counselling, one might logically conclude that premarital or preconception clinics might help to avoid the first detection of a high-risk situation when pregnancy is already underway. This does not seem to have evolved as a widespread practice in the UK, though it is likely that a considerable amount of information on possible tests in pregnancy is appropriately given in primary care and community health clinics, as well as through the media. As with genetic counselling overall, and indeed in medicine generally, it is likely that the educated and articulate minority are more likely to access genetic services early, while those from deprived communities more often have unplanned pregnancies and are lacking information on genetic risks and services in advance.

The timing of genetic counselling, and associated genetic testing, for children and adolescents in relation to an adult onset disorder such as Huntington's disease is discussed in the next chapter; while there is a general consensus that genetic testing of young children should be avoided unless there are benefits from their treatment, the situation for adolescents is more difficult to make clear guidelines on.

GENETIC COUNSELLING FOR ETHNIC MINORITIES

When genetic counselling started to develop in Britain during the 1950s, the UK was a relatively homogeneous population, both culturally and genetically; differences between the Celtic West and the East of the country for common disorders such as neural tube defects existed but were not clear-cut. In America race was a major issue for workers like Sheldon Reed – a common cause for referral was whether an adopted mixed-race child would 'pass for white' – but the concept of providing services specific for the black community had yet to arise.

The catalyst for change was, as in so many aspects of medical genetics, the disorders of haemoglobin, in combination with the large-scale movements of populations from the Caribbean, former African colonies and the Indian subcontinent. It gradually became clear that conditions such as sickle cell disease and the thalassaemias were no longer rare and exotic disorders but were frequent in those parts of Britain with significant ethnic minority populations. Existing medical genetics services were unprepared for this, as indeed were medical services generally.

Initially, the prevalent view was that these populations were not receptive to genetic counselling, or to proposed screening for the heterozygous carrier state, but this was soon shown not to be the case when community-based programmes were started that could provide services within the cultural framework of the specific populations involved, which differed considerably between themselves. The developments for beta thalassaemia from the work of Aamra Darr and Bernadette Modell have been described in Chapter 5, and the corresponding work on sickle cell disease was likewise pioneered by a forceful woman worker, in this case Elizabeth Anionwu. As with so many badly needed developments for often disadvantaged minority communities, an activist approach was required, a contrast perhaps to overall genetic services, which have in general responded to perceived need rather than campaigning actively.

Elizabeth Anionwu (see Figure 4.9) has given a fascinating account of how sickle cell disease services developed over the last quarter of the twentieth century in her powerful and frank autobiography (Anionwu 2016), which shows also how important and necessary was her background in community nursing, as well as being part of, though not restricted to, the London black community. One difficulty she rightly highlights is the traditional separation of haematology and medical genetics services, something also mentioned in my interviews with Bernadette Modell [70] and David Weatherall [30]. The strong link formed by Elizabeth Anionwu with Marcus Pembrey at the Institute of Child Health clinical genetics unit was thus especially valuable in this respect.

Although the development of genetic counselling and related services first developed in areas of Britain with large minority populations, there are few parts of the country now where these needs are not present and a pattern has evolved where specific genetic counsellors, often but not always based in genetics centres, provide a service not only for haemoglobin disorders but for other wider genetic issues met frequently in these populations. This includes the genetic risks potentially arising from consanguinity, where a careful and sensitive balancing of these alongside the cultural advantages is needed.

GENETIC COUNSELLORS

One of the most important features of genetic counselling, and indeed of medical genetics overall, during the past 30–40 years has been the development of graduate genetic counsellors as a specific group of professionals, distinct from clinical geneticists and others in the field. Being so recent, the history of this process in Britain has not yet been written, but hopefully it will be documented soon, while the founders are still living and able to provide first-hand evidence. This is all the more important since the only historical book on the topic so far, Stern's *Telling Genes. The Story of Genetic Counseling in America*, confines itself entirely to America, with almost no reference to the very different patterns that have developed in Europe. Its title is also misleading, since it is essentially a history of *genetic counsellors*, not of *genetic counselling*, in America, largely excluding and ignoring the long, distinguished and continuing contributions of American medically trained geneticists to genetic counselling. Having worked in both continents (admittedly a long time ago in America), I found it difficult at times to recognise the isolated picture of genetic counsellors in America painted by Stern, having always found them closely linked to and appreciative of clinical geneticists, the converse equally applying. Having made these criticisms, the book does give a valuable and detailed account of the work of Sheldon Reed, and of the founding and development of the Sarah Lawrence Master's degree course in genetic counseling, based in New York.

In Britain the influence of the Sarah Lawrence School has also been strong, and furthermore extremely positive, possibly because of the very different history of medical genetics services in general (see Chapter 8), which has seen develop a varied but largely integrated mixture of professional groupings, usually with responsibility for a defined regional population, and which has allowed the development of a new group, that of genetic counsellors, in a progressive and generally harmonious manner. With virtually no involvement of the private sector or commercial interests, and none of the problems concerning financial reimbursement which seem to have dogged its development in the United States, the forging of a new discipline has been able to occur with broad professional support from the other, longer established groups such as clinical geneticists.

Returning to the early years of the field, we have already seen that medical geneticists across the country were based in teaching centres, but in very small numbers, commonly one or two per centre initially for a population of several million. With rapidly expanding possibilities for both services and research, it was clear from the outset that help was needed, and this came in different forms that have changed over the years. Thus Cedric Carter's colleague Kathleen Evans (see Figure 2.8b), whose background was in social work, was principally involved in the various family studies, but, as we saw in Chapter 2, was essential in providing the 'counselling' element in Carter's genetics clinic. I myself was fortunate in having a similarly exceptional social worker, Audrey Tyler, involved in the Cardiff work on Huntington's disease, who was able to extend both the research and the service aspects into areas far beyond my own capacity and expertise.

The professional group outside medicine most involved in genetic counselling during the 1980s and 1990s was that with a nursing background, often from community nursing and usually with no previous experience of genetics. Frequently they carried much of the responsibility for organising the network of genetics clinics outside the main teaching hospital and medical genetics centre, which rapidly grew as families and referring clinicians became more aware of the need for and value of genetic counselling. The experience of running a series of 'outreach' clinics in Northern Ontario was vital, for example, in allowing the later development by Helen Hughes of comparable clinics across the isolated rural communities of North Wales (see recorded interview [90]). A role closer to traditional nursing-related activities has been as part of multidisciplinary clinics for specific genetic disorders, already mentioned, where the provision and coordination of medical needs, rather than genetic counselling, are the main objectives.

A major reason why nurses became part of the medical genetics structures in Britain was because the nursing profession already existed, with posts for specialist nurses in a variety of other fields widely accepted, so that comparable 'genetics nurse specialist' posts could often be created without the necessity for separate funding, training schemes or new professional structures, these all coming later. Most of the key people involved in the initial UK development of genetic counsellors in fact had a nursing background and Figure 6.2 shows two of them, Heather Skirton and Christine Patch. This predominance can also be seen in the titles of the new UK Society when, with the strong support of medical geneticists, it was actually formed. Initially it was 'Genetics Nurses and Social Workers Association', later 'Genetic Nurses and Counsellors Association' (see Skirton et al. 1997, 2013).

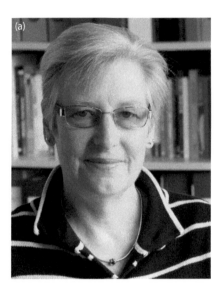

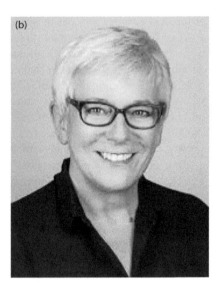

Figure 6.2 Some early UK genetic counsellors with a nursing background. **(a)** Heather Skirton. (Courtesy Heather Skirton.) **(b)** Christine Patch. (Courtesy Christine Patch and King's College London.)

As the numbers of staff grew, so did their role and responsibilities; having been seen initially as 'assistants' or 'associates' for clinicians, they have progressively become professional colleagues of equal standing. This necessitated a radical reshaping of training, with nursing no longer a sufficient basis, but increasingly becoming one of a number of basic 'first degree' specialties acting as an entry point to specific higher degree courses in genetic counselling. This was facilitated by the initiation of specific MSc degrees, as in America; first in Manchester (1992), pioneered by Sarah Lawrence graduate Lauren Kerzin-Storrar (Figure 6.3); then in Cardiff (2000), founded by clinical geneticist Angus Clarke (see Figure 7.1) and genetic counsellor Heather Skirton (Figure 6.2a). These between them have trained around 200 individuals over the past 25 years (personal communication 2018 from Angus Clarke). Currently in the UK some of the structures are being revised in the light of genomic developments, and of health service devolution, but there is little doubt that this now sizeable group of Master's degree genetic counsellors is setting the ethos and pattern for the role of genetic counsellors in Britain.

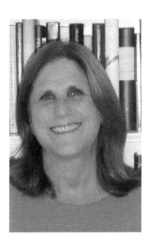

Figure 6.3 Lauren Kerzin-Storrar, originator of the Manchester genetic counselling MSc degree course. (Courtesy of Lauren Kerzin-Storrar.)

It is interesting, and encouraging, that there seem to have been few problems so far in finding jobs for these new graduates, as indeed was also the case for the first trainee clinical geneticists (see Chapter 8). Many have found places in established regional medical genetics centres, working alongside clinical geneticists, often taking on specific roles in such areas as prenatal diagnosis and cancer genetics. Rather fewer have entered posts in other specialist centres, and very few so far in primary care, despite pressure for the 'mainstreaming' of medical genetics to involve general practice. None in the UK, to my knowledge, have become 'free-standing' practitioners or joined commercial healthcare companies.

Looking at the patterns for genetic counsellors across the rest of Europe, developments have been very variable in different countries, but generally much slower, with the exception of France. This was fortunate to have as health minister a medical geneticist, Jean-François Mattei, from Marseille, who was able to establish, among other things, a defined and recognised standing for genetic counsellors (see Harper 2018). The British experience has also been influential in other countries, largely thanks to the close mutual contacts forged through the European Society of Human Genetics (ESHG), despite problems arising in some countries from the legal necessity of a medical training for undertaking particular responsibilities. The UK training schemes for genetic counsellors have been especially helpful in this process of harmonisation.

It can be seen from what I have written here that the overall development of genetic counsellors in Britain has gradually and partially converged with that seen in America, but without the need for what seems to have been, at times, painful (and perhaps unnecessary) distancing from clinical geneticists seen there. It is greatly to be hoped that changes recently imposed by the Health Department (England) in the light of genomic developments will not damage this pattern of progressive, professionally led evolution that has served UK genetic counselling and overall medical genetics services well since its beginnings.

GENDER AND GENETIC COUNSELLING

With the majority of genetic counsellors in Britain coming from a background in nursing, and the image of genetic counselling shifting from a purely scientific field to forming part of the 'caring professions', it is not surprising that the great majority of graduates from the genetic counselling Master's degree courses should be women, but this shift has also occurred in medical genetics as a whole, and indeed in medicine and science generally. Around three-quarters of those working in clinical genetics are now female, but this has not caused any significant difficulties, at least to my knowledge, perhaps because even when the majority of clinical geneticists were men, there were relatively few showing what might be considered excessively male characteristics by comparison, for example with specialties such as surgery. Clinical genetics, with its large component of genetic counselling, and with reproductive issues prominent, might naturally be considered as a largely feminine field, regardless of the gender of those practicing it.

A second reason why this major shift in gender has occurred without disturbance to the specialty is undoubtedly the high calibre of many of its female members since the beginning. This has long been clear in the laboratory and research field, with early cytogenetics being the clearest example, but molecular genetics is now comparable. In clinical genetics, the progressive introduction of flexible training and the removal of career barriers have allowed many able women to take on leadership roles in both research and service activities that were considerably more difficult for their counterparts in the first generations of medical geneticists in the 1960s and 1970s. This, like many other topics that I have flagged in different chapters, would make a good historical project for someone to examine in detail.

CONCLUSION

I hope that I have made it clear in this chapter that genetic counselling is a complex and to some extent a composite activity, depending on the input and interactions of several professional groups. It needs to rest on firm clinical and genetic foundations, but to extend beyond these to fulfil an educational, psychological and supportive role for families with genetic disorders. Equally it needs to utilise but not be dominated by the laboratory aspects of medical genetics which, as discussed in Chapter 10, are rapidly changing. On the whole in Britain, this difficult and dynamic balancing act has resulted in a high-quality genetic counselling service, responsive to the widely differing situations that arise in medical genetics practice and equitably distributed across the country. Until now it has evolved steadily and organically as the result of professional interaction and cooperation between the groups involved, without the need for 'top down' direction, and it is to be hoped that this will continue whatever laboratory advances occur. Looking back over the history of genetic counselling, the major needs for families and the issues arising from these have actually changed relatively little over the past half century, and they will probably still remain largely the same into the future regardless of any changes in the technology underlying medical genetics.

SOME BOOKS ON GENETIC COUNSELLING

These books, arranged approximately chronologically, give a good picture of how the field has evolved over the past 60 years. I have deliberately made the list worldwide, rather than confining it to the UK, since the influence of both writing and practice across boundaries has been great.

Reed SC. 1955. *Counseling in Medical Genetics*. Philadelphia: WB Saunders. The first book on the subject and still worth reading, especially to gain an idea of the main problems then seen.

Fuhrmann W, Vogel F. 1969. *Genetic Counselling: A Guide for the Practising Physician*. New York: Springer. Fuhrmann was the first person to establish genetic counselling in post-war West Germany (see interview with Friedrich Vogel [05]).

Stevenson AC, Davison BC, Oakshott MW. 1970. *Genetic Counselling*. Philadelphia: Lippincott. This book, based on the experience of Stevenson and his Oxford MRC unit, gives one of the first accounts of the use of Bayesian risk analysis in genetic counselling.

Murphy EA, Chase GS. 1975. *Principles of Genetic Counseling*. Chicago. Yearbook. This book emphasises the risk analysis and especially Bayesian aspects, but was probably too mathematical to have been widely appreciated.

Lubs HA, de la Cruz F. 1977. *Genetic Counseling*. New York: Raven Press. This is a multi-author volume based on a workshop held in 1976 and is valuable for showing how many different aspects of genetic counselling were being actively followed at this time. It also documents the debate in America over who should do genetic counselling.

Kessler S. 1979. *Genetic Counseling: Psychological Dimensions*. New York: Academic Press. The first book to document the key psychological aspects of genetic counselling.

Harper PS. *Practical Genetic Counselling* (1981) 1st edn. Bristol: John Wright. 7th edn. 2010 London: Hodder Arnold. An 8th edition (2020) written by Angus Clarke, will appear shortly.

Clarke AJ. (ed.). 1994. *Genetic Counselling: Practice and Principles*. London: Routledge.

Weil J. 2000. *Psychosocial Genetic Counseling*. New York: Oxford University Press.

Evans C. 2006. *Genetic Counselling: A Psychological Approach*. Cambridge: Cambridge University Press.

Uhlmann W, Schuette J, Yashar B. (eds.). 2009. *A Guide to Genetic Counseling*. New York: Wiley-Blackwell.

Stern AM. 2012. *Telling Genes - the Story of Genetic Counseling in America*. Baltimore: Johns Hopkins University Press.

REFERENCES

Adams J. 1814. *A Treatise on the Supposed Hereditary Properties of Diseases*. London: Callow.

Anionwu E. 2016. *Mixed Blessings from a Cambridge Union*. London: ELIZAN.

Bateson W. 1909. *Mendel's Principles of Heredity*. Cambridge: Cambridge University Press.

Bundey S. 1978. Calculation of genetic risks in Duchenne muscular dystrophy by geneticists in the United Kingdom. *J Med Genet*. 15(4):249–253.

Carter CO. 1978. Genetic counselling. *Br J Hosp Med*. 19(6):557–562.

Carter CO, Roberts JA, Evans KA, Buck AR. 1971. Genetic clinic. A follow-up. *Lancet*. 1:281–285.

Clarke AJ. 1997. The process of genetic counselling. Beyond non-directiveness. In: Harper PS and Clarke AJ (eds.). *Genetics, Society and Clinical Practice*. Oxford: Bios, pp. 179–200.

Fraser FC. 1974. Genetic counseling. *Am J Hum Genet*. 26:636–659.

Harper PS. 2018 Jul. Conversations with French medical geneticists. A personal perspective on the origins and early years of medical genetics in France. *Clin Genet*. 94(1):115–124.

Harper PS, Reynolds LA, Tansey EM. 2010. *Clinical Genetics in Britain: Origins and Development*. London: Wellcome Trust Centre for the History of Medicine at UCL.

Kelly TE. 1980. *Clinical Genetics and Genetic Counseling.* Chicago: Year Book Medical Publishers.

Kessler S. 1979. *Genetic Counseling: Psychological Dimensions.* New York: Academic Press.

Kevles DJ. 1985. *In the Name of Eugenics: Genetics and the Uses of Human Heredity.* New York: Knopf.

McGrayne S. 2012. *The Theory That Would Not Die.* New Haven: Yale University Press.

Mohr OL. 1934. *Heredity and Disease.* New York: Norton.

Murphy EA, Chase GS. 1975. *Principles of Genetic Counseling.* Chicago: Yearbook.

Murphy EA, Mutalik GS. 1969. The application of Bayesian method in genetic counseling. *Hum Hered.* 19:126–51.

Roberts JAF. 1940. *An Introduction to Medical Genetics.* London: Oxford University Press.

Skirton H, Barnes C, Curtis G, Walford-Moore J. The role and practice of the genetic nurse: Report of the AGNC Working Party. *J Med Genet.* 1997;34(2):141–147.

Skirton H, Kerzin-Storrar L, Barnes C, Hall G, Longmuir M, Patch C, Scott G, Walford-Moore J. 2013. Building the genetic counsellor profession in the United Kingdom: Two decades of growth and development. *J Genet Couns.* 22(6):902–906.

Young ID. 2000. *Introduction to Risk Calculation in Genetic Counseling.* Oxford: Oxford University Press.

7

Genetics, ethics and society

ABSTRACT

Both practice and research in medical genetics encounter numerous ethical issues, something that is inevitable given the many personal and sensitive aspects involved. Since medical genetics turned its back on eugenics after World War II, beginning with the example of Penrose and the Galton Laboratory, those working in the field have mostly been highly sensitive to these ethical aspects and have led the way in identifying and analysing them, and later in alerting those in other countries and other fields of medicine to their existence. Prenatal diagnosis and issues surrounding termination of pregnancy arose in the 1970s, but the most difficult have been those involving molecular genetic testing from the 1980s on, especially prediction of late-onset genetic disorders such as Huntington's disease. Extensive studies of these problems led to increasing involvement and collaboration of those in the social sciences and humanities, and to the creation of formal bodies such as the Human Genetics Commission and Nuffield Council on Bioethics, with numerous valuable reports influencing both government and professionals, in Britain and abroad. A related important development has been the growth of numerous lay societies for genetic disorders, often working closely with medical geneticists.

BACKGROUND

Ethical issues, rightly, are now central to the practice of all branches of medicine, and for research, too. But it was not always so, and while ethical considerations have guided medical practice since the time of the Hippocratic oath, it was only following the second world war, in the light of the terrible abuses seen in Nazi Germany, but also prevalent in the USSR and elsewhere, that the ethical conduct of medical research was codified in the 1964 Declaration of Helsinki (World Medical Association 1964), itself based on the earlier (1947) Nuremberg Code.

One of the most important initial questions to be considered in charting the development of UK medical genetics is, how did it shed its eugenic origins? Eugenics was a prominent feature of late nineteenth and early twentieth century genetics, with ethical aspects given little consideration and abuses frequent during World War II and previous decades, not only in Nazi-dominated Germany but in other countries such as America. This forms a sharp contrast with modern post-World War II medical genetics. The reasons for this are complex, but the fact remains that current medical genetics practice is now one of the most ethically aware areas of medicine, that British medical geneticists have played a leading role in this transformation, and that they continue to do so. Some readers outside the field may question this statement, so it is worth examining in some detail, starting at the beginning.

We have already seen that human genetics research, particularly in Britain, was already becoming strongly developed by the 1930s, with the principal UK workers in the field mostly opposed to eugenics and often outspoken on the subject (e.g. Hogben, Penrose and, to a lesser extent, Haldane). Even RA Fisher, who in his largely theoretical writings had expressed support for eugenics, was ambivalent to the extent of publicly splitting with the UK Eugenics Society over its unscientific attitude. It has already been mentioned (Chapter 1) that applications to the MRC Human Genetics Committee showed a complete absence of proposals related to eugenics.

After the war, Penrose's appointment to the Galton Chair and his worldwide influence in shaping human genetics were key factors in ensuring that both research and practice in the field would have a sound ethical basis during the critical years of its rapid development, when medical aspects were for the first time starting to become prominent. His presidential address to the Third International Human Genetics Congress in 1966 is an example:

At the moment we are only scratching the surface of this great science and our knowledge of human genes and their action is still so slight that it is presumptuous and foolish to lay down positive principles for human breeding. Rather each person can marvel at the prodigious diversity of the hereditary characters in man and respect those who differ from him genetically.

Penrose 1967

This was also an implicit criticism of the 'genetic enhancement' views of Hermann Muller, advocating sperm banks based on eminent men, given in a talk at the same congress. Despite Muller's eminence (and his Nobel Prize), it was Penrose's views that were to predominate in setting the ethos for the newly developing medical genetics.

It is doubtful whether the early medical geneticists involved with patients and families were particularly aware of specific ethical aspects of their own field during these early years, certainly not as theoretical or philosophical principles. I put this to Dr Frank Clarke Fraser of Montreal, whose own unit began in 1950, and he agreed. My own view is that the early medical geneticists were mostly fundamentally decent people and good medical doctors, keenly aware of the sufferings imposed by genetic disorders and of how little they could often do to help, but also of how valuable to patients and families was the ability to listen to concerns and to provide accurate information without imposing their own views. Perhaps the most important aspect of all was the opportunity to give adequate time to a consultation, something that was to become, and which has remained, an essential attribute of genetic counselling, as described in Chapter 6.

ETHICAL ISSUES IN GENETIC TESTING

In the early years of medical genetics, the limited number of possible interventions meant that there were few areas raising ethical difficulties, even when serious disorders or high genetic risks were identified. How to convey bad news sensitively has always been an important aspect of medicine generally but is especially prominent in genetic counselling. It is often not appreciated though that considerably more people receiving genetic counselling are able to be given a low risk than a high one, many of whom were until then assuming that the risks for a future child would be high.

A new situation arose when prenatal diagnosis became feasible in the early 1970s, the 1967 UK Abortion Act having already made termination of pregnancy legal in limited circumstances. This raised difficult questions such as which disorders might justify termination, and whether professionals or patients should be the arbiters of this. As has frequently happened in medical genetics, time has allowed many of these dilemmas to resolve spontaneously, especially where therapy has proved effective. Thus, although prenatal diagnosis for phenylketonuria has been technically feasible for a long time, demand for prenatal diagnosis or pregnancy termination has been virtually nonexistent; in my own 30-year experience of involvement with a phenylketonuria clinic, I never encountered a request for this, in contrast to the more numerous disorders where the results of therapy are limited or nonexistent. In general, the more benign or treatable a disorder is, the lower is the proportion wishing for prenatal diagnosis, showing how unwise it is to make rigid laws on this, given the rapid rate of progress.

An even greater change occurred when DNA-based genetic tests allowed for the first time prediction for a wide range of inherited disorders where previously no testing of any kind had been possible. Huntington's disease (HD) has provided a paradigm for this new situation (Harper 1996), perhaps in part because it gives an extreme example, as a devastating brain disorder of adult life causing both physical and mental symptoms, with high genetic risks to relatives and until now no effective therapy. This combination of problems forced itself early into the awareness of those involved in research on the disorder, mainly geneticists and neurologists, and it is fortunate that this international community had already allied itself closely with lay groups providing support and promoting research on the disease, by the time that genetic prediction for the condition became possible in the mid 1980s.

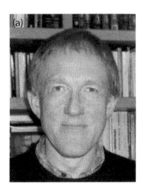
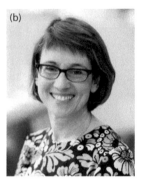
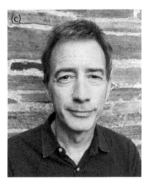

Figure 7.1 Some UK clinical geneticists who have made major contributions to ethical aspects of genetics in medicine. **(a)** Angus J Clarke (born 1954). Recorded interview [96] 10/10/2013. Angus Clarke was one of the first clinical geneticists to recognise the major ethical consequences of molecular genetic testing, especially in relation to prediction of disease in late onset disorders. His close links and training in the social sciences, along with his incisive books and other writing, have been largely responsible for the productive and sustained collaborative studies in this area. **(b)** Anneke Lucassen, member of Nuffield Council on Bioethics and developer, with Michael Parker, of clinical ethics committees. (Courtesy of Anneke Lucassen and University of Southampton.) **(c)** Michael Parker (born 1958) was responsible for founding the Oxford Centre for Clinical Ethics, and for developing the concept of 'clinical ethics committees'. (Courtesy of Michael Parker and Ethox Centre, Oxford.)

A whole series of ethical dilemmas immediately arose from this advance and, again fortunately, the international HD community, with UK workers in the forefront, decided to pool its experience in identifying both practical and ethical problems by documenting and analysing them fully, even though they might not always be able to avoid them. Since in the UK medical geneticists were the principal people who actually delivered presymptomatic testing for HD to those at risk who requested it, this was a further step in making workers in this field ethically aware, and correspondingly to become leaders in ensuring that those in other specialties became equally aware of these and comparable ethical issues in their own fields of practice (Figure 7.1).

A considerable number of practical ethical problems arose in the initial years of HD presymptomatic testing, and a remarkably large proportion of these proved to be avoidable or soluble, *provided that they had been thought about beforehand.* The first of these was that most people at risk, after careful thought and discussion, proved *not* to want to be tested, the proportion of around 20% actually having testing being much less than earlier surveys before prediction was possible had suggested, and showing the importance of avoiding inadvertent or 'lab only' testing. The pattern of genetic counselling that evolved for HD also emphasised the need for an interval between first discussion of the topic and undergoing the test, to allow reflection and the possibility of changing an initial decision. The pooled data also showed that suicide or other serious harmful effects were rare, largely allaying the fears of many professionals, some of whom had previously even suggested that testing should not be allowed because of the risk of harmful effects.

Completely new issues also arose, notably those surrounding the presymptomatic testing of children for late-onset disorders, which had barely crossed the minds of most workers in medical genetics, or other medical specialties, until they were confronted by requests for it in relation to HD (Harper and Clarke 1990).

Genetic testing for late-onset disorders in childhood has proved a particularly important and informative area where ethical issues could only be satisfactorily worked through in the context of real-life examples. When the issue first arose in the context of HD, it took medical geneticists and others by surprise, as mentioned, and soon proved more complex than it had first appeared. In particular, two different scenarios, the testing of young children unable to give consent, and testing of adolescents themselves requesting this, raised very different issues, which initially were often confused. Large studies in the UK and Netherlands showed that where professionals and families disagreed, careful discussion could resolve the situation in almost all cases (see Harper and Clarke 1990 for full references on these studies).

A further unforeseen issue was the testing of those at 25% risk for HD, where an abnormal result would inevitably also affect the intervening currently healthy but at-risk parent of the person tested, who had not requested this for themselves and might even be unaware of their own risk. It is of interest, and highly relevant to guidelines for best practice that, as with childhood testing, extensive studies showed that these difficult situations could almost always be resolved by careful discussion prior to testing.

As a result of these studies of ethical issues, based on hundreds of actual case situations, it became possible to draw up a series of clear guidelines for good practice in relation to predictive genetic testing, without the need for any specific law on the topic. The UK was again particularly suitable for this, since essentially all testing was done by laboratories and medical geneticists working through the NHS, with negligible involvement of the private sector. These guidelines for good practice proved especially important internationally, since in some countries professionals were initially largely unaware of the problems.

Within a few years of the development of predictive genetic testing for HD, this also became possible for a range of other late-onset genetic disorders; workers involved with these soon realised that the issues identified and analysed for HD were not unique for it but also applied to these other conditions, especially inherited neurological disorders, but also familial types of cancer. While there were significant differences, notably those relating to the possible availability and effectiveness of therapy, it became clear that most of the ethical problems were general ones, having been identified for HD first because they showed themselves here in especially clear-cut form.

Until this point it is probably fair to say that most of the medical geneticists and others involved with genetic testing had given little or no thought to formal ethical principles; most indeed may not have known that such principles existed, yet this had not stopped them from using them, pragmatically but effectively, in practice, especially in genetic counselling, as described in the previous chapter. Now, however, a valuable two-way collaboration began to develop, as an increasing number of philosophers, ethicists and others in the humanities and social sciences began to become aware of the important ethical problems in medical genetics that were actually arising in practice, not just as theoretical concepts. The Nuffield Council on Bioethics and the Human Genetics Commission (HGC; see below) proved to be two bodies that were especially important in bringing the different disciplines together.

The broad principles that genetic testing issues have helped to illustrate include *confidentiality* (is there a right or duty of professionals to share information that may have implications for other family members? Do employers or insurers have a right to know genetic test results?) and *ability to consent* (testing of young children and those who are mentally incapacitated), which is also a general principle; so is the relationship between research and service (is there a duty to give back research results to participants?).

Most of these workers in the humanities (see Figure 7.2) had previously been just as unaware of medical genetics as geneticists had been of them, but once the connection had been made, particularly at the level of individual collaborative groups, it became clear that both areas had much to offer each other. This was

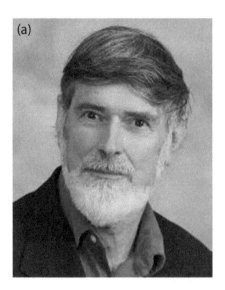
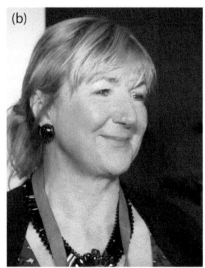

Figure 7.2 Workers from the social sciences and humanities making important early contributions to ethical aspects of medical genetics. Theresa Marteau (London) has been pictured in Chapter 5. **(a)** Martin Richards (born 1940). Director, Centre for Family studies, Cambridge. (Photo courtesy of Martin Richards.) **(b)** Ruth Chadwick (Lancaster/Cardiff). Philosopher and director of the Cardiff/Lancaster ESRC Centre.

encouraged by the possibility of funding for work in the field, thanks largely to European Union and American human genome project initiatives, but also by the UK research councils and Wellcome Trust. The ethical and social aspects of genetics were also brought to the attention of the wider public by the reports and other activities of specific organisations, as described below.

These cross-disciplinary links have required a readiness to adjust to very different academic traditions and cultures. The humanities and social sciences as academic disciplines previously had little connection with genetics, and virtually no awareness of medical genetics; their meetings and societies had little common ground or shared membership with geneticists, while even their reading and publishing was (and still is) largely separate, the humanities relying mainly on books and book chapters, while scientists and medical workers, including geneticists, have used the peer-reviewed journal as the main channel for disseminating their results. Collaboration, an essential feature throughout genetics, was much less prominent as a tradition in the humanities.

Indeed there is still a tendency for some social scientists (and their funding bodies) to regard medical geneticists simply as 'providers of material' rather than as true collaborators. Thus the various bodies and committees mentioned below, along with their counterparts in other countries, proved to be among the few forums where the disciplines could meet and learn from each other. Historians have been one of the slowest groups to become aware of the importance of genetics in medicine for their own field, but this has fortunately begun to change rapidly during the past few years, as described in Appendix 2 of this book.

ETHICAL ISSUES IN RESEARCH

Most of the ethical issues raised so far have related to the practice of medical genetics, in particular genetic testing, but the Declaration of Helsinki and similar developments were concerned primarily with the conduct of research. Not surprisingly, genetics research has given rise to a number of problems too, not unique to the field but often more conspicuous than in other areas of biomedical research. Indeed there are some areas of genetics research that by their very nature raise ethical problems.

A notable example is research on the genetic basis of psychiatric illness and on behavioural disorders and characteristics, such as intelligence (see Chapter 4). It seems self-evident that any work in this important but highly sensitive area is bound to raise major ethical concerns which need to be addressed before the work is carried out. The chequered history of early work in the field (see Chapter 1) makes this all the more imperative, yet some workers, mostly outside Britain, have gone ahead with studies that are inherently almost impossible to make free from bias and other confounding variables, and which will inevitably be interpreted by many people as more conclusive than they really are.

A further problem of a general nature is what, if any, of the results of a research study should or should not be fed back to participants. In the United States it appears that there are legal constraints that make this almost mandatory, which seems a flawed policy, fortunately not applying to Britain or most other countries. Since research results are by definition provisional until confirmed (which they frequently are not), it seems most unwise to give detailed results to individuals such as those having genetic tests as part of research, unless this has been clearly justified in advance. Not only may a supposed abnormality turn out to be a harmless variant in the light of further work, but a research laboratory may lack the strict quality standards required for being an accredited service provider. Furthermore, it may not be clear which participants in the research do or do not wish to receive their results, or if they are fully aware of their nature and potential consequences.

It may seem obvious that these aspects should be made clear when the research is designed, not at a late stage, yet this has sadly not always been the case. I remember an example of such lack of clarity arising during a somewhat belated consultation session on the proposed UK Biobank sample collection, when one of the principal investigators seemed quite uncertain whether or not specific research results would be fed back to participants. After somewhat reluctantly agreeing that they should not, he added, 'unless of course they showed something really important'(!).

Since then a report on genetic testing for late onset disorders from the UK Advisory Committee on Genetic Testing (2003) started a wider debate on this topic, which has resulted in greatly increased awareness and clarity, and may have avoided a considerable amount of harm from otherwise valuable genetic projects. Since the ethical issues for whole genome testing are essentially the same, it is to be hoped that those undertaking genomic projects will learn from the now extensive experience with those based on testing of single genes.

Of course, the boundaries between research and service are not always clear-cut and, for rare disorders especially, service-related testing may initially be delivered by research laboratories, but the issues mentioned above need careful consideration before this is embarked on.

PATENTING AND GENETIC TESTS

This provides an important practical example of ethical issues colliding with commercial interests and not only illustrates the importance of the NHS in ensuring that research advances can be translated into patient services without hindrance, but also the value of concerted international action to uphold this. The long tradition in genetics of mutual cooperation and exchange of knowledge and resources had ensured that molecular testing resulting from the isolation of the genes for numerous rare disorders was made freely available worldwide, so when American proposals to severely restrict use of the breast cancer susceptibility (BRCA) genes were applied to Europe also, there was an immediate reaction on both ethical and medical care grounds, coordinated by Gert Matthijs in Leuven and strongly supported by UK research institutes and lay organisations as well as medical geneticists generally.

The role of the Institute of Cancer Research, London, in making the use of genetic tests available across Europe is mentioned further in Chapter 11 and was an important part of the invalidating of broad gene-related patents. This outcome, belatedly followed by the United States Supreme Court, has ensured that patenting restrictions have not played a significant role in genetic test delivery in Britain, an outcome that might have been very different had it been in the hands of commercial organisations, as in the United States.

FORMAL BODIES CONCERNED WITH ETHICS AND GENETICS

The Nuffield Council on Bioethics

Many countries now have an official or semi-official body that advises their government on important ethical issues arising from medical advances or developments in biological research, but when this was initially suggested for Britain it was firmly turned down by the government of the day.

Eventually a compromise was reached by which an independent bioethics body was funded by the charity Nuffield Foundation, with contributions from Medical Research Council and Department of Health. The resulting Nuffield Council on Bioethics, established in 1991 (nuffieldbioethics.org), thus began life with a high degree of independence, free from government restrictions and influence, and able to choose for itself which topics should be investigated. It could also choose its own members, who were appointed for their own specific expertise rather than to represent a particular interest, a contrast with, for example, France, which has a large and somewhat unwieldy National Ethics Council (www.ccne-ethique.fr).

The subject for its first report was 'genetic screening' (Nuffield Council on Bioethics 1993) and it is not surprising that various genetic topics have formed a considerable proportion of the more than 30 reports produced over the past 25 years; some of those most relevant to genetics are listed in Table 7.1. These

Table 7.1 The Nuffield Council on Bioethics: Reports on topics relevant to genetics and medicine

Date	Topic
1993	Genetic screening: ethical aspects
1998	Mental disorders and genetics
2000	Stem cell therapy
2002	Patenting DNA
2002	Genetics and behaviour
2003	Pharmacogenetics
2006	Genetic screening (update)
2012	New techniques for the prevention of mitochondrial DNA disorders
2016	Genome editing
2017	Noninvasive prenatal genetic testing
2018	Genome editing and human reproduction: social and ethical issues

reports have had a wide readership and influence, especially internationally, while in Britain they have highlighted major issues that might have become contentious and divisive had they not been thoroughly and objectively explored and debated at an early stage by the Nuffield Council working groups.

One reason for the value of the Council's work has been the high calibre of those involved, including the support staff, and also the interdisciplinary links involving both the humanities and the sciences. Despite the reluctance of central government to be directly involved, it has mostly acted on, or at least not disowned, the reports' various recommendations, even though they carry no legal standing. It is high time for a full history to be written of this important body and for the key people involved to be interviewed while still living.

The Human Genetics Commission

While many of the Nuffield Council reports addressed genetic topics, the first official UK body with a remit to focus specifically on ethical, social and regulatory aspects of human genetics was the Human Genetics Commission, established in 1999. It had been recommended by the government's cross-party Science and Technology Committee in 1995 (UK House of Commons Science and Technology Committee, 1995), but was initially rejected, the government instead creating the more narrowly based Advisory Committee on Genetic Testing, which produced valuable reports on 'Genetic Testing for Late Onset Disorders' (2003) and on 'over-the-counter' genetic testing, but wider genetic issues were outside its remit. Not satisfied with this, the Science and Technology Committee again recommended a broader based body, and the Human Genetics Commission started its work in 1999 under the chairmanship of the redoubtable and highly influential human rights lawyer Helena Kennedy (Figure 7.3). Reports from the Commission and from the Advisory Committee on Genetic Testing (ACGT) can be found on the HGC archived website (see references).

Specific topics addressed included a further report on commercial 'direct to consumer' genetic tests (2003, updated 2010) and examination of the newly established forensic DNA database (2009); as with the Nuffield Council reports, wide-ranging and expert membership resulted in considerable and widespread influence. The Commission also held regular meetings, open to the public, in different parts of Britain, and was frequently critical of existing government policies (or lack of them). Importantly, it opened up to wider scrutiny areas where major ethical issues had never been considered; for example the then National Forensic Science Service (since privatised) proved, when visited by the Commission, to have no mechanisms to take into account ethical aspects of either its research or the National DNA Database for which it was responsible, despite the controversial nature of much of this work; after the visit, these were introduced.

Possibly as a result of its forthright and independent approach, the Human Genetics Commission was abolished in 2010, but its 12 years of active work have helped greatly to ensure that new genetic developments and applications receive detailed public and professional scrutiny and are not hidden under either commercial or governmental secrecy. Its work, and that of the Nuffield Council on

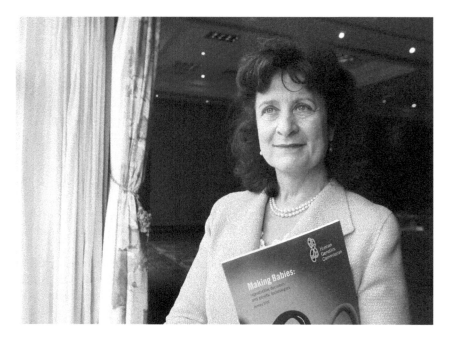

Figure 7.3 Helena Kennedy, Chair of the Human Genetics Commission 1999–2015. (Getty Images.)

Bioethics, also emphasise the value and effectiveness of these bodies in identifying likely future problems and defining codes of good practice before rather than after unwise or harmful applications have already occurred or become widespread, something that has helped to maintain trust between professionals and the public in a rapidly changing and inevitably controversial field, and a providing a striking contrast to the situations arising for genetically manipulated foods, or the debacle over the bovine spongiform encephalitis (BSE) epidemic.

One way in which the UK differs markedly from some other countries, most notably France and Germany, is in its reluctance to pass laws related to difficult ethical issues, including most of those mentioned above in relation to genetics. It does not seem that this lack of legal framework in the UK has actually hindered the development of good practice, or that abuses have occurred as a result; laws may in fact create problems through their imperfect drafting and are difficult to change once passed. This is especially relevant in the field of genetics, where developments have been so rapid, and where problems can often be avoided by ensuring that professional guidelines are carefully followed, as in the examples described above for Huntington's disease.

GENETIC TESTING AND INSURANCE

This has proved to be a particularly contentious issue, and one not entirely resolved yet. In the UK arguments have revolved mainly around life insurance rather than, as in the US, health insurance, though that could change if commercial health companies were to replace the work of the NHS. The possible use of genetic tests in altering disease risk for inherited conditions was first raised many years ago, in the 1930s, by RA Fisher and others (see Chapter 1), but it was only half a century later that it became a reality with the analysis of DNA. Widespread concern was raised by the possibility that healthy individuals might be obliged to disclose the results of their predictive genetic tests and be penalised by this, even though testing might relate to illness many years ahead and might bring them real health benefits through early therapy, as has already been seen with a number of the familial cancers.

The life insurance industry initially stuck to the mantra of genetic test results being 'no different from other medical information', ignoring the fact that it was healthy individuals under consideration and that they already had access to details of family history, so that any losses through 'adverse selection' were likely to be minimal (Harper 1997). When detailed actuarial studies confirmed this (MacDonald 1997), the insurers eventually conceded that they would not be disadvantaged by having no access to genetic data, apart from policies involving extremely large sums, leaving an uneasy stand-off that could well rear its head in future, particularly in the context of widespread whole genome screening. Yet again it was British medical geneticists who were in the forefront of this debate and caused the issue to be raised across Europe.

LAY SOCIETIES FOR GENETIC DISORDERS

Many genetic disorders now have a specific lay society which affected families can turn to, whether for social and medical support or for promotion of research. This is a major change from 50 years ago, when few existed and those that did were mostly broad, generic 'children's charities' or small, often fragmented support groups. It is not only their number that has increased greatly, but their remit and complexity. Also they increasingly work as partners with professionals such as medical geneticists and give independent advice to government policy makers. Here I look briefly at some of the main UK lay societies and charities that have been prominently involved in genetics over the past half century, but it is a topic that deserves a thorough historical study.

Starting with the oldest and largest, Britain has lacked the long tradition of philanthropy on a large scale that has underpinned much American medical research; a good example of this is the March of Dimes, begun as the National Foundation for Infantile Paralysis, with the target of eliminating poliomyelitis, and largely transferred to the field of birth defects and genetics when the original target had been achieved. Some major American charities directly benefited Britain from an early stage; thus the Rockefeller Foundation, under its scientific director Warren Weaver, contributed to early genetics research in the UK and across Europe, largely because of the possibilities offered by the stability of health systems and populations by comparison with the US.

In the UK itself the pre-eminent large charitable body involved in medical research has been the Wellcome Trust, whose massive income, derived originally from the pharmaceutical firm Burroughs Wellcome, now allows it to function as essentially a second but more flexible Medical Research Council. While its remit is not specific to genetics, this has been a high priority in recent decades, including its major contribution to the Human Genome Project (Chapter 12) and to subsequent programmes at the Wellcome-funded Sanger Institute, as well as its Oxford Centre for Human Genetics. A comparable broad genetics focus has also developed for the major cancer research charities.

The remarkable early achievement of the UK Spastics Society (now Scope) in funding not only Paul Polani's genetics research but an entire institute for this has already been mentioned (Chapter 2). It is an outstanding example of how the independent sector, with a scientific committee led by a few exceptionally far sighted individuals, and free from bureaucratic controls, can mobilise a large sum of money for a long-term goal. With a wise and energetic director like Polani, this high-risk strategy paid off handsomely, especially since Polani deliberately put some of the funding towards service application, thus attracting NHS investment, as described in Chapter 8. Another broadly based 'children's charity', Action Research for the Crippled Child, also had a major early focus on genetic topics.

Turning to more disease-specific charities, these inevitably have a difficult balancing act between funding research and providing services for affected patients, especially as successive governments have increasingly attempted to shift their responsibility for these services towards charities. The balance has naturally tended to vary over the years, but examples where UK lay society funding for research has made major research contributions include the Cystic Fibrosis Trust (https://www.cysticfibrosis.org.uk), Muscular Dystrophy UK (https://www.musculardystrophy.org) and Tuberous Sclerosis Association (www.tuberous-sclerosis.org). In return, many workers in medical genetics, basic scientists as well as clinical geneticists, have contributed much time and expert advice to these societies and their members.

Most lay societies for genetic disorders are small, often very small; indeed, one of the strong motivations leading to their formation has been the isolation of affected families and the feeling that nothing is being done to help their particular problem. The greatest contribution of these many societies has been to end this isolation and to provide practical support based on the problems faced by their members, though promoting research and especially the contribution of key samples and family data have often been highly effective activities too. Development of the internet and of social media has facilitated this process. Links with medical geneticists have been extremely fruitful, with laboratory workers benefiting not only from access to samples but often becoming highly motivated as a result of actually meeting affected patients and seeing their problems at first hand. From my personal experience of working on conditions such as Huntington's disease and myotonic dystrophy I have seen the value of these links, which in these instances have resulted in the evolution of a mixed community of clinicians, basic laboratory workers and families, with strong long-term bonds.

Many small lay societies and support groups are originally founded by one or a few highly motivated people, often patients or parents, and usually with

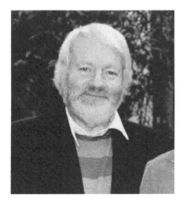

Figure 7.4 Alastair Kent, leader of Genetics Alliance UK and its predecessor Genetic Interest Group (GIG) from 1993 to 2017. (Courtesy of Alastair Kent and Genetic Alliance UK.)

strong personalities. As the societies grow and the founders age, problems of succession can prove difficult, as can confusion due to multiple opinions. An important strand in development of the field has thus been the formation of 'umbrella groups' or alliances bringing together numerous small individual societies so that they can have greater numbers and influence than would be possible on their own. In the UK the organisation Genetic Interest Group, now Genetic Alliance UK [https://www.geneticalliance.org.uk], founded in 1988 as a group of 12 societies and now representing over 180, has been extremely effective in achieving this, being led for most of this time by Alastair Kent (Figure 7.4); again it is time that a full history of this is written and key players interviewed while they are still alive.

GENETICS, MEDICINE AND THE LAW

Apart from DNA fingerprinting and the vexed question of the national DNA database, discussed in Chapter 10, the law has had until now surprisingly little interaction either with medical genetics or with wider aspects of genetics in medicine in the UK. I say 'surprisingly' because as a field of both medical practice and research dealing regularly with sensitive and at times controversial aspects of life, with numerous new applications appearing over the years, one might have been expecting much more legal involvement. At a personal level, over a period of more than 40 years in the practice of medical genetics, I have only set foot once in a court of law, and that was as a witness on behalf of a colleague in another centre.

This represents a considerable difference from the USA (Milunsky 1976), which seems to be more litigious generally (possibly due to an overabundance of lawyers); but also from France, where many controversial areas have been enshrined in law, as mentioned in relation to its National Ethical Committee. In the UK (in this respect Scotland is no different apart from tighter restrictions on use of the DNA database) there are fewer laws to be broken, giving less scope for legal action. Having said that, however, I think that there are some real differences between medical genetics practice and that of most other UK medical specialties in relation to the law, some of which reach a long way back into history.

The first of these is the long-standing association of medical genetics with risk estimation and the fact that medical geneticists have always been comfortable with handling uncertainty in a quantitative manner (see Chapter 6). It has been rare for patients or relatives receiving genetic counselling to be given an impression of certainty, even at the present time when accurate genetic tests are often available. Terms such as 'impossible' are avoided when discussing recurrence, and given a background level of around 2% for anyone having a child with a significant birth defect, this is clearly wise. By contrast, many other specialties are reluctant to admit uncertainty in their practice, even when it is obvious that it exists, leaving them open to legal action when the inevitable rare adverse event eventually happens.

A second reason why legal problems are infrequently encountered in medical genetics is undoubtedly the standard practice of giving those seen a written letter setting down what has been discussed, again a contrast with other specialties. Such letters are a valuable permanent record for families following genetic counselling, as discussed in Chapter 6, and avoid the problem of any subsequent debate over what was or was not said. A final reason, perhaps most important of all, is the adequate time given in a consultation for listening to those seen and ensuring that their questions are fully answered.

When genetic tests and related laboratory issues are considered, a key factor is their interpretation by medical genetics professionals who are aware of the limitations of the tests and of their context. This may well become a bigger issue with increased whole genome testing and especially the screening of those not at high risk. Most legal problems that do arise at present are no different from those occurring in other fields of laboratory medicine, such as sample mix-up or mislabelling, which can be minimised by rigorous quality control (see Chapter 10) and by the use of accredited laboratories.

CONCLUSION

Overall, considering the general sensitivity of the field and the numerous specific pitfalls encountered on a day-to-day basis in the practice of medical genetics, I feel (even though inevitably biased) that it is fair to say that those involved in UK medical genetics have done a creditable job in recognising the numerous ethical issues involved and in avoiding most of the pitfalls. They have also done a service to colleagues in other specialties, and for medical genetics internationally, by analysing these problems rigorously, and by pointing out that most of them are not unique to genetics but can arise in many other areas of medicine. Thus the lessons learned, often from hard experience, by medical geneticists, are now being incorporated, with the help of others, into the general fabric of medical ethics. This process will need to be continued and increased into the future, as genetics becomes increasingly part of the practice of medicine overall.

REFERENCES

Advisory Committee on Genetic Testing. 2003. *Report: Genetic Testing for Late onset disorders.*

Comité Consultatif National d'Ethique pour les Sciences de la Vie et de la Santé (CCNE). (www.ccne-ethique.fr)

Genetic Alliance UK. https://www.geneticalliance.org.uk

Harper PS. 1996. *Huntington's Disease*, 2nd edn. Oxford: Oxford University Press.

Harper PS. 1997. Genetic testing, life insurance, and adverse selection. *Philos Trans R Soc Lond B Biol Sci.* 352(1357):1063–1066.

Harper PS, Clarke AJ. 1990. Should we test children for 'adult' genetic diseases? *Lancet.* 335(8699):1205–1206.

Human Genetics Commission. webarchive.nationalarchives.gov.uk/

Human Genetics Commission. 2009. Nothing to hide, nothing to fear? Balancing individual rights and the public interest in the governance and use of the National DNA Database. London: Department of Health.

Human Genetics Commission. 2010. A common framework of principles for direct-to-consumer genetic testing services. London: Department of Health.

MacDonald AS. 1997. How will improved forecasts of individual lifetimes affect underwriting? *Philos Trans Roy Soc B.* 352:1067–1075.

Milunsky A. 1976. *Genetics and the Law.* New York: Springer.

Nuffield Council on Bioethics (nuffieldbioethics.org).

Nuffield Council on Bioethics. 1993. *Genetic Screening: Ethical Issues.* London: Nuffield Council on Bioethics. (Supplement published 2006.)

Penrose LS. 1967. Presidential address: The influence of the English tradition in human genetics. In: Crow JF, Neel JV (eds.). *Proceedings of the Third International Congress of Human Genetics.* Baltimore: The Johns Hopkins University Press; pp. 13–25.

UK House of Commons Science and Technology report. 1995. *Human Genetics: The Science and the Consequences.* London: HMSO.

World Medical Association. 1964. WMA Declaration of Helsinki - Ethical Principles for Medical Research Involving Human Subjects.

8

Making an impact on health: Medical genetics and the UK National Health Service

ABSTRACT

Medical genetics in Britain began at around the same time as the UK National Health Service (NHS) and remains an integral part of it, something that has been valuable in allowing equitable development across the country and avoiding duplication or developments of doubtful value. The first post-war medical geneticists were university funded, but NHS posts, both laboratory and clinical, progressively became the majority as academic funding declined. Governance and training in the field were largely the responsibility of the Royal Colleges and specialist societies, who worked together flexibly and efficiently and oversaw the steady growth of the network of regional centres. While this model has worked well for specialist hospital-based services, the development of medical genetics in primary care and in public health medicine has been slower. Recent years have seen increasing and at times unwise politicisation of both service and policy developments, notably those related to genomic medicine, while devolution of health care for Scotland and Wales has also resulted in unevenness of developments, raising major issues for the future of the field.

The UK National Health Service (NHS) was established in 1948, now over 70 years ago, and has remained the main provider of medical services to the entire country since that time, despite recurring financial problems, reorganisations (mostly misguided or fruitless) and political attempts to replace or even abolish it. Although in some areas of medicine private or insurance-based services have grown up alongside it, they have until now had little direct effect on the development of medical genetics services, so that these, both clinical and laboratory based, have been almost entirely provided under the NHS since the beginning of the specialty, if one takes the 1946 initiation of the first genetic counselling clinic at Great Ormond Street Hospital, London, as the starting point.

This is a truly remarkable achievement, considering that the field of medical genetics was initially nonexistent in terms of a service when the NHS was launched, was completely unfamiliar to clinicians generally, and still had the legacies of eugenics, and later a perceived association with abortion, to contend with in terms of public and political perception. It is worth looking more closely at how this could have and did come about.

There are more general lessons to be learned too from this transition of genetics in medicine from research to medical service, which can be applied to other areas of science, and which deserve the attention of historians in the form of detailed studies. So far very few have been made, the work of William Leeming (2004) on genetic services in Manchester and in Canada being the most significant.

Earlier chapters have shown how the initial post-war advances in human and medical genetics were mainly research orientated; this was in part because there were few soundly based applications that were feasible, as Penrose had emphasised in his presidential lecture to the Third International Human Genetics Congress in 1966, with the previous disastrous abuses of eugenics very much in mind. I quoted this in Chapter 7 (page 168) and it can be regarded as the touchstone for modern medical genetics.

Penrose's emphasis on strengthening scientific foundations and respect for variation was indeed a wise one, quite apart from any question of eugenics, but already there was some demand for genetic counselling in relation to serious inherited disorders; John Fraser Roberts had set up the first UK genetic counselling clinic in 1946 (see Chapter 6), and the new medical genetics posts starting to be established around the country, mostly university-based, generally included a modest provision for this among their other activities. The advent of diagnostic chromosome analysis and the growing awareness, especially among paediatricians, that it might greatly modify genetic risks, sharply increased the need for skilled clinicians with a specialist knowledge of genetics and an aptitude for genetic counselling; hence a number of the first NHS consultants in medical genetics, in contrast to the original founders, often came from a paediatric background. Since these were usually based in existing medical teaching centres, often alongside university-based workers, this reinforced the developing pattern of regional medical genetics centres, with research and service, laboratory and clinical staff interacting closely. A further stimulus from the 1970s was the introduction of prenatal diagnosis, which required not only service cytogenetic laboratories but also genetic counselling, which most obstetricians were reluctant to devote sufficient time to.

Paul Polani's London unit, originally funded largely by medical charities and research grants, provides a good early example of how a transition from research to service might be managed, both for clinical and for laboratory services.

PSH: Can I ask, in terms of getting the NHS involved, because I mean that was a real achievement ..., that you seem to have got this very early involvement of the NHS, and not just in London but the whole of the South-east region. Was this something that happened easily or did you have really to put a lot of effort into getting that to happen?

PEP: I think the secret was the 'proof of the cake'. In this sense ..., that to do the clinical side, the application side, genetic counselling and any prenatal diagnostic things which were in the offing, because I mean it was something that was only just being considered, we had to demonstrate its usefulness, or at least its feasibility first of all and then its usefulness. And I argued therefore that, given that we had enough money from the Spastics Society, that we should invest a proportion of that money into the practical uses, and so we did and for two or three years, I forget now exactly how many, we ran a service, a genetic service with research money.... So that was a pump-priming operation, in a sense, which then, when it turned out to be useful, we convinced the Department of Health that here they could have something going and should contribute. So that was the first step.

Interview with Paul Polani 12/11/2003 [01]

John Hamerton, who had previously worked with Charles Ford at Harwell, joined Polani in 1960 and led the cytogenetics laboratory for the next decade, forming a vital part of the transition:

PSH: So coming back to Guy's, at what point did the cytogenetics work start becoming a diagnostic service as well as a research area?

JH: I would say in the late sixties. I think it was a diagnostic service for certain things that we were interested in for research right through; Down's syndrome, Turner's syndrome, Klinefelter's syndrome. We did quite a bit of work on chromosomes in one or two surveys of the mental retardation population, things like that, but certainly as an official NHS service it was much later, in fact it was towards the end of my time at Guy's. Like so many other things, the service was done, but as part of...

PSH: On the back of research.

JH: On the back of research, as it was here [Winnipeg, Canada] when I came here.

PSH: So it must have been a very, everybody I have spoken to says it was an exciting time, those first years of human cytogenetics.

JH: Oh fascinating. I mean you found something new every day virtually. You never knew when you were going to find something new.

Interview with John Hamerton 26/10/2004 [21]

Polani's key factor for success was, as he states above, that because he had already invested some of his research funds in service applications, he had been able to show their importance and effectiveness; when applying for NHS funding he thus already had evidence to give the NHS authorities. Having John Hamerton as an exceptionally able scientist colleague, involved in both cytogenetics research and services, was an equally essential part of the equation.

What Polani does not mention in the interview is that he had already taken the time and trouble to build good relationships with senior NHS managers, regarding them as key allies rather than 'the opposition'. A comparable building of links also proved fruitful in Manchester, and in Cardiff and Glasgow, where it was often easier than in London to identify a single key person in policy making as responsible. This is again a general topic relevant to other fields besides medical genetics, worthy of detailed study not only because it highlights the value of these links but also in showing how the more recent 'politicisation' and seemingly perpetual re-organisation of the NHS can so easily destroy them, as described later in this chapter.

Once it became clear that medical genetics was becoming an established clinical specialty, the important questions began to arise of how standards of clinical and laboratory practice should be established and maintained and, equally, how new recruits to the field should be attracted and trained. We have already seen that the initial generation of medical geneticists was a disparate group, with backgrounds in a range of clinical fields and their experience of genetics largely derived from research, rather than from clinical practice. This was fine if their function was to found and develop academic units, but not always satisfactory if they were to be responsible for clinical or laboratory services. Likewise, the founders of the field, with whom many of the first generations of practicing clinical geneticists (Table 8.1) had trained, were inspiring individuals but not themselves service orientated, and there were no formal training programmes at the time.

Yet most of the expansion of posts and funding during the 1970s and 1980s was service related, and while some of this was channelled through established university departments, most new posts were NHS based; there was a marked absence of the situation common across continental Europe, where clinical genetics services were often just an appendage of an academic institute. During most of these early and formative years, the NHS itself took a relatively 'hands off' approach to detailed management, leaving this mainly to professional bodies. Medical genetics was no exception, once it had been formally recognised as a distinct specialty. Hence the regulation of this new group of medical geneticists practicing in the NHS became largely the function of the 'Royal Colleges', which in turn linked closely with the relevant specialist societies.

TRAINING, GOVERNANCE AND REGULATION

The Royal College of Physicians

Taking clinical geneticists first, the Clinical Genetics Society (see Chapter 9) set up a committee to consider training in 1975, while the Royal College of

Table 8.1 British medical geneticists trained with the original UK founders of the field (italicised)

Cyril Clarke, Liverpool
David Price Evans
Peter Harper
Rodney Harris
Richard McConnell
Marcus Pembrey
Michael Pope
David Weatherall

Cedric Carter, Great Ormond Street Hospital, London
Michael Baraitser
Sarah Bundey
John Burn
Anne Child
Marcus Pembrey
Joan Slack

Paul Polani, Guy's Hospital, London
Caroline Berry
Marcus Pembrey

Lionel Penrose, Galton Laboratory, London
Eric Blank
George Fraser
Alan Johnston
Paul Polani

Physicians (RCP) London was also early and proactive in taking measures to ensure high standards, setting up its Clinical Genetics Committee in 1984, not long after medical genetics had been recognised as a full specialty in 1980. The first chairman was Rodney Harris (Manchester) with Alan Johnston (Aberdeen) as Secretary. This was in part because they were adult-trained physicians, closely involved in the general activities of the College. Harris in particular was very effective in understanding and utilising the sometimes arcane ways by which the RCP functioned and also in generating a valuable series of reports (see Table 8.2), which, emanating from the College itself, often proved influential in extracting new funds from sometimes reluctant regional health authorities. They also provided models for delivering genetic services in many other countries across Europe, even those where the structure and funding of healthcare generally might be different from that in the UK.

Initially no separate college of Paediatrics existed, but when it became clear that one would be formed (as late as 1996), the question would inevitably arise, which College should be responsible for medical genetics? By this time I had become the

Table 8.2 Some reports on medical genetics from the Royal College of Physicians

Prenatal diagnosis and genetic screening: community and service implications
Report of a working party (1989)

Teaching genetics to medical students: a survey and recommendations
Report of a working group of the Clinical Genetics Committee (1990)

Ethical issues in clinical genetics
A report of a joint working party of the College Committee on Ethical Issues
   in Medicine and the College Committee on Clinical Genetics (1991)

Clinical genetics services in 1990 and beyond
Report of the Clinical Genetics Committee (1991)

Purchasers' guidelines to genetic services in the NHS: an aid to assessing the
   genetic services required by the resident population of an average health
   district
Report of a working group of the Clinical Genetics Committee (1991)

The retention of medical records in relation to genetic diseases
A report of a working group of the Clinical Genetics Committee (1991)

RCP Clinical Genetics Committee Chair, so I suggested that an informal ballot be held of all UK clinical geneticists, the result of which was unanimous in preferring to remain with the Royal College of Physicians, this including those whose initial training had been mainly in Paediatrics. I think that this decision reflected the general concept held by UK clinical geneticists, that it was a specialty crossing all age groups, again a contrast with much of continental Europe and also with Australia, where the specialty was almost exclusively paediatric for many years. This independence of age was something that would greatly help its acceptance, as adult areas such as cancer genetics and neurogenetics grew progressively more important.

Incidentally, at the following meeting of the Clinical Genetics Committee, the then Secretary of the College, David Pyke, seemingly unaware of the ballot, announced that following an informal meeting he had had (over lunch) with a paediatric member, they had decided that the two colleges should jointly control the specialty, a suggestion that sank without trace after he learned of the ballot, but illustrating the persistence of the old 'wheeling and dealing' approach of the College of Physicians!

Clinical Consultant training programmes in medical genetics have been the responsibility of a separate training committee (initially a subcommittee of the paediatric committee) of the Royal Colleges as a whole; in practice the two committees worked closely and harmoniously together under the aegis of the Royal College of Physicians, giving a professionally led and forward looking leadership for the new specialty which had considerable influence internationally, as well as in the UK.

Thus, during the critical period from the mid 1970s through the 1990s, when medical genetics was beginning to develop rapidly and was becoming a distinct specialty, it had a comprehensive and relatively democratic system of governance involving the Royal Colleges and professional societies, that was able not only to ensure that workers in the field across Britain felt listened to and represented, but was able to provide carefully argued and realistic proposals that regional health authorities and the Department of Health centrally could seriously consider for funding.

The resulting structure of medical genetics services has proved both effective and durable, and has also been capable of incorporating the radical advances made possible by clinical molecular genetics and the introduction and development of non-medical genetic counsellors (see Chapter 6). It is worth noting, too, that in terms of professional structure it has been notably 'flat' in the sense that there have never been attempts for a single centre to become dominant over the others, as has been seen in France and in some smaller countries; nor for the service aspects to be regarded as subsidiary to a more important academic structure. Indeed, there has been a long tradition, among clinical geneticists in particular, for academic staff to play a considerable role in clinical services, while NHS medical genetics staff have had a correspondingly large and at times distinguished role in research. The geographical distribution has also become increasingly 'flat', with clinical genetics services dispersed relatively uniformly over individual districts, following the laudable aim of equity of access regardless of where one lives. (Equally sensible has been the aim of centralising laboratory genetics services within a region to maximise efficiency and quality.)

Needless to say, these admirable principles have not always worked out so well in practice. One reason for this was that the initial academic expansion of the field begun in the late 1950s came to an abrupt halt in the 1970s, just as the NHS developments were increasing. This meant that almost no purpose built and fully funded university departments of human or medical genetics were created after 1980, as noted in Chapter 3; junior academic posts at university lecturer level likewise almost disappeared, so that the lack of a clear academic career structure meant that promising young clinical research workers, who might later have led the field nationally and internationally, were mostly forced to take service-related NHS posts instead. Often they were initially single handed and overstretched; it is a credit to them how much they have achieved, but it is sad that even the most research minded of them have had to contend with little or no support, with perhaps the token award of a personal Chair (often NHS funded) late in their career as their only recognition. There can be no doubt that the lack of a substantial academic career structure has blunted the research contributions of many British medical geneticists.

Trainees and training posts

Until the late 1970s there was no organised system in the UK – nor for that matter elsewhere in Europe — for training in medical genetics as a specialty. The Galton Laboratory under Penrose had been the centre for gaining theoretical and research experience, attracting people from across Europe and from America, as well as from UK (see above and Chapter 2), but there was no organised training system at the Galton, though independent-minded people could and did find a wealth of talented workers in and around the centre to learn from. The MRC offered a series of training Fellowships, most of them attached to its own units, but again these were research orientated.

The first NHS-based clinical training posts (officially classified as 'senior registrars') were created in 1978 and, while few in number (initially three), were important in providing the start of a career structure in medical genetics. Based in Manchester, Cardiff and London, they attracted outstanding candidates and indeed the first generations of trainees as a whole (see Figure 8.1) produced a series of able leaders for the profession over the following decades. (I still find it difficult to accept that they in turn are now retiring or have already retired!) By 1998, 20 years on, the number of trainees had risen to over 50.

A thorough four-year training programme was drawn up by the Royal College of Physicians committees, those in the posts being expected to have already had a wide clinical experience and to have taken the College membership exam (MRCP). There was a rocky period initially during which it was not clear whether there would be any permanent NHS (consultant) posts for these individuals after completion of their training, but fortunately these were created just in time and a close balance has been maintained ever since, largely avoiding the sudden swings in demand and supply that have characterised some other specialties.

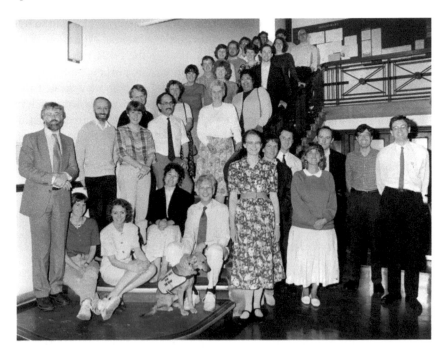

Figure 8.1 An early group of clinical genetics trainees (Circa 1991 in Cambridge) with Rodney Harris (Manchester) and John Yates (Glasgow and Cambridge). (Photo courtesy of Frances Flinter.)

As a further anecdote which may perhaps be relevant to other 'new' specialties, the areas considered necessary as part of a training programme in medical genetics were contributed to by numerous people with varied interests, with the inevitable result that it was soon realised that completing them all would take at least a decade of training! Fortunately this was recognised before deterring too many potential recruits, and was largely solved by replacing the term 'essential' by 'desirable' for many of the requirements in the job description.

LABORATORY GENETICS SERVICES AND THE NHS

Early laboratory research in human and medical genetics has been discussed in Chapter 2 and in more detail in the author's previous book, *First Years of Human Chromosomes* (Harper 2006), while more recent developments are covered in Chapters 10 and 11. During the period of the 1970s and 1980s laboratory as well as clinical genetics services were also rapidly expanding and evolving; these came largely under the care of the Royal College of Pathologists, founded in 1962, which also developed a genetics committee, linking especially with the laboratory-based professional societies (see Chapter 10), the Association of Clinical Cytogeneticists (ACC) and later the Clinical Molecular Genetics Society (CMGS). These merged in 2012 as the Association for Clinical Genetic (now Genomic) Science, and form one part of the 'umbrella' organisation, the British Society for Genetic Medicine (BSGM). It is not surprising that this proliferation of laboratory and clinical bodies began to cause confusion, so it was a welcome development when a merged Genetics Services Committee was formed in 1999 that allowed the various bodies, laboratory and clinical, to give unified advice to the NHS regions and the UK Health Department. (This has now been followed by a Joint Committee on Genomics in Medicine.)

One particular area in which the UK laboratory genetics services have played a leading role has been that of quality assessment and accreditation. Initially many local cytogenetics services had begun as research laboratories; this was even more the case for molecular genetics laboratories, which often mixed research with service applications and, at times, lacked the rigour required for providing a reliable service. The introduction of National External Quality Assessment Service (NEQAS) criteria, along with accreditation systems (now mostly mandatory for NHS laboratories), produced a consistently high quality across the UK and again provides an example of how this has influenced services over Europe as a whole when European quality assessment systems were developed under the auspices of the European Union and European Society of Human Genetics.

There was a downside to this separation of service labs from research though, in that the culture of innovation characterising research laboratories tended to be lost, especially in cytogenetics, with a few notable exceptions; indeed this is one of the reasons why molecular geneticists, remaining closer to their research origins, preferred to keep their identity distinct when forming their own Society.

The need for and value of genetics services seems generally to have been more appreciated by regional health authorities, which at that time had considerable independence over funding new developments, than by the Department of

Health centrally, which was for many years largely indifferent to genetics and where it was often not clear under whose responsibility the new field was. It is fortunate that some of the key early research leaders, notably Paul Polani and Cedric Carter in London and Malcolm Ferguson-Smith in Glasgow, were active in obtaining NHS funding to support not only their services but also in convincing their health authority colleagues that this was important across the country as a whole. In time, the support and leadership coming from the RCP, became a further powerful factor.

GENETICS AND PRIMARY CARE

General practice and related primary care activities are in many ways well placed to play a major role in delivering medical genetics services, especially in the NHS where everyone is registered with a specific GP and access is free of charge. It also has the potential to provide a continuity of care and an involvement with family groupings across the generations which helps in the detection of inherited disorders following mendelian inheritance. It should be remembered that George Huntington was a family doctor, and that the description of the disorder bearing his name resulted from the combined observations of himself, his father and his grandfather in the same practice on Long Island, New York State (Harper, 1991).

A small but enthusiastic number of GPs, including Hilary Harris (Manchester) and Nadeem Qureshi (Nottingham), have indeed made systematic efforts to identify patients in their practice populations with serious genetic disorders and to develop systems that can be followed by their colleagues, but there have been major hindrances to this becoming generalised. Foremost among these is that GPs are already overloaded with many other duties, some valuable but others more administrative, often producing a stressed situation where there is little time or energy left to give thought to genetic services outside the context of a particular family. Despite repeated government exhortations that medical genetics should move more into primary care, the overwhelming majority of practitioners continue to see it as a specialist service, generally one that they are happy with, but one to refer to rather than be closely involved with providing themselves. Likewise, few of the genetic counsellors graduating from the MSc programmes described in Chapter 6 have so far associated themselves with primary care.

Not surprisingly, most of the referrals from GPs to genetics services are related to relatively rare mendelian or chromosomal disorders, rather than to common conditions, where there has mostly been little obvious benefit or demand for genetic counselling until now. Occasional flurries of demand from patients result from media publicity or genetic disorders among celebrities (e.g.: genetically determined cancers) but in general the most productive approach from primary care has come from an alertness to familial disease and willingness to refer to specialist genetic services. It is difficult to see this pattern changing much unless specific funds are injected to allow a more active and systematic approach.

GENETICS AND PUBLIC HEALTH

Public health medicine has had a difficult time over the past 30 years in defining what its overall role should be, having changed from being responsible for classical population-based fields of disease prevention such as infectious diseases, clean water and smoking prevention to controlling the commissioning and funding of services, including medical genetics, at a district and regional level. This uncertainty of roles and the associated reorganisation of boundaries and posts has meant that genetics has not generally been high in the priorities of those working in the public health field. In general, those working at the 'regional' level, dealing with populations commonly of 3,000 000–5,000 000, a comparable level to many medical genetics services, have been most appreciative of their value. But in the successive reorganisations this 'regional' tier of organisation has often been downgraded or abolished, with policy and funding decisions becoming made at a more local level, where those involved are more concerned with local acute and short-term aspects.

Apart from these organisational issues, there are other reasons why public health medicine and medical genetics have not developed a closer and more constructive relationship. First has been the lingering legacy of eugenics, with both medical geneticists and public health medicine staff uneasy lest this raise its head again in the guise of genetic prevention, especially in relation to prenatal screening programmes. Added to this is the concern that, while usually not stated explicitly, at least in the UK, genetic advances may be viewed through the lens of 'cost effectiveness' at a population level rather than of their benefit to individuals themselves.

A further problem is that any teaching or training in genetics for those entering public health medicine has been minimal or absent, despite their longstanding shared basis in statistics and epidemiology; I remember being asked by one professor of epidemiology and public health running a two-year MSc course on the subject, whether a single one-hour lecture would be sufficient to cover genetics! From this ignorance of genetics has grown a widespread view (though there are a few exceptions) that 'proper epidemiology' is concerned solely with the environmental factors in disease, not the genetic aspects too, 'genetic epidemiology' (or epidemiological genetics) being considered as something entirely separate. I have likened this to astronomers thinking that because the 'dark' side of the moon has not been visible until recently, it could safely be ignored, or even considered not to exist. Such an attitude might have been defensible until it actually became visible, as increasingly have the genetic aspects of disease. By contrast, geneticists have from the earliest years always considered the genetic and environmental aspects of disease, particularly for common disorders, to be complementary and balanced, rather than opposed or mutually exclusive.

A final factor to be considered is that public health physicians are generally attuned to preventive measures where large numbers of people (often entire populations) are involved, giving only small changes of risk at the individual level. By contrast, most work, and the greatest advances in medical genetics until now, have begun at the level of the individual or individual family, only spreading later, and in selected instances, to the population level.

This difference in perspective, where neither side is necessarily 'right' or 'wrong', may in part explain the slow development of preventive services for the condition familial hypercholesterolaemia (FH), already mentioned in Chapter 4. UK workers in public health medicine and primary care had rightly become sceptical of the value of serum cholesterol as a population measure for preventing coronary heart disease,; but they had ignored the very real value of detecting those with the highest levels due to the mendelian and treatable FH, where the great majority of affected individuals remained unrecognised, and where 'cascade screening' of families, working outward from the initial affected proband, could detect family members at risk without the need for whole-population screening with its attendant false positives and other drawbacks. After the slow start, this approach, mainly led by medical geneticists working closely with clinical biochemists and lipid specialists, now provides a good example of how medical genetics services, generally starting from small numbers of people where a major risk alteration can be achieved, can complement the public health approach which involves large numbers with individually small risk changes. A comparable situation has also developed with the recognition of mendelian subsets involving a small proportion (often 5%–10%) of common cancers.

The creation of a unit for Public Health Genetics in Cambridge, in 1997 under an enthusiastic director, Ronald Zimmern (Figure 8.2) (succeeded by Hilary Burton up to 2017), developed, after some initial reticence, strong links with medical geneticists, and indeed with most clinical specialties – Public health medicine itself proved the most difficult to convince, older entrenched attitudes remaining

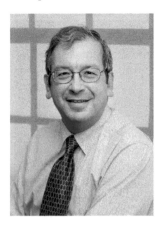

Figure 8.2 Ronald Zimmern, first Director of the Public Health Genetics Unit, Cambridge. (Courtesy of Ronald Zimmern.)

strong until recently; the small numbers of those in the field with an active appreciation of genetics have received little encouragement from most of their colleagues and it remains to be seen to what extent this will change with the new developments occurring in genomic medicine.

The unit itself, now rebranded as the Public Health Genomics (PHG) Foundation, and classified as a charity affiliated to Cambridge University, has a 'timeline' on its website (www.phgfoundation. org) that gives some useful landmarks. It also lists some valuable and at times critical reports, notably on 'Genomics in mainstream clinical pathways' (2018), which emphasises the key role of clinical assessment and medical genetics expertise in genomics and concludes that it will be a considerable time before widespread genomic testing is ready to enter 'mainstream' clinical practice.

POPULATION SCREENING FOR GENETIC DISORDERS

The word 'screening' is used in a number of different ways in relation to medical genetics, often imprecisely or inaccurately. 'Genetic screening' may refer not just to genetic disorders but to the use of genetic technologies in relation to non-genetic conditions, or the term may be used incorrectly for the testing of individuals rather than populations. Most of the general public make no distinction between 'screening' and any kind of testing. To avoid confusion, I shall use 'genetic screening' in the sense of population or large group testing for genetic disorders, regardless of the technology used.

The history of population screening for genetic disorders goes back a long way, beginning with newborn screening for phenylketonuria (PKU) in the 1960s. Introduced first in America by Robert Guthrie (Guthrie and Susi, 1963) but soon adopted in Britain. PKU was in many ways an excellent candidate for screening; it was severe if untreated, dietary therapy was effective, while a simple, sensitive and specific test for a raised blood phenylalanine level was possible on a dried blood spot and could be confirmed by a more accurate biochemical test. The fact that the condition was genetic was largely incidental.

The extension of newborn screening to congenital hypothyroidism was likewise uncontroversial, but as it became clear that many other disorders were potentially detectable on the same sample, particularly with the use of tandem mass spectroscopy, the technology began to run ahead of any proven benefits. Fortunately, in the UK there were already established bodies within the NHS for assessing population screening generally, notably the National Screening Committee, which determines whether a new screening programme, genetic or otherwise, should be funded by the NHS. Here medical geneticists found themselves largely on the same side as Public Health Medicine in taking a cautious and critical approach, even though initially the National Screening Committee contained no genetic expertise. This has formed a strong contrast to how the area has developed in America, where a combination of lobby groups has resulted in widespread newborn screening programmes of uncertain value.

When population screening became feasible for cystic fibrosis, the situation became considerably more debatable. The main aim of carrier screening for pregnant women, couples or adults generally was not to improve treatment but to allow termination of affected pregnancies; also it was far from clear what proportion of women or couples actually wanted it. Several British pilot programmes were undertaken, which gave a broad consensus that carrier screening was generally acceptable but that there was little spontaneous demand for it. As therapy for cystic fibrosis improved, the case for newborn screening also became stronger. Currently there is no uniform consensus as to which approaches are optimal at a population level.

Down's syndrome screening during pregnancy has already been mentioned in Chapter 5, and the situation is changing rapidly with the introduction of noninvasive prenatal testing (NIPT) as a population screening measure. The use of ultrasound in early pregnancy, now almost universal, likewise gives challenges.

Finally, the history of population screening for genetic disorders has been strongly influenced by the experience with minority populations showing a particularly high frequency of specific conditions. Thalassaemias and sickle cell disease form striking examples here and are in many ways very different from each other, as well as from the situation of Tay Sachs disease in the Ashkenazi Jewish population. The experience of Bernadette Modell and her colleagues (Chapter 5), both laboratory and community based, for thalassaemia shows how if any programme of combined screening, prenatal diagnosis and therapy is to be successful it must have a strong community base and support. The same is true for population-based screening for sickle cell disease in the UK Afro-Caribbean population, for which Elizabeth Anionwu in London, with a community nursing background, has played a leading role (see Chapter 6).

Carrier screening for the severe and currently untreatable recessively inherited disorder Tay Sachs disease has been much less prominent in Britain than in America, with its much larger Ashkenazi Jewish population; learning from the earlier pioneer studies there it has been introduced quietly as an 'opt in' programme for the Jewish community, coordinated from London and delivered through the NHS.

Altogether the topic of population screening in relation to genetic disorders is much too big to deal with adequately here, and deserves a detailed and impartial historical study, — yet another to add to the list of valuable projects still to be done (Appendix 2). With the possibility of widespread genomic testing and screening now technically feasible, such a study is urgent if we are to avoid making errors comparable or worse than have occurred with population screening in the past.

POLITICS, THE NHS AND MEDICAL GENETICS

For the first decades after the NHS was set up, the politicians of successive governments took a relatively 'hands off' approach to the practical aspects of organising and delivering the various parts of the service, leaving this largely to the various regions and to the Royal Colleges. Fortunately this was the time when medical genetics services were developing across the country and, while workers in the field may have felt neglected by central government, they could not complain of interference. The past 20 years have seen a radical change in approach, so that one may indeed invoke the maxim 'be careful what you wish for'. Now governments, and individual politicians within them, find it difficult (impossible?) to avoid creating grandiose and often unrealistic plans and reorganisations, often with minimal or no consultation with those working in the area. The NHS overall has suffered greatly in recent years from such interference and micromanagement, though for medical genetics the results have been more mixed. The often quoted and possibly apocryphal lament of a Roman general 2000 years ago is just as relevant for those working in medical genetics today.

> We trained hard — but it seemed that every time we were beginning to form up into teams we were reorganised. I was to learn later in life that we tend to meet any new situation in life by reorganising,

and what a wonderful method it can be for creating the illusion of progress while actually producing confusion, inefficiency and demoralisation.

Attributed (probably incorrectly) to the Roman general
Gaius Petronius Arbiter (AD 27-66)

The first example of this affecting medical genetics came in the form of two reports produced for the NHS Research and Development board (Department of Health, 1995a,b), issued simultaneously but very different, in fact largely contradictory, in character. The first, written by a working group chaired by Martin Bobrow, gave a factual statement of the benefits achieved from medical genetics to date, recommending modest and affordable further developments based on these, but no radical change. The second report, focusing on common diseases, foresaw an impending 'genetic revolution' that would require restructuring of the entire system and probably necessitate extensive involvement of the commercial sector. The reason for two such different reports being issued simultaneously was apparently that the government of the time felt that the initial report was insufficiently 'exciting'. In the event, the promised revolution of the second report was postponed for another decade or more, giving all concerned (including the private sector) time to look at the likely future more soberly.

Martin Bobrow, in an interview with the author, puts the situation from the viewpoint of one directly involved:

PSH: …. in terms of what you might call Department of Health policies, you really have had an important role in keeping the Department of Health on the one hand anchored in reality and on the other hand still convinced that genetics is important.

MB: I wonder!

PSH: OK but…

MB: I often wish that I was a more effective diplomat and might actually have been able to achieve what you've just said. I think that I often spoke a bit too clearly for the Department of Health and, I believe I was right in what I said, but I don't think that isn't an excuse for saying it. In some senses I suspect that I irritated the Civil Service rather more than was actually necessary.

PSH: But the two reports which stick in my mind are your 'First report to the R&D Group' and then your laboratory services report. It's fair to say without those two reports, things might have gone terribly wrong, because there were other groups pushing in very very different directions weren't there?

MB: Well certainly that 'First report to the R&D Group' as you again know, was well underway when the Director of R&D decided that the rather pragmatic and downbeat messages coming out of this were so far from what he wanted that he was constrained to set up a rival working group, without initially telling me about it, and you are quite right that our working group essentially said that what we ought to do for the next 5 years, which was our brief, was to try to make things like Down's and Fragile X and one or two others of that ilk work properly, because we were some little distance from that and that we should worry about common diseases as and when it became reality. Yes, well the five years have passed haven't they? [This interview was in 2004!]

PSH: I also remember when those two reports came out, which I think were more or less simultaneous.

MB: Oh yes, they were published together.

PSH: And at the time the Department of Health had that meeting in London, the second report had more or less collapsed spontaneously, at least in the eyes of everybody at that meeting I think, but if it hadn't been for your report being out there with it, there wouldn't have been anything to hold to.

MB: I think a lot of people contributed to and continue to contribute, which I don't now because I'm no longer that welcome down there, to try to make the Department of Health concentrate on health delivery rather than the fantasy of the year after tomorrow. They do love to fantasise and I understand why. Politicians need to fantasise to an extent, and I don't object to them saying fantastic things. I really do object to them spending very large amounts of money, when money is a very tight commodity, on things that are just not going to work and they get perilously close, well not perilously close; they have just done it again the year before last with the 'White Paper'. I calculate that about a third of the money in that White Paper was spent on things that were complete Never Never Land; which is, you know, two thirds was spent on really good things, so one should be duly grateful.

Interview with Martin Bobrow 2004 [24]

As a second example of politicisation of the NHS affecting medical genetics may be given the unintended consequences of redrawing regional boundaries and re-organising various tiers of NHS administration, often resulting in the loss of personal contacts and of patterns of referral and practice which had been built up painstakingly over many years. These changes were particularly damaging for medical genetics, as a specialty built upon defined populations and areas, and with strong traditions of epidemiological research.

A third and, on balance, more positive government initiative was that referred to by Martin Bobrow above, the 2003 'White paper' (an arcane term for a specific plan for action as opposed to a 'green paper' indicating for discussion only), entitled 'Our Inheritance, our Future', which made a series of mostly valuable recommendations promoting genetics in medicine, with funding attached. It included a series of 'Gene Knowledge Parks' for which competitive tenders were invited (the successful centres were Cambridge, Cardiff, London, Oxford,

Manchester and Newcastle) to encourage the translation of research into service and to enhance awareness of the public, also a National Genetics Education Centre based in Birmingham. In addition, two NHS reference laboratories (in Manchester and Salisbury) to develop molecular genetics techniques were created, as well as some less well thought-through ideas such as the possible genetic profiling of all newborns (again apparently added as an afterthought to make things more exciting), which in the event did not get further than the discussion stage.

This initiative gave a real boost to UK medical genetics, especially to the network of previously underfunded molecular genetics laboratories; it is probably no coincidence that the then health minister had his constituency base in Newcastle on Tyne, which had a flourishing medical genetics service led by a politically astute clinical geneticist, John Burn.

DEVOLUTION AND MEDICAL GENETICS

Equity of provision of genetic services across the UK has always been a key aim of the medical genetics community, though inevitably some regions have always been more advanced than others; indeed Scotland and Wales had led the way in a number of developments in both research and services, most notably the Scottish Consortium model for molecular genetic testing (Kelly et al. 2002). However, following devolution, health became totally devolved to each country, both as regards policy making and funding. This radical step has had major consequences for the NHS overall, creating in essence four separate systems with the potential for increasing divergence, especially since the governments involved have had widely differing overall policies and ideology.

This political development has already had significant effects on medical genetics. Coming just as the 'white paper' developments were being implemented, it resulted in Scotland missing out on them entirely at the time, while in Wales partly separate funding had to be sought. (A senior Department of Health official told me at that time that any application from Wales would be a waste of time, since it would go straight into the bin! They had not read the detail, though, which stated clearly that short-listing would be decided on quality alone). Devolution also resulted in a wider change of attitudes, with many civil servants in the London Department of Health taking it as a signal that that they could ignore the other 'home countries'. This has had serious consequences as, with its much larger population and thus amount of available funding, England has had the ability to initiate new developments, such as in genomics, requiring large amounts of capital that are less readily available to smaller populations. Fortunately, most of the organisations and professional societies in medical genetics have been set up on a UK basis, while research council units are likewise currently not devolved, so that the overall medical genetics community remains firmly united.

Not all the effects of devolution have been negative. Scotland has for a long time had wise policy guidance (see Chapter 3), while in Wales close personal links and supportive government, much easier to achieve in a smaller population, have also been fruitful despite the constraints of limited funding. Both have also been free from the wider flights of ideology that have at times characterised the more politically controlled Health Department in England. Some of these differences were explored in a recent 'Witness Seminar' (Harper et al. 2010).

Finally it is perhaps worth noting that none of the prominent British medical geneticists, whether in the early years or more recently, have become involved in more general politics, a remarkable contrast to France (Harper 2018), which has seen a medical geneticist as Health Minister (Jean-François Mattei [94]), another a presidential advisor to President Nicolas Sarkozy (Arnold Munnich [93]), while the founder of the field (Robert Debré), was father of the Gaullist prime minister Michel Debré, who apparently used to telephone him each Sunday to discuss difficult problems. Whatever one's views may be on their wider politics, there is little doubt that medical genetics benefited from their influence. It is of interest to speculate which of our more charismatic medical geneticists might have filled such roles and what the results might have been!

At the time of writing, the British NHS has just celebrated its 70th birthday and is still largely intact, as are medical genetics services, though continuing 'top down' developments in genomics as well as the natural evolution of the field look set to create further major changes, notably the reorganisation of laboratories into a small number of 'genomic medicine centres'. Since this is primarily a historical book I shall not try to cover these very recent events, though the scientific basis of some of them is documented in several thorough and readable recent accounts, mostly American orientated, that follow both the technology and the more human aspects of the field up to the last few years (Mukherjee 2016, Hogan 2016).

Hopefully, those involved in devising and implementing policies for medical genetics services and genomics, and for the wider involvement of genetics in medicine generally, will listen to those already in the field and also spare a little time to see what has happened in the past and what can be learned from both previous successes and mistakes.

REFERENCES

Department of Health. Leeds: DoH, NHS Research and Development Directorate. 1995a. First report to the NHS Central Research and Development Committee on the new genetics.

Department of Health. Leeds: DoH, NHS Research and Development Directorate. 1995b. The genetics of common diseases: A second report to the NHS Central Research and Development Committee on the new genetics.

Guthrie R, Susi A. 1963. A simple phenylalanine method for detecting phenylketonuria in large populations of newborn infants. *Pediatrics*. 32:338–343.

Harper PS (ed.). 1991. *Huntington's Disease*. London: WB Saunders.

Harper PS. 2006. *First Years of Human Chromosomes*. Oxford: Scion Press.

Harper PS. 2018. Conversations with French medical geneticists. A personal perspective on the origins and early years of medical genetics in France. *Clin Genet*. 94:115–124.

Harper PS, Reynolds LA, Tansey EM. 2010. *Clinical Genetics in Britain: Origins and Development*. London: Wellcome Trust Centre for the History of Medicine at UCL.

Hogan AJ. 2016. *Life Histories of Genetic Disease: Patterns and Prevention in Medical Genetics*. Baltimore: Johns Hopkins University Press.

Kelly KF. 2002. The Scottish molecular genetics consortium – 15 years on. *Health Bull (Edinb)*. 60(1):83–90.

Leeming W. 2004. The early history of medical genetics in Canada. *Soc Hist Med*. 17:481–500.

Mukherjee S. 2016. *The Gene: An Intimate History*. London: Vintage.

National Screening committee https://www.gov.uk/government/groups/uk-national-screening-committee-uk-nsc

Public Health Genomics Foundation. 2018. *Genomics in mainstream clinical pathways*.

UK Government White Paper. 2003. *Our Inheritance, our Future: Realising the Potential of Genetics in the NHS*. Norwich: HMSO.

9

The wider context: Medical genetics as a community

ABSTRACT

Medical genetics, like other fields of science and medicine, functions within the context of a diverse community of workers and a series of activities outside the core remit of research, teaching and services. For Britain these have been exceptionally productive, and influential worldwide. A long series of books, from 1940 to the present, has played a major role in defining the field, and has included introductory and more advanced textbooks for medical students and others, monographs and practical handbooks, all given increased influence by the international use of the English language. British scientific journals have also been prominent, with the *Journal of Medical Genetics* being the first in the field worldwide. A series of professional societies has represented British medical genetics, the Clinical Genetics Society being the first of these. Strong international links, both with other European countries and with North America, have always characterised the field; in the early years a series of important workers came to Britain as refugees from fascism, while the Galton Laboratory was an international focus for many who became leaders of medical genetics in their own countries. Later, a number of British medical geneticists trained in America, notably with Victor McKusick in Baltimore.

As a new field of science or medicine grows and matures, a range of activities develops as part of it, whose main function is to maintain and enhance communication. These activities include textbooks for those learning the subject or already in the field, monographs synthesising knowledge on a particular topic, journals for disseminating original work, and congresses or smaller meetings allowing people to meet and to exchange ideas personally. Without these activities it is difficult for any field to flourish and to develop cohesion and a specific identity. British medical genetics has shown a wide range of them, some of considerable international importance.

These activities in genetics and medicine have occurred across the world, not just in Britain, with valuable and often lasting effects resulting from international congresses, training fellowships and individual career moves both from and to the UK, as well as within it; they have all been major factors in moulding the character of British medical genetics over the past 60 years, so I make no apologies for devoting a chapter to this 'wider context'.

BOOKS

Books have traditionally been the bedrock of most scientific fields, and medical genetics is no exception. Perhaps the first may be Joseph Adams' 1814 *Treatise on the Supposed Hereditary Properties of Diseases*, mentioned in Chapter 1, but the first British book clearly devoted to modern genetics in medicine was John Fraser Roberts' *An Introduction to Medical Genetics*, published in 1940 by Oxford University Press (Figure 9.1a). Aimed primarily at physicians (the author was medically trained but never practiced medicine), and possibly also medical students. It set a precedent by stating firmly in the introduction that:

> Plant and animal examples have been completely excluded. This may seem an unduly rigid limitation. But the expounders of genetics to medical men have gone so far to the opposite extreme that it seemed wiser to deny oneself the luxury of an occasional plant or animal example, if only to show that the subject can be explained without any of them.

Fraser Roberts' book, despite its wartime publication, proved successful and durable; taken on later by Marcus Pembrey, it had reached its 12th edition by 1986 (Roberts and Pembrey 1986). It is interesting to note that at the time of the first edition, Roberts was working at the Stoke Park unit for mental handicap, Bristol, and was honorary lecturer in human genetics at Bristol University – it would be another 40 years until Bristol appointed a full-time medical geneticist and the university has never created an academic medical genetics unit!

Next in succession as an introductory book, and more clearly medical student orientated, comes Alan Emery's *Elements of Medical Genetics*, Emery 1968 first published in America, but transferred to Livingstone of Edinburgh when the author moved there (see Chapter 3). The book has been continued by a series of authors up to the present 15th edition. Clearly publishers like to retain the name of a successful author even long after the originator has handed over! Another successful book from Scotland has been Connor and Ferguson-Smith's *Essential Medical Genetics*, first published in 1984 (Connor and Ferguson-Smith, 1984).

Turning from textbooks to more 'practice-based' handbooks, Britain has been the source of several of the most widely used books internationally of this type, some of which are listed in Table 9.1. It is notable that several of these have a strongly practical emphasis, including Read and Donnai's *The New Clinical Genetics*, (2007), Firth and Hurst's *Oxford Desk Reference: Clinical Genetics* (Firth and Hurst 2005, first edition), and from a laboratory perspective Strachan and Read's *Human Molecular Genetics*, 2004.

(a)

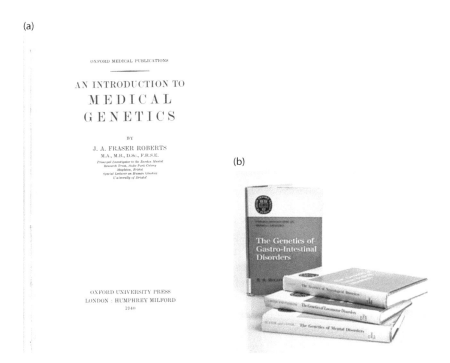

(b)

Figure 9.1 Key early books on medical genetics. **(a)** The first edition (1940) of John Fraser Roberts' book *Introduction to Medical Genetics*. **(b)** Some of the early volumes of the *Oxford Monographs on Medical Genetics* series. (From Harper, 2013, courtesy of Genetics and Medicine Historical Network.)

Table 9.1 Some general 'Working' books on medical genetics by British authors

	First published
Roberts JF. *Introduction to Medical Genetics*	1940
Clarke CA. *Genetics for the Clinician*	1962
Emery AEH. *Elements of Medical Genetics*	1968
Harper PS. *Practical Genetic Counselling*	1981
Connor JM and Ferguson-Smith MA. *Essential Medical Genetics*	1984
Young ID. *Introduction to Risk Calculation in Genetic Counselling*	1991
Strachan T and Read A. *Human Molecular Genetics*	2004
Firth H and Hurst J. *Oxford Desk Reference Clinical Genetics*	2005
Read A and Donnai D. *The New Clinical Genetics*	2008

Note: See Chapter 6 for books on genetic counselling.

It is perhaps not immodest to say that my own *Practical Genetic Counselling,* (Harper, 1981) while not the first on the topic (see Chapter 6), has played a significant role in helping the development not only of genetic counselling itself but also of clinical genetics overall. When originally written in 1980 I had aimed the book at practising general hospital clinicians and family doctors, and was surprised when medical geneticists found it useful, as they clearly did around the world. So also have non-medical genetic counsellors, as they developed as a specific professional group, even though my views on the nature of genetic counselling may have seemed unorthodox and politically incorrect to some of them. Almost 40 years (and eight editions) on, *Practical Genetic Counselling* has now taken on a new lease of life under my friend and colleague Angus Clarke, and I wish it well. People have often asked me why it has remained popular, and I think that the main reason is that it has remained small, despite growth of the field, and is simply written. It has certainly made me a lot of friends, and one of the great pleasures of my life has been to feel that foreign translations, especially in countries with authoritarian regimes (e.g.: Russia, China, Iran, East Europe [in past times]), may have helped a more humanistic and non-directive approach to genetic counselling to emerge and become established.

Many of the books mentioned here have gone through multiple editions over a long period, giving scope for interested historians to see how the field of medical genetics has changed during the past 50 years, though it is interesting to see how many of the key aspects have altered relatively little. This is one reason why the *Human Genetics Historical Library* (see below and Appendix 2) aims to keep a copy of each edition.

Writing a book is a very different activity to writing and publishing research papers, and requires a temperament which only a minority possess. Very few people are prolific authors; JBS Haldane in the early years was one example, while Alan Emery has been another from more recent times. In my view an essential factor in this is that one should enjoy writing, and be able to write simply and clearly; also that one is prepared to regard it as largely an 'out-of-hours activity' and that one's family should be able to tolerate this. As with other 'creative arts' it can intrude excessively into wider life unless it is kept under some degree of control. Its main advantage to the writer is that it allows a high degree of independence from peer review and the conventional structure of scientific papers, so that to a large extent one can write what one wants, in the way that one wants. A few years ago I thought that the writing of books and their appearance in print might be a dying art, but this does not now seem to be the case and the printed book seems to be regaining favour over the 'e-book' in many situations.

Book series

Books published as a series tend to develop an identity and character over and above that of the individual volume, and the collecting streak in many of us probably helps their sales too. In medical genetics there is no better example of this than the Oxford University Press *Monographs in Medical Genetics* series, begun in 1963 and based in Britain for the first 20 years of its existence, though always international in its approach. I have written a brief informal article on the series (Harper 2013) which contains a complete list, free from the spelling errors that have crept into the publisher's version. Figure 9.1b shows some of the early volumes. Each monograph was free-standing, but the plan was to cover all of the main clinical areas of medical genetics, as well as to provide authoritative accounts of various special fields; the first numbered volume was Richard McConnell's 1966 *Genetics of Gastrointestinal Disorders* (see Figure 2.10b for a photograph of McConnell). Thanks to the high quality of its authors, a hard-working panel of editorial advisors and some able editors at Oxford University Press (OUP), it certainly succeeded in its aim and became the most immediately recognisable series in the field. The initial series editor was John Fraser Roberts, and his *Introduction to Medical Genetics* was taken as the starting point so that authors of the later books could assume a knowledge of basic genetics from the readers; he was followed by Cedric Carter, and then a panel consisting of Arno Motulsky, Martin Bobrow, Peter Harper, and later Charles Scriver and Judith Hall. By the time of its 50th anniversary in 2013 the series had reached over 60 volumes.

A further distinguished series is the *Society for the Study of Inborn Errors of Metabolism* volumes, representing the annual conferences of this Society, international but British based, and providing valuable accounts of a variety of individual conditions, or groups of inherited metabolic disorders. The prime movers here were mainly medical biochemists rather than medical geneticists, with a few key individuals like Charles Scriver providing a bridge between the two. The series began in 1963 and the Society still flourishes, with its proceedings now supplements to the *Journal of Inherited Metabolic Disease* rather than free-standing volumes.

Reference books, catalogues and databases

The days of large and weighty reference books in print are now over, and these are now mostly online (e.g.: *Online Mendelian Inheritance in Man (OMIM)* (originally *Mendelian Inheritance in Man, McKusick, 1966*), and *Metabolic and Molecular Bases of Inherited Disease* [Scriver et al. 2001]). Both of these were American in origin, though universally used across Britain and the rest of Europe, and with British contributors; the only example with a major British contribution known to me is *Emery and Rimoin's Principles and Practice of Medical Genetics* (Rimoin et al. 2007). An especially valuable resource that has been electronic from the outset has been the *London Dysmorphology Database*, one of the cornerstones in the development of the area of dysmorphology as part of British medical genetics (see Chapter 4) (Winter and Baraitser 1987).

'Popular' books

A brief note must suffice for the long and distinguished tradition of books written for the wider public by both medical and non-medical geneticists. JBS Haldane has already been mentioned as an early example, while Steve

Jones has maintained the tradition at University College London. As well as general popular books, there are numerous examples relating to specific genetic disorders, aimed mainly at patients and family members, the Oxford University Press series *The Facts* being notable. Again, these books have not been superseded by the internet.

Book collections

Identifying individual books on medical genetics in libraries, other collections or online is usually possible but not always easy, since the topic overlaps into so many different fields. But it is also important to be able to get a feel for the broad range of books being written and being read by those working in medical genetics, and this has until recently been close to impossible. A few historic collections based on specific workers exist, such as the libraries of William Bateson and Cyril Darlington at the John Innes Institute archive, Norwich, but there is now a resource available that gives a picture of the field overall through its books – the *Human Genetics Historical Library*.

Begun in 2004 as one of the activities of the recently formed *Genetics and Medicine Historical Network*, this collection started with the donation of what had originally been the library of the Oxford MRC Clinical and Population Genetics Research Unit (see Chapter 2). Two other major donations followed as bequests – the entire libraries of Professors John Edwards (Oxford) and Paul Polani (London), together with numerous smaller donations from individuals and departments. Fortunately the collection has been professionally curated from the outset and detailed cataloguing data are available online. For those wishing to know more, a published article has been written on it (Harper and Pierce 2010), as well as numerous progress reports in the newsletters of the Genmedhist Network. The collection now numbers almost 4000 volumes and continues to grow, with interest and donations coming from across Europe as well as from within Britain (Figure 9.2).

(a)   (b)

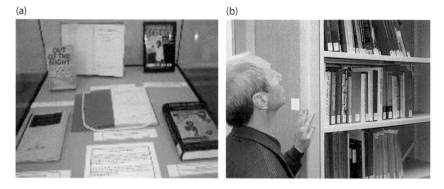

Figure 9.2 The Human Genetics Historical Library **(a)** Exhibit, 2010, at Cardiff University Special Collections and Archives. **(b)** Part of the collection with archivist Peter Keelan. (Courtesy of Genetics and Medicine Historical Network.)

JOURNALS

If one wishes to form a picture of what has been happening in any field of science or medicine, not just genetics, one can do no better than to look at the major journals in the field. This is particularly true for the second half of the twentieth century, when journals had largely supplanted books as the principal form of communication, but had not yet been overtaken by the electronic age.

Of course, really major discoveries have, both then and now, tended to be reported in high profile, international general journals such as *Nature* and its offshoots (for basic science research) or *Lancet* (for clinically orientated work). These have carried numerous articles relevant to medical genetics over the years. But it is the medium-level journals that give a flavour of the type and range of work going on around the country. For America, a good analysis of this has been given by James Crow (2005), but no account of how British medical and human genetics has related to its journals has yet appeared, to my knowledge.

Journal of Medical Genetics

First published in September 1964, with Arnold Sorsby as editor, this journal was the first internationally to be devoted to medical genetics, marking the specialty's arrival as a distinct field. As Sorsby's opening editorial noted in the first issue:

> ...the *Journal of Medical Genetics* is the first to be exclusively medical and to be broadly based.

But other areas were not to be discouraged either, such as pathology and laboratory aspects of genetic disorders, and relevant animal models.

There were of course journals already existing that published some clinically orientated articles, notably the *American Journal of Human Genetics* and *Annals of Human Genetics*, but none were aimed specifically at medical workers. Sorsby was an ophthalmologist, one of a number internationally who have played a distinguished role in early medical genetics (see Chapter 4). He was based at the Institute of Ophthalmology in London, but he had close links with the major genetics units of the time, as well as with the still small number of clinicians involved in genetic research. The contents of issues (four per year) from the first years of the journal reflect the wide range of topics, and contributors to the initial issue came from virtually all the active UK groups and individuals. All the early issues are freely accessible via the journal's archive. A notable contributor in these first years was George Fraser (see interview [32]) who at the time was working with Sorsby as research fellow.

In addition to original papers, the journal published case reports (one of the first to recognise the value of this), and its medical base was emphasised by it forming part of the *British Medical Journal*'s series of 'specialist journals', something that gave valuable technical and publishing support, though it may have been an adverse factor in the perception of the journal from across the Atlantic, where it was for a long time regarded and referred to as the '*British*' *Journal of Medical Genetics*. At this point, editorials were rare but book reviews were abundant, though sadly tending to be brief.

In December 1970, the editorship passed to Cyril Clarke, then Chair of the Department of Medicine at Liverpool University, and a practising physician as well as a pioneer clinical geneticist (see Chapter 2). Clarke edited the journal for 15 years, with Cedric Carter as assistant editor, and saw it grow to six issues a year and become an integral part of the British medical genetics scene. The journal also published abstracts of early meetings of the Clinical Genetics Society, and gives a good indication of the high quality of many of the contributions.

I took on the editor's role in 1985 and aimed both to increase the journal's profile and reduce its publication time, but also to give it a more 'rounded' character, so that each issue would be enjoyable to read as a whole, not just for a particular article that it contained. Maintaining a balance between general and specific aspects was not easy, but I was greatly helped by a series of exceptionally able section editors, including Kay Davies for molecular genetics, Patricia Jacobs for cytogenetics and Michael Conneally for American papers.

Ten years on, the journal had become monthly, with a larger format and content more than doubled, so I felt it was time to hand over, first to Martin Bobrow and then Eamonn Maher, following which it has crossed the Atlantic to Canada, where it continues to flourish based at McGill University, though still forming part of BMA journals.

Annals of Human Genetics is another UK-based journal of relevance to medical genetics, though its dubious past has always caused most medical geneticists to maintain a respectful distance. Originally founded as *Annals of Eugenics* as part of Francis Galton's endowment, it contained a mixture of papers on eugenics with valuable contributions on inherited disorders, as well as statistically orientated articles (Karl Pearson and then RA Fisher were the first editors). Traditionally the editor was always the Galton Professor; when Penrose was appointed in 1945, he purged the eugenics aspects, though it took another 20 years to change the name from *Annals of Eugenics* to *Annals of Human Genetics*. As the 'house journal' for the Galton Laboratory, it became progressively less clinical after Penrose retired, reflecting the biochemical genetics interests of his successors, Harry Harris and Elizabeth Robson, but of limited interest to medical geneticists, apart from those involved in human gene mapping and enzyme polymorphisms.

The other general journal, again more of scientific than of clinical appeal, that has now become UK based is *Human Genetics*, originally founded by Friedrich Vogel in 1964 as *Humangenetik*, as described in the interview with him in the Genmedhist series [05]. Although initially it was mainly German language based, it progressively converted to English and had from the outset Arno Motulsky, a close friend of Vogel, as the American editor. When Friedrich Vogel retired and David Cooper became its editor in the UK (Cardiff), there was some initial consternation in Germany, fortunately soon overcome, that the country was losing something precious; such factors count for little today, though, in the current global and highly competitive world of scientific publishing.

As medical genetics developed its range of special interests, so journals were started that reflected this, all essentially international but some British based, including *Human Molecular Genetics*, *Nature Genetics* and *Clinical Dysmorphology*. The continuing British strength of scientific publishing and the now almost universal use of English as the international scientific language has encouraged close involvement of British workers, both clinical and scientific, as editors and contributors to many journals.

MEDICAL GENETICS SOCIETIES

As it had been with journals, Britain was also slow by comparison with America in developing societies specific for medical geneticists. The long established Genetical Society, (now Genetics Society), founded by William Bateson in 1919 (see Chapter 1) and currently celebrating its centenary, was always open to medical people, but it remained focused on general, especially plant genetics, as did its journal, *Heredity*. Likewise the Eugenics Society, off-putting to most on account of its past and its name, was not a suitable forum for modern medical geneticists, even though its symposia became valuable meetings, with published proceedings, largely devoid of any eugenic views. An attempt was made in the 1990s to reform the Eugenics Society, but this succeeded only in changing its name (to the confusing Galton Institute), its original character remaining largely unchanged. It has to be admitted, though, that in its early years the Clinical Genetics Society accepted funding from the Eugenics Society for printing some of its reports.

Abroad, the American Society of Human Genetics (ASHG) had been founded in 1948 and the European Society of Human Genetics (ESHG) in 1967, but neither were readily accessible, especially to impecunious younger British workers; the latter's activities were limited in the early years to holding an annual conference, but it did build 'frugality' into its constitution (Harper 2017a).It is not surprising then that by the end of the 1960s the growing community of British medical geneticists, whether clinicians or laboratory workers, felt the need for a more specific society with which they could identify; this gave rise in 1970 to the Clinical Genetics Society.

The Clinical Genetics Society

The prime mover in founding and establishing the Clinical Genetics Society was Cedric Carter, ably assisted by his colleague Sarah Bundey, both then based at the Institute of Child Health, London. In January 1970 they sent a circular letter to British medical geneticists and to others who might be interested, inviting them to a meeting at the Institute of Child Health to discuss the formation of a 'medical genetics group'; this was duly held on 1st May 1970, consisting of a scientific presentation ('The genetics of spina bifida' by CO Carter) followed by a business meeting.

The Society was duly established, and a constitution drawn up, with the name agreed as 'Clinical Genetics Society' and the principal aim being:

> To encourage contact between medical geneticists in the United Kingdom and to learn of their current interests, research projects and clinical experience.

This was confirmed at a second meeting in Edinburgh on 16th October, 1970, also preceded by scientific presentations by Alan Emery and others.

A pattern developed of twice-yearly meetings in different centres around the country, particularly valuable for the regional centres now beginning to establish medical genetics in their area (not always an easy process). This helped to set the precedent of a geographically dispersed network of medical genetics centres, usually based in the relevant university teaching hospital, rather than a London-focused specialty. It also confirmed the clinically orientated nature of the society; indeed, at some early meetings patients with genetic disorders were presented in person, something that initially gave rise to debate since non-medical people were also present.

British Society for Human Genetics

As the laboratory aspects of medical genetics developed, in particular cytogenetics, other genetics professionals understandably felt the need for a forum more specifically tailored to their own needs and formed the Association of Clinical Cytogeneticists (ACC); in due course Clinical Molecular Genetics Society followed, as did Genetic Nurses and Social Workers Association (see Chapter 7). Their coming together in 1996 to form the British Society for Human Genetics (BSHG) was prompted by the fragmentation that was beginning to occur, partly in terms of advice to the Department of Health, but also in the picture of medical genetics given overall, to other medical fields. Creating and maintaining this unification was a far from easy process and considerable credit must be given in particular to Peter Farndon, Andrew Read and Martin Bobrow for their efforts in achieving this. The resulting annual meetings proved of extremely high quality, despite the reluctance of most workers in the large basic research institutes to become involved in the society, taking their cue largely from the persistently somewhat dismissive attitude of the leaders of these to applied and clinical research, something already touched on in Chapter 3.

As medical genetics grew as an overall field, it became increasingly clear that the great majority of BSHG members had a medical affiliation of some type, whether scientific or clinical, and in 2013 the society renamed itself as British Society for Genetic Medicine (BSGM), having already gained sub-groups, such as the Cancer Genetics Group. The new title was intended to highlight that the society's activities were increasingly incorporating colleagues from non-genetics specialities who were involved in research and clinical applications of genetics in medicine. The annual meetings have subsequently evolved to concentrate on the applications of genomic medicine. BSGM has an increasing number of members from other medical disciplines who have an interest in the clinical applications of genomics, including bioinformatics.

This fluidity of membership and character is a natural feature of professional and scientific societies in any rapidly evolving field and is not confined to Britain; comparable changes have occurred in the European Society of Human Genetics, while in America they resulted in the American College of Medical Genetics evolving out of American Society of Human Genetics for the representation of medical geneticists.

Informal groups and meetings

Perhaps the most valuable of all types of meetings in cementing and developing the different aspects of medical genetics in Britain have been those of the smaller, often not formally constituted groups based around a particular topic. These were generally open to anyone interested and not confined to medical geneticists, though they predominated in those mentioned here. Some of them proved transient, others evolved into a full-sized meeting. Commonly they were held once or twice a year on the day before (or after) a larger meeting, to minimise travel costs.

The Dysmorphology Club (see also Chapter 4) is a good example of this second category, and its development is well described in the interviews with some of its founders, such as Dian Donnai [63], Michael Baraitser [33] and John Burn [100]. Beginning around 1985 as a lunchtime meeting to discuss unusual syndromes at Institute of Child Health, London, it soon developed into a forum where clinical geneticists could bring photos of individual cases and discuss them with others who might have seen similar patients. When people started to travel to it from elsewhere, it was converted to a half-day meeting and eventually a full day, though it has never become formally constituted. Not only was this the place where many specific syndromes were identified, usually well before they had any clear genetic or molecular basis, but it was also valuable for trainees, especially those with a strong paediatric background. In addition, it provided an example of how valuable it was to share information with others, both at a national level and later internationally, as workers across continental Europe began to realise the importance of such sharing.

A second valuable example has been the UK Huntington's Disease Prediction Consortium, which began soon after molecular prediction, initially by linked genetic markers, became feasible. The sharing of anonymous data on results, and especially on problems encountered, was a powerful factor in helping clinical geneticists and genetic counsellors avoid the numerous potential pitfalls in this totally new form of predictive medicine, giving rise to patterns of good practice that were a great help and support to those in isolated centres, as well as deterring others from approaching this difficult area casually or without consideration of the many wider issues. As prediction increasingly became feasible for other progressive neurogenetic disorders, and later for the familial cancers, it became clear that the 'Huntington's model' was applicable to a wide range of late-onset genetic disorders, and that the issues that were initially thought to be specific to HD were in fact general ones (see Chapter 7). The extensive shared and published experience attracted ethicists, psychologists and others from the humanities and social sciences, who realised that these issues, based on real-life experience, could be as valuable, if not more so, as the purely theoretical concepts that many of them were more used to considering. They also could attract more funding!

It is not surprising that this area of predictive testing progressively became the province primarily of non-medical genetic counsellors as their specialty developed, given the importance of counselling skills in comparison to clinical and diagnostic aspects. Interestingly there was very little friction between the different types of professionals who were or might have been involved in this area, perhaps reflecting the generally good relations that had been built up previously. The new diagnostic molecular laboratories were also highly collaborative, partly because they recognised the practical advantages of working closely with clinical geneticists and genetic counsellors in avoiding the pitfalls that a 'lab result only' service might produce.

Other informal UK groups and meetings have included the Genethics Club, (see Chapter 7), while what began as the Cancer Families Study Group has become part of the British Society of Genetic Medicine, as the Cancer Genetics Group.

TEACHING MEDICAL GENETICS

For almost all established university staff in medical genetics, and for many NHS clinical genetics staff too, teaching is one of their key activities. Indeed, the term 'medical genetics' was originally used in the context of teaching general genetics to medical students by Madge Macklin in Canada and the United States in the 1930s, before medical genetics was thought of as a specific field in its own right. Early European books, such as that of Mohr (1934), mentioned in Chapter 6, likewise focused on accounts of basic genetics for medical staff and students, so that John Fraser Roberts' 1940 *Introduction to Medical Genetics* was an exception in using only human examples.

As research and applications of genetics to medicine steadily increased from the 1960s onwards, human- and disease-orientated teaching became easier in both lectures and written teaching material; mathematical aspects (always off-putting to medical students) decreased correspondingly. Nonetheless, despite reports from the Royal College of Physicians (see Chapter 8) and other bodies, and a range of books referred to above (Table 9.1), it remained a struggle in many centres to find time in the medical curriculum to cover medical genetics adequately, by comparison with the abundant hours given to older and more established departments such as anatomy and biochemistry.

As medical genetics has radiated outwards in its scope to involve medical postgraduates, laboratory staff, nurses and genetic counsellors, so the character of the various courses has changed, and with it the background to those responsible for teaching them. This was reflected in the National Genetics Education Centre established in Birmingham as part of the 'Genetics White Paper' initiative mentioned in Chapter 8. The Centre asked health professionals across all disciplines what genetics knowledge and skills were important for their roles, translating these into learning outcomes and workforce competences, supported by online resources and e-learning. In addition, the Centre organised courses for trainers on how to support learning outcomes.

With rapid research advances often radically changing the field, it could be difficult for courses to keep up to date, as can be seen from the experience of Muriel Lee, working as Patricia Jacobs' technician in the early years of human cytogenetics in Edinburgh.

I was going to night school at that time and I was being taught that there were 48 chromosomes. The human number was 48, and I was going to work the next day and counting 46 and it was just so exciting, because we were right in there at the beginning, you know.

Interview with Muriel Lee, 2004 [12]

Fortunately now most teaching in medical genetics and related areas is now done, and should be, by those working at the forefront of their field.

THE INTERNATIONAL DIMENSION

Genetics overall has been a highly international field of science since its beginnings, and medical genetics equally so, both for clinical and laboratory aspects. The early British prominence in pre-war human genetics research and the virtually total destruction of the field across continental Europe meant that it was natural for European countries to look initially to Britain when building or rebuilding the field. While America might be a magnet for basic laboratory research, with its abundant funding, it had been slow to take up human genetics, many of its workers having been put off the field by the pre-war influence of eugenics. The international influence of Germany had been completely abolished for the near future; indeed, post-war German scientists found it difficult to work on human genetics in their own country for the next several decades.

Penrose's reformed Galton Laboratory in London thus became the premier centre in Europe for human genetics, as described in Chapter 2, even though it was not particularly well organised for this role, with few laboratory facilities and no specific system for teaching apart from the existing lectures by university staff. It seems as if it was this very lack of structure, along with Penrose's character, that attracted the series of able and independent-minded people from across Europe and further, some listed in Table 9.2, and helped by a remarkably wide range of other workers in allied fields at University College London. This influence of Penrose and his colleagues was brought up repeatedly in my own series of interviews with the early founders of medical genetics across continental Europe, as seen below.

International conferences were another area of early British prominence; although the first International Congress of Human Genetics in 1956 was held in Copenhagen under Tage Kemp, Penrose was President for the third, held in Chicago in 1966, (Crow and Neel, 1967) and I have mentioned his important Presidential Address in Chapter 7. JBS Haldane had been originally chosen as President, but died shortly before the congress. British workers were also much involved in the founding of the European Society of Human Genetics in 1967, as I have described in an article on its early history (Harper, 2017a).

By the time that medical genetics had begun to differentiate itself from human genetics in the 1960s, training opportunities for medical workers hoping to

Table 9.2 Early international links. Medical geneticists from outside the UK trained in human genetics at the Galton Laboratory, London

Workers from continental Europe

Jean Frézal	Paris
Herman VandenBerghe	Leuven
Jan Mohr	Oslo/Copenhagen
Marco Fraccaro	Pavia
Renata Laxova	Brno
Marcello Siniscalco	Italy

American and other visiting workers

Barton Childs	Baltimore
Victor McKusick	Baltimore
Charles Scriver	Montreal
Arno Motulsky	Seattle
David Danks	Melbourne
Alick Bearn	New York
Samuel (Ned) Boyer	Baltimore
Park Gerald	Chicago
Arthur Veale	Dunedin

enter the field as a career were becoming more promising in America, where the founding departments had more extensive and organised training programmes, with funding open at that time to those from outside America.

From the perspective of the UK, much the most relevant of these was that based at Johns Hopkins Hospital and led by Victor McKusick, originally a cardiologist but appointed to head the 'chronic diseases' division of the Department of Medicine, which he converted into a unit for medical genetics (McKusick 2006). Being part of an already established structure had many advantages, notably the existence of training posts; McKusick had already made close links with the UK, especially with Cyril Clarke in Liverpool, so the 1960s and early 1970s saw a steady flow of British clinicians, most trained or training in adult internal medicine, many but not all being from Liverpool (see Table 9.3). This greatly boosted the numbers of people who could take up senior posts in medical genetics after their return home; surprisingly few remained in the United States, though some took posts in neighbouring Canada (Harper, 2012).

This two-way flow of skilled personnel, experienced in both clinical medicine and genetics, made an indelible mark on UK medical genetics in its early decades, contributing to its broadly based nature in terms of its medical specialties of origin. Those people trained with McKusick, whether from Britain or elsewhere, have retained a remarkable degree of loyalty and identity over the years and have transmitted at least some of this to younger generations, in a similar way to those

Table 9.3 UK medical geneticists trained in Baltimore with Victor McKusick, 1960–1975

Name	Main future UK place of work
Sarah Bundey	London/Birmingham
J Michael Connor	Glasgow
Alan Emery	Manchester/Edinburgh
David Price Evans	Liverpool
Malcolm Ferguson-Smith	Glasgow
Peter Harper	Cardiff
Alan Johnston	Aberdeen
F Michael Pope	London
David Siggers	Southampton
David Weatherall	Liverpool/Oxford
RS (Charles) Wells	London

who worked with Penrose. Other transatlantic centres, such as Seattle, Boston and Toronto, also developed UK links, but these have been less frequent for clinical geneticists by comparison to laboratory scientists.

One of the most damaging changes in recent UK NHS clinical training programmes has been the reduction in opportunities for research, and in particular for research and more general experience abroad. This has only partly been alleviated by the development of short-term courses such as the European School of Medical Genetics and other European Union initiatives and has made it more difficult for those in training to obtain an all-round experience not confined to a single specific centre.

The British medical genetics diaspora

In addition to the international links just described, the close links between medical genetics centres across much of the world, at least the anglophone world, has given opportunities for UK medical geneticists to take up long-term positions abroad, often of a clinical academic nature. Language proficiency is an especially important skill for genetic counselling and related clinical activities, something that has greatly limited until recently workers from countries such as France. Table 9.4 shows that 'old Commonwealth' countries such as Australia and Canada are well represented, helping to maintain these international links. In the other direction, the Indian subcontinent has more recently contributed considerably to the body of UK medical geneticists, probably in line with other medical specialties. This list is almost certainly incomplete, but it is perhaps surprising that I can find no record of clinical geneticists from Britain moving permanently to the USA; it does not include scientists moving for research purposes but is limited to those whose work has involved wider medical genetics.

Table 9.4 The British medical genetics diaspora

Australia

George Fraser[a]	Adelaide
John MacMillan	Brisbane
David Ravine	Perth/ Melbourne
Bob Williamson	Melbourne

Canada

Stephen Bamforth	Edmonton
Peter Bowen	Edmonton
George Fraser[a]	Newfoundland
Helen Hughes[a]	Toronto
Elizabeth Ives	Newfoundland
Philip Welch	Halifax

Netherlands

Martin Bobrow[a]	Amsterdam
George Fraser[a]	Leiden
Peter Pearson	Leiden

South Africa

Peter Beighton	Cape Town
Trefor Jenkins	Johannesburg

[a] Indicates eventual return to UK.

Refugees

The important early contribution made by refugees from fascism in the late 1930s has already been described in Chapter 1; this contribution was mostly to research in human genetics, since medical genetics as a specialty did not exist at the time. For those later arrivals taking up clinical genetics, the English language was an important factor. Just a few examples are given here but I have addressed the topic more fully in a recent paper (Harper 2017b).

After the war, Renata Laxova [55] came to Britain as a refugee from Czechoslovakia and worked with Penrose before later moving to Wisconsin, recording her experiences in a memoir and in her autobiography (Laxova 1998, 2001). She had originally come as a child before the war on the Kindertransport, becoming fluent in English, but after returning found that this marked her out by the communist regime as undesirable and she was forced to flee the country; her memorable account of her reception by the Penroses after arriving with her husband as penniless refugees is heartwarming.

It is Friday, mid-morning. You are about to leave the city for a long weekend in the country when you find yourself opening your front door to four bedraggled political refugees. It is difficult for you even to recognize the weary man, woman, and two girls as people whose casual acquaintance you had made on a single previous occasion about two months ago, during a brief 3 day work-related visit to their country. You invite them in, show them around and, 15 minutes later, the dazed visitors, now ensconced in your home, are waving good-bye to you as you leave for your weekend in the country. How many people are there among us who would be willing to entrust their homes, in their absence, to practically complete strangers arriving on their doorstep from a foreign country?

That morning in late August 1968, in answer to my telephone call intended merely to inform them that we had escaped from our country, which had been invaded by Soviet forces, Lionel and Margaret Penrose invited my husband, daughters, and me for what we thought would be a polite cup of tea. They met us at the door and, to our amazement, instead of a handshake they handed us their house keys, their only set; characteristically, the spare keys were nowhere to be found.

Laxova, 1998

Other refugees have included Ursula Mittwoch (see Chapter 2), George Fraser [32] and Michael Laurence [13]. Sadly, one has to wonder how these people, so valuable to British life and to science and medicine in general, would have been welcomed today.

South Africa provides an interesting more recent example, though these were mainly voluntary migrants rather than enforced refugees. Martin Bobrow [24] and Michael Baraitser [33], in their interviews, give their perspective from the viewpoint of the incomer:

Michael Baraitser:

PSH: And then when you came to this country, was that to a neurology post initially?

MB: No, we took great chances. My wife woke up one day and she said we just cannot stay in this country any longer. We had four young kids to educate and so we decided on the spur of the moment to emigrate. My wife's father was a well-known psychiatrist in Johannesburg and he knew Sir Martin Roth, the psychiatrist in the UK, and Martin Roth knew Roger Gilliat, the neurologist, and so it was arranged for me to go for 6 months to Queen's Square and see if I could find my feet.

Matters proved not entirely straightforward though:

…And so I went to interviews here for the rheumatology job, which I never got, and they said 'what have you published?' I said, 'I've published a couple of books on antique furniture'. Boom. Finished. I was out like a shot!

Fortunately, medical genetics, with Cedric Carter, was more welcoming (see Chapter 2).

Martin Bobrow also came to Britain from South Africa:

PSH: Growing up in South Africa, and being yourself part of a minority in South Africa, how much did that shape your outlook?

MB: Scientifically, not much I suspect. I think it shaped my political views very strongly. I was left with all the obvious aftermath of someone who just didn't like the society in which they were growing up, and from as far back as I can remember I was pretty plain that I needed to get out of it. I didn't see, I saw no way in which I believed I could influence what was going to happen. I saw a future which I thought was going to be cataclysmic; turns out fortunately that I was wrong, but I have to say looking back on it I still think the odds were on the way I was looking at it and I just didn't want to be there on either side.

The second thing is that, although less so today, Britain is a pretty class-ridden place. Coming from outside of the country enables one to bypass many of the class distinctions that native-born people find themselves grouped by. Us colonials, ex-colonials, just are not expected to know how to behave properly; we don't behave properly and it doesn't seem to have formed as much of an inhibition as it might have done for other people.

It can be seen that there has been extensive mobility among medical geneticists between different countries, something that has considerably influenced the character of the field, almost certainly to its great advantage. This movement has also occurred for laboratory geneticists and is particularly well illustrated by the large number of workers trained in molecular techniques at the London unit of Bob Williamson (see Chapter 10), who have gone on to make outstanding careers in various aspects of medical genetics research across the world.

Medical genetics and the European Union

While many, perhaps most. international links and exchanges have been initiated by the individuals involved and the host departments, they have been greatly facilitated by a range of funding initiatives from the European Union. For medical geneticists the most fruitful have probably been the support for collaborative research projects involving multiple centres, which usually funded the collaborative aspects rather than the primary research itself. Small workshops or other meetings have likewise been highly effective in bringing colleagues from across Europe together. Britain has from the outset been a leading player in all these activities; should it be excluded from them because of political changes, as seems all too likely at the time of writing this, the result will be extremely damaging for all concerned.

REFERENCES

Adams J. 1814. *A Treatise on the Supposed Hereditary Properties of Diseases.* London: Callow.

Connor JM, Ferguson-Smith MA. 1984. *Essential Medical Genetics.* Oxford: Blackwell.

Crow JF. 2005. Early American genetics journals (essay). *Nat Rev Genet.* 6:715–720.

Crow JF, Neel JV (eds.) 1967. *Proceedings of the Third International Congress of Human Genetics, Plenary Sessions and Symposia.* Baltimore: The Johns Hopkins University Press.

Emery AEH. 1968. *Elements of Medical Genetics.* Edinburgh: Livingstone.

Firth HV, Hurst JA. 2005. *Oxford Desk Reference: Clinical Genetics,* 1st edn. Oxford: Oxford University Press.

Harper PS. 1981. *Practical Genetic Counselling,* 1st edn. Bristol: John Wright.

Harper PS. 2012. Victor McKusick and the history of medical genetics. In: Dronamraju K, Francomano C (eds.). *Victor McKusick and the History of Medical Genetics.* New York: Springer, pp. 145–161.

Harper PS. 2013. Oxford Monographs on Medical Genetics: A piece of genetic history. *Newsletter of the Genetics and Medicine Historical Network.* 17:9–11.

Harper PS. 2017a The European Society of Human Genetics: Beginnings, early history and development over its first 25 years. *Eur J Hum Genet.* doi: 10.1038/ejhg.2017.34.

Harper PS. 2017b. Human Genetics in troubled times and places. *Hereditas.* 155:7.

Harper PS, Pierce K. 2010. The Human Genetics Historical Library: An international resource for geneticists and historians. *Clin Genet.* 77:214–220.

Laxova R. 1998. Lionel Sharples Penrose, 1898–1972: A personal memoir in celebration of the centenary of his birth. *Genetics.* 150:1333–1340.

Laxova R. 2001. *Letter to Alexander.* Cincinnati, OH: Custom Editorial Productions.

McConnell RB. 1966. *The Genetics of Gastrointestinal Disorders.* Oxford: Oxford University Press.

McKusick VA. 1966. *Mendelian Inheritance in Man: Catalogs of Autosomal Dominant, Autosomal Recessive, and X-Linked Phenotypes,* 1st edn. Baltimore: The Johns Hopkins University Press.

McKusick VA. 2006. A 60-year tale of spots, maps and genes. *Annu Rev Genomics Hum Genet.* 7:1–27.

Mohr OL. 1934. *Heredity and Disease.* New York: Norton.

Read A, Donnai D. 2007. *New Clinical Genetics,* 1st edn. Oxford: Scion.

Rimoin DL, Connor JM, Pyeritz P, Korf BR (eds.) 2007. *Emery and Rimoin's Principles and Practice of Medical Genetics,* 5th edn. London: Churchill Livingstone, pp. 3–32.

Roberts JAF. 1940. *An Introduction to Medical Genetics.* London: Oxford University Press.

Roberts JAF, Pembrey M. 1986. *An Introduction to Medical Genetics*, 12th edn. Oxford: Oxford University Press.

Scriver CR, Beaudet AL, Sly WS, Valle D (eds.). 2001. *The Metabolic and Molecular Bases of Inherited Disease*, 8th edn. New York: McGraw-Hill.

Strachan T, Read AP. 2004. *Human Molecular Genetics*, 3rd ed. London: Garland.

Winter RM, Baraitser M. 1987. The London Dysmorphology Database. *J Med Genet*. 24:509–510.

10

The laboratory basis
of medical genetics

ABSTRACT

Medical genetics is a hybrid discipline, depending on the interaction between laboratory and clinical workers, but most of its key advances over the past half century have depended on laboratory discoveries. Cytogenetics was the first laboratory field to have practical applications; after the initial recognition of human chromosome abnormalities from 1959, a series of technical advances, most notably chromosome banding, saw it largely change from a research to a service area, usually linked with clinical genetics and stimulating this through the need for diagnostic interpretation and genetic counselling. Biochemical genetics also advanced but in Britain stayed less closely connected with medical genetics. From around 1980 human molecular genetics developed a major impact, pioneered by molecular analysis of the haemoglobin disorders, but then allowing the understanding, diagnosis and prediction of many other mendelian disorders, principally through the isolation of the genes involved through gene mapping and positional cloning. Important mendelian subsets of some common disorders, such as cancers, were found, and the close collaboration between molecular and clinical geneticists led to rapid development of molecular diagnostic services. During this time computing developments enabled the development of both laboratory and clinical databases, facilitating both research and service applications.

As a clinically orientated medical geneticist I am not perhaps best placed to give a detailed analysis of the evolution of the laboratory aspects of medical genetics, but I should begin this attempt by stating that almost all of the key advances in the field have resulted from major developments in technology and in laboratory research. This has been true for other fields of medical science, too, such as medical biochemistry and haematology, but it is fair to say that medical genetics is one of the best examples of a 'hybrid specialty', where the close interaction between clinical and laboratory workers has benefited all concerned, not least the patients and families with genetic disorders.

This chapter focuses on the applied aspects of laboratory medical genetics, rather than on more basic research advances, some of which will be described in the following chapter. But it should be recognised that in this rapidly moving field, the boundary is a fluid one, with research techniques moving quickly into service applications and being adapted accordingly. Laboratory workers have moved frequently between research and service work, and major units have frequently contained groups involved in each. The dominant role of the National Health Service (NHS) in delivering medical genetics services in Britain, described in Chapter 8, has applied just as much to laboratory genetics services as it has to clinical genetics, in contrast to America and some other countries where private and commercial laboratories have been prominent in providing testing services as well as in the provision and development of equipment and reagents.

Since human chromosomes were the first area of laboratory medicine to make a significant impact on medical genetics, it is appropriate to start with them, and to indicate how clinical cytogenetics evolved from the early research described in Chapters 1 and 2 to become for many years the key laboratory service underpinning medical genetics as a whole. Table 10.1 shows some of the landmark advances involving human chromosomes up to the late twentieth century. Bangham and de Chadarevian (2014) give a valuable historical account of this period, while the close relationship to radiation risks is analysed by de Chadarevian (2006).

We saw in Chapter 1 how many of the first discoveries of chromosome abnormalities in human disorders came from Britain and France, with few American contributions initially. But this soon changed in the early 1960s, especially as the diagnostic possibilities increased. The fact that the co-discoverer of the correct human chromosome number, JH Tjio, had moved from Europe to Denver, Colorado stimulated the holding of the 'Denver Conference' on human chromosome nomenclature there in 1960, though the original idea had come from Charles Ford of Harwell (Denver Conference 1960). Of the three British participants, Charles Ford, Patricia Jacobs [06] and David Harnden [08] (out of a total of only 13), I was able to interview the last two, and the transcripts make it clear what a valuable, though at times difficult, process it was to obtain agreement on a nomenclature that inevitably meant that everyone had to give up part of their preferred system (Figure 10.1).

The convenor, Theodore Puck, has given a graphic account (1994), as has pioneer cytogeneticist TC Hsu (1979); I have tried to convey some of the atmosphere in my own earlier book *First Years of Human Chromosomes* (Harper, 2006). Fortunately, a unanimous agreement was eventually reached, as recounted by TC Hsu:

> The meeting lasted four days. Progress was made despite many heated disagreements. It was amazing to witness the emotional involvement over minute details..... The participants worked hard to reach a sensible, yet flexible, nomenclature system, and proceeded to write a report. The draft was read and reread, corrected and

Table 10.1 Laboratory landmarks in early human cytogenetics

Date	UK	Elsewhere
1949		Sex chromatin body discovered (Barr and Bertram)
1956		Correct human chromosome number determined (Tjio and Levan)
1959	First sex chromosome anomalies (XXY, Jacobs and Strong; XO, Ford et al.)	Trisomy 21 in Down syndrome (Lejeune, Gautier, Turpin)
1960	Trisomy 18 (Edwards syndrome) XXX syndrome (Jacobs) Use of cultured fibroblasts (Harnden)	Trisomy 13 (Patau syndrome) 'Philadelphia' chromosome in chronic myeloid leukaemia (Nowell and Hungerford) Chromosomes from peripheral blood culture using phytohemagglutinin (Moorhead)
1961	X chromosome inactivation (Lyon)	Denver nomenclature conference
1963		5p – (Cri du Chat) syndrome (Lejeune et al.)
1965	XYY syndrome (Jacobs)	4p – (Wolf-Hirschhorn) syndrome High frequency of chromosome anomalies in spontaneous abortions (Carr)
1967		Mouse-human cultured cell lines for human gene mapping (Weiss and Green)
1969	Hamerton's *Human Cytogenetics* (vol. 1)	Chromosome banding (Zech and Caspersson) Fragile X syndrome recognised (Lubs)
1970	Y chromosome specifically identified by fluorescence (Pearson; Bobrow)	In situ hybridisation using autoradiography (Pardue and Gall)
1971	Giemsa banding (Seabright)	
1977		de Grouchy and Turleau's *Clinical Atlas of Human Chromosomes*
1984	Meiotic chromosome studies (Hulten; Chandley)	
1991	Fluorescent in situ hybridisation (Malcolm et al.)	
1992	Chromosome painting (Ferguson-Smith)	Comparative genome hybridisation (CGH)

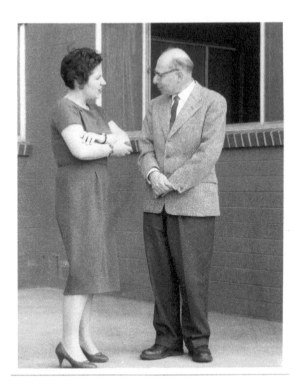

Figure 10.1 Patricia Jacobs and Curt Stern at the Denver Conference, 1960 (Courtesy of David Harnden.)

recorrected, and, by the afternoon of the third day, it was complete. The participants felt a sense of relief, as if a historic document was being written. Indeed it was; but thinking in retrospect, I could easily appreciate the difficulty of the American forefathers in arriving at the nation's constitution. Here we were worrying about how to name the 23 pairs of human chromosomes, not the welfare of the country and its people, yet it took three days to reach some agreement.'

Hsu 1979

The Denver nomenclature, shown in Figure 10.2a after incorporating the comments of TC Klaus Patau, who had not been present, stood the test of time well, largely because it gave rise to the International System for Cytogenetic Nomenclature (McGowan-Jordan et al. 2016), which revised it in the light of numerous technological developments and produced reports at regular intervals over the next 50 years (see Figure 10.2b).

Next the challenge was how to convert this exciting research into something that could be used clinically outside major research units. Top of the list was to

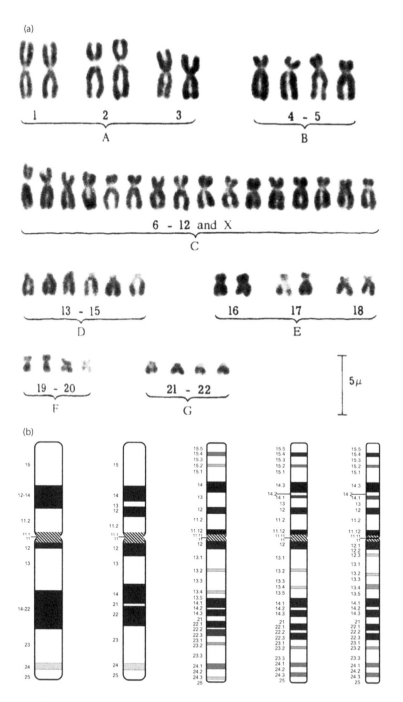

Figure 10.2 Chromosome nomenclature arising from the 1960 Denver conference and the establishment of the ISCN system. (a) The original Denver system incorporating comments by Klaus Patau. (b) ISCN half a century on. The 2009 version for Chromosome 11. (Courtesy Karger Publishers and Nicole Chia.)

find techniques that did not require invasive approaches. It is easy to forget that initially chromosome analysis depended on testicular biopsy or bone marrow analysis, neither of them comfortable procedures. Malcolm Ferguson-Smith's early Klinefelter work had depended on collaboration with a Glasgow urologist to provide testicular tissue from infertility patients, while Patricia Jacobs used bone marrow from leukaemia and other patients, taken using sternal puncture by clinician Michael Court Brown, head of the unit, which was not without its problems. As her technician Muriel Lee [12] remembers:

ML: I can remember so many times going there to the ward and he was taking it from the sternum and young nurses kept fainting. And I remember that quite clearly.
PSH: What about the patients, did they faint?
ML: No, the patients they were quite OK mostly. They were quite OK. They were flat on their backs and they couldn't really see what was happening so much.
PSH: No, and they couldn't faint if they were flat on their backs.
ML: Exactly. They were flat on their backs so that was quite... But many's the nurse I had to help off the floor.

A step in the right direction came when David Harnden [08] in Harwell and John Edwards [14], then in Birmingham, found that a small pinch biopsy of skin could produce cultured fibroblasts for chromosome analysis (Harnden 1960). Figure 10.3 shows Harnden's 'self portrait' using this technique, and many of the older generation of medical geneticists (myself included) still carry the small scars that form a permanent record of its use. It was quickly superseded for chromosome analysis when methods utilising peripheral blood were devised, but has remained useful in detecting mosaicism, as well as for the diagnosis of enzyme defects.

The finding that peripheral blood contained cells that could be induced to divide was a major advance. Originally discovered by Russian workers in the 1930s (Chrustschoff et al. 1931, Chrustschoff and Berlin 1935), but then 'forgotten' for almost 30 years, despite being published in a major Western journal, it was then reintroduced in 1960 by Moorhead et al. (1960) in America, with the mitotic stimulant phytohemagglutinin as the agent. When put together with the use of air drying and hypotonic solutions to spread chromosomes, this resulted in a simple and reliable technique that could be used diagnostically on large numbers of blood samples. It could also be used for research on populations, such as the Edinburgh studies of first adults and then newborns, pioneered by Patricia Jacobs and her colleagues, which gave the first accurate estimate of the true frequency of chromosome abnormalities (Brown et al. 1965, Ratcliffe et al. 1970); this is perhaps an appropriate point at which to emphasise the importance of Shirley Ratcliffe's longitudinal studies of an unselected cohort of sex chromosome anomaly patients followed from birth. The studies on spontaneous abortions, initially by Carr in Canada, showed how frequent non-viable chromosome defects were as a cause of these (Carr 1963).

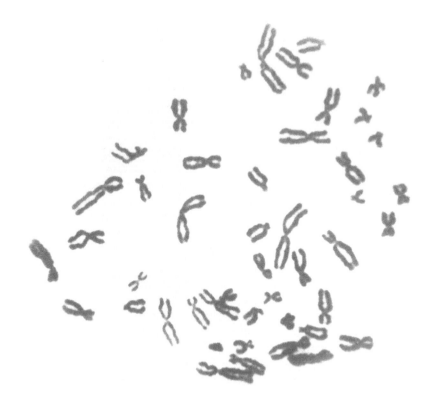

Figure 10.3 David Harnden's 'chromosomal self portrait' of cultured cells from a small skin biopsy (Courtesy of David Harnden.)

The next 10 years produced a wealth of data, and medical workers became accustomed to seeing photographs of mounted karyotypes in laboratory reports and in journal articles (particularly *The Lancet*), contributing to a steady rise in referrals of both samples and patients to genetic clinics, as much for interpretation and diagnosis as for genetic counselling. This decade of progress was well put together in the two-volume book by John Hamerton [21], *Human Cytogenetics* (Hamerton 1969, 1971), written just as he was leaving Britain for Winnipeg, Canada. This also marked the point at which the next major technological advance, chromosome banding, became part of clinical cytogenetics.

It is easy to forget that before 1970 most human chromosomes (including the X and Y) could not be individually distinguished but had to be placed in groups (A–G according to the Denver classification). The situation was radically transformed by the discovery of Lore Zech [28], working in Torbjorn Caspersson's laboratory in Stockholm, that quinacrine mustard staining techniques produced a banding pattern on fluorescence for human and other chromosomes that was unique for each chromosome (Caspersson et al. 1970, 1971). British workers, notably Peter Pearson and Martin Bobrow, in Stevenson's Oxford unit at the time, rapidly extended this work and also showed that the Y chromosome could be detected in non-dividing cells (Pearson et al. 1970), akin to the X chromatin body for females, already known for many years, having been discovered by Canadian workers as long ago as 1949 (Barr and Bertram 1949) [23].

As Martin Bobrow explains:

....we used quinacrine dihydrochloride, which was much easier to handle, and that made quite a big difference, because, although the banding probably in retrospect isn't as good, it was good enough and it was easy to use in the lab. It wasn't carcinogenic in the same way. So we introduced that, we made the observations, particularly Peter made the observations on interphase fluorescence, made observations on the meiotic process in man and looked at sex chromosome pairing, and then started working our way into the question of what these banding patterns might mean.

Interview with Martin Bobrow [24]

A further important advance, made by Marina Seabright of Salisbury (see Figure 3.26), was that the banding patterns could also be seen clearly and more stably after Giemsa staining (Seabright 1971), giving a technique that was much more suitable for routine diagnostic use.

The new techniques also allowed much smaller changes in chromosome structure to be recognised, so that a series of new chromosomal malformation syndromes could be defined when combined with careful clinical assessment. This work, much of which resulted from studies in the Paris laboratories of Lejeune and de Grouchy, was brought together in the classical book of de Grouchy and Turleau (1977), *Clinical Atlas of Human Chromosomes* (see the interview with Catherine Turleau [42]). It also became an important part of the development of the field of clinical dysmorphology, as described in Chapter 4.

By the early 1980s, after 20 years of unchallenged predominance as the laboratory basis for medical genetics, clinical cytogenetics had begun to settle down into a reliable and widespread medical service but had lost much of its impetus as a field of research, apart from in a few centres. Interestingly, in the UK, these were principally those of the original research cytogeneticists of the 1960s, including Patricia Jacobs, who returned from America in 1988 to succeed Marina Seabright in Salisbury, Malcolm Ferguson-Smith [03], who moved from Glasgow to Cambridge in 1987, and Peter Pearson, who had moved from Oxford to Leiden, as well as Maj Hulten [10], who had moved from Stockholm to Birmingham in 1974, where she continued to pioneer research on meiotic chromosomes, as also did Ann Chandley in Edinburgh. This small group of workers helped to form a bridge between the 'old' cytogenetics and the 'new' molecular genetics which was now starting to transform medical genetics as a whole, and to ease the somewhat difficult transition, described below.

First, though, it must not be forgotten that there were several important advances which cytogeneticists were responsible for during this period. Notable among these was the recognition of several disorders showing chromosome breakage as a cytogenetic finding, with cancer predisposition as a prominent feature. These included the recessively inherited Bloom syndrome and ataxia telangiectasia, the latter worked on extensively in Britain by David Harnden and Malcolm Taylor in Birmingham (Harnden 1994).

Cancer cytogenetics in general was also starting to progress again, after a long period of disappointment following the initial excitement of chronic myeloid leukaemia being associated with the 'Philadelphia' chromosome fragment, which was shown by the work of Janet Rowley, while in Oxford, to be the result of a translocation between chromosomes 9 and 22, involving the site of a specific oncogene (Rowley 1973). The renewed progress was mainly a result of the ability of banding techniques to distinguish the often complex patterns of rearrangement involving specific regions of individual chromosomes, and the coordination of the findings of different centres internationally through Felix Mitelman's *Cancer Chromosome Database* (both primarily Swedish achievements).

Following the development of chromosome banding, a later technique that would help to bridge cytogenetics and human molecular genetics was in situ hybridization, initially using autoradiography to detect radioactive probes for repetitive DNA sequences, by Pardue and Gall (1970) in America, then progressively refined to detect single copy sequences, using fluorescent rather than radioactive labels. Multiple probes allowed 'chromosome painting', pioneered by Malcolm Ferguson-Smith and colleagues, by now based in Cambridge; this proved especially useful in comparative cytogenetic studies of different species, where patterns of chromosome segment rearrangement could often indicate their evolutionary lineage. Ferguson-Smith (2015) has outlined the successive developments in this transition period.

A third area which would link cytogenetics with clinical molecular genetics at both service and research levels was the study of fragile sites, in particular fragile X syndrome. This condition had long been recognised clinically, first in 1943, by J Purdon Martin and Julia Bell, as a specific X-linked disorder causing mental handicap and some other distinctive features, but in 1969 Herbert Lubs, at that time in America, noted the association with apparent fragility of the terminal part of the long arm of the X chromosome. Initially searches for this in other patients with X-linked mental handicap proved negative, but after it was realised by Grant Sutherland [60] and others (Sutherland and Ashforth 1979) that the fragile site was only visible if specific culture media were used, it became clear that it was considerably commoner than thought originally to be the case, and that the inheritance pattern was unusual, with transmission through clinically normal males, not to be expected from an X-linked disorder. As molecular gene mapping and isolation advanced, a major international initiative developed, in part collaborative, in part competitive, which included several UK members including the laboratories of Kay Davies and Patricia Jacobs, while the original suggestion of a two-step process including a premutation, to explain the anomalous inheritance, came from Marcus Pembrey and Robin Winter in London (Pembrey et al. 1985). The final recognition of DNA instability as the underlying mechanism in this and a series of other disorders is described in the next chapter.

THE TRANSITION FROM MICROSCOPY TO MOLECULAR ANALYSIS

During the 20-year period from 1960 when human chromosomes formed the sole laboratory diagnostic aide for genetic disorders, they proved especially valuable in the recognition of a number of malformation syndromes and for prenatal diagnosis to detect or exclude these, but the great majority of mendelian or common multifactorial disorders showed no such abnormalities, even with the newer techniques, so that their diagnosis remained essentially clinical. During most of this time, even the idea that one might directly be able to detect mutations in specific single genes seemed implausible, though mendelian principles allowed accurate risks to be estimated for genetic counselling and 'empiric risks' were available for a number of common disorders (see Chapter 6).

Clinical cytogenetics had originated, as described earlier, from a long and distinguished tradition of microscopy, stretching back to the nineteenth century and even before. This was a tradition shared with much of general biology, including cell biology, and many human cytogeneticists began their careers as zoologists or botanists. The microscope was the central point around which cytogenetics as a discipline was focused and it had essentially changed very little in its general design apart from progressively increased resolution, though with numerous ancillary but important techniques such as those allowing spreading of chromosomes, mitotic arrest, chromosome banding techniques, photomicrography and automated analysis, some of which have already been described.

The microscope had also become the principal 'icon' for scientific research in genetics, both for people and for societies; eminent workers were normally photographed at their microscope (see Figures 2.4, 2.6, 12.1b), even if they might have long since ceased to use it, and it was a powerful symbol for scientific progress and for fund-raising. The major microscope manufacturers, such as Zeiss and Leitz, developed close associations with cytogenetics and supported scientific meetings and other activities, which also generated good custom intended for them. In the Edinburgh MRC Human Genetics Unit, there was considerable research into automated approaches to the analysis of cytogenetic images by Denis Rutowitz and colleagues.

It is not surprising then that considerable adjustment was needed, both practical and psychological, for laboratory workers in clinical cytogenetics, when the microscope was forced first to share, then to abandon its dominant position in the life and structure of medical genetics by the growing power of molecular genetics, nor that the transition should have been so protracted. The origins of the two fields have indeed been very different, though to a considerable extent complementary. Most early workers in human molecular genetics had a background in basic molecular biology, chemistry or biochemistry, with very few having microscopy expertise. This inevitably made the conversion of cytogeneticists into molecular geneticists difficult, sometimes impossible, especially for those NHS service– based workers whose entire career had been based on microscopy. The laboratory training programmes and the social networks of meetings and societies likewise were very different. As a result of these major differences the process of change must have felt at times more like a takeover than a progressive evolution.

Cytogeneticists fought a spirited rearguard action; the striking visual images that human chromosomes produced, especially when combined with molecular techniques, were also an advantage for them, being particularly convincing for non-scientists, in contrast to the small tubes and their invisible contents used by the molecular geneticists, which sceptics might be reluctant to accept really contained DNA! Fluorescent in situ hybridisation (FISH) provided a valuable field where the two could find common ground. In the end, the disciplines became satisfactorily fused, though only to be overtaken recently by automated and whole genome sequencing. De Chadarevian (2018) provides a historical perspective on the transition, while Ferguson-Smith (2006; 2015) documents the evolution of cytogenetics from the viewpoint of one who has taken part in the field of human cytogenetics from its beginnings. Jacobs (2014) has likewise given a vivid autobiographical account of her life and work in the field over the past 50 years.

It must be emphasised that while microscopy may no longer form the dominant part of laboratory genetic services, it remains important in the detection of chromosome rearrangements and is an essential part of research on the detailed three dimensional structure and function of chromosomes in the cell nucleus, especially in developmental genetics, as mentioned in Chapter 11.

HUMAN BIOCHEMICAL GENETICS

Before looking at human molecular genetics in more detail, it is important not to omit the field of human biochemical genetics, which had been developing steadily, though in relative isolation from the rest of medical genetics, during this time. Starting from Garrod's seminal work and ideas at the beginning of the twentieth century, the concept of 'inborn errors of metabolism' had extended with the discovery of enzymes and the recognition that many, indeed most mendelian metabolic disorders were due to defects or deficiencies in these. Crucial to this recognition was the Cambridge-based work of Frederick Gowland Hopkins and his colleagues, notably JBS Haldane, already mentioned, and Joseph Needham, whose work on the chemical basis of development complemented that of Waddington in Edinburgh. Needham's three-volume book *Chemical Embryology* (Needham 1931) contains a definitive history of the field up to 1930, though after 1940 he became, in his own words, 'seconded as it were to another universe' and embarked on the work over the next 50 years that would underpin his monumental *Science and Civilisation in China* (Needham 1954 et seq.). Haldane's prolific writing and incisive mind, as seen in his books *Enzymes* (1930) and *The Biochemistry of Genetics* (1954), helped to ensure that the new field of biochemistry did not drift too far away from genetics.

In the post-war years, a major British role in the area of inherited disorders was played by Charles Dent, strategically located at University College Hospital adjacent to Penrose's Galton Laboratory unit, facilitating links with such workers as Harry Harris and also Charles Scriver [56], whose subsequent work in Montreal was based on these London foundations. But in such landmark volumes as *The Metabolic basis of Inherited Disease*, edited originally by Stanbury, Wyngaarden and Fredrickson (1960) and subsequently by Scriver and colleagues (2001), it is clear that the majority of work in this field was now originating from America rather than from Britain. Likewise, if one looks at the series of volumes produced by the Society for the Study of Inborn Errors of Metabolism, mentioned in Chapter 9, most contributors have an affiliation to medical biochemistry rather than to medical genetics units.

Despite the close early links provided by the work of Garrod with Bateson, and then Haldane, Harry Harris and others, the field of inherited metabolic disease in Britain never developed the close links with medical genetics overall that characterised cytogenetics and later human molecular genetics, nor did it become part of the training or practice of medical genetics services to a significant extent, except in relation to prenatal diagnosis. In this it differs sharply from countries such as the United States, France and Australia, where medical geneticists are often closely involved in the diagnosis and management of these disorders. At the laboratory level, likewise, they have remained largely separate; as molecular techniques have been adopted for metabolic disorders they have tended to take their place alongside enzyme analysis, rather than to replace it.

HUMAN MOLECULAR GENETICS

While human cytogenetics began with the belated (1956) recognition of the human chromosome number, and advanced through being able to detect progressively smaller abnormalities, though still involving scores of genes, it remained largely a 'whole genome downwards' process. By contrast, human molecular genetics began essentially as a 'single gene upwards' approach, with the microscopically invisible individual gene as the focal point and a very different tradition, mainly derived from chemistry.

Although the establishment of the structure of DNA by Watson and Crick in 1953 preceded the recognition of the correct human chromosome number by several years, it actually had no significant immediate or practical effects on human and medical genetics (Olby 2003), nor did it greatly influence the thinking as to how these fields might develop. This was largely because the technology at the time, and for the next 20 years, gave no possibility of utilising in mammalian cells the microbial and biophysical approaches that had been so productive for simpler organisms in detecting the structure of DNA and the nature of the genetic code. By contrast, the move from establishing the normal human chromosome number to the initial medical applications of cytogenetics had required no significant change in technology.

The molecule that held the key to molecular biology entering the field of medicine generally and medical genetics in particular was haemoglobin, with its disorders the thalassaemias and other haemoglobinopathies. Numerous workers across the world have studied different aspects of its structure, function, pathology and genetics, but among UK contributors several stand out. First and foremost is Max Perutz, whose work begun in Cambridge during the 1930s, using x-ray crystallography to analyse its molecular structure, culminated 20 years later in its full amino acid sequence and arrangement. The phrase 'interrupted by the war' is especially apt for Perutz who, as a refugee from Nazi-controlled Austria, was interned and transported from Cambridge to the internment camp on the Isle of Man and then to Canada, as memorably told in his essay *Enemy Alien* (Perutz 1998). Perutz then collaborated with another refugee scientist, Herman Lehmann, in the study of different human variants of haemoglobin.

The UK leader of the next phase of research, understanding the mechanisms of molecular pathology of the two specific globin genes involved, was David Weatherall (see also Chapter 3 and Figure 3.24), using as the starting point patients with thalassaemias and other haemoglobinopathies encountered during his compulsory military service in the Far East. Ironically Lehmann had advised Weatherall not to base his research on haemoglobin;

> ....shortly after I got to Taiping I found a child with a fast moving haemoglobin and so I think I just wrote to him [Lehmann] and said could I send you a sample of this just to see if you agree, and after that I sent him one or two samples and then, when I finished in the army, I went dutifully to see the great man at Bart's [St Bartholomew's Hospital, London], who told me that I shouldn't continue in that field because there was nothing left to do, and should go and work on red cell enzymes, but he was very helpful. He was a delightful character.

> *Interview with David Weatherall [30]*

Working with biochemist John Clegg, initially in Baltimore but then in Liverpool and finally Oxford, Weatherall and Clegg were able to analyse first the synthesis of the globin chains, then the globin RNA, and finally the cDNA, which allowed direct study of the molecular basis of the various haemoglobinopathies, including the thalassaemias. Discovery of deletion of the alpha globin chains in the lethal newborn form of alpha thalassaemia was a particularly notable step.

Once the genes for globin had been isolated, it soon became clear that the range of molecular pathology was far greater than had been thought likely from previous protein studies, and disorders of haemoglobin became a paradigm for mendelian genetic disorders as a whole in illustrating the numerous possible types of defect at the molecular level. Weatherall expressed this in an interview with me, and in more detail in his influential book *The New Genetics in Clinical Practice* (1982)

PSH. I seem to remember at one point you said something along the lines that, almost all the abnormalities or what we have learned in the molecular basis of human disease had been based on the haemoglobin disorders, or at least could be, and there wasn't going to be much to learn once one went outside those. Do you think that is still a reasonable view or...?

DJW. No, I think that very exciting time in the late 70s early 80s, when these mutations were pouring out by the week, and you got this kind of whole spectrum, from regulatory mutations to what you'd expected from microbial genetics and so on, that it was going to be a reasonable kind of preview of what would turn up in other diseases. Perhaps I overstated it, but of course if you look at the totality of molecular pathology, OK, it didn't certainly disclose the kind of single gene neurological diseases with those boring extensive bits of DNA, and obviously there have been lots of other exciting molecular mechanisms, but I suppose what it did at the beginning, it showed the extraordinary diversity at the molecular level. I didn't do a countdown over time but within about four years or so, there had been about 60 different mutations found in the thalassaemias – there are now over 300!'

Interview with David Weatherall, 2004 [30]; see also Chapter 3 for details of Weatherall's life and links with Liverpool and Oxford.

In my 2004 interview, now 15 years ago, David Weatherall also emphasised the complexity of the molecular basis of monogenic disorders, voicing doubt as to whether the same approaches would work so well for common non-mendelian diseases. He was also sceptical on the feasibility of 'personalised medicine'.

So when I think of the gruesome complexities of monogenic disease and then transport that to common diseases, I have a problem. It seems to me that the epidemiologists and public health people, the W.H.O. has now got sensible targets for trying to reduce risk factors; nobody knows how successful that will be but it probably is worth tackling the genetics of multigenic disease, particularly where you haven't the faintest idea what the molecular pathology may be, just for hints.

...The genome hunt? Well I'm persuaded, particularly for the diseases where we haven't a clue still, that it really is worth a go and that that may give us some clues in the long term about the molecular pathology of diseases. That also could perhaps direct the pharmaceutical industry in the right direction. But given the enormous complexity of genotype and phenotype I think it will be a slow cutting away at those diseases, but as I say there may be some useful fallout. But the kind of broader picture of personalised medicine I would have thought very unlikely. Well very unlikely in the foreseeable future.

I do not know how far these views might have changed 15 years on, before Weatherall's recent death in 2018, but their cautious nature still seems to me well founded.

At the same time as David Weatherall was approaching the analysis of the globin genes from the starting point of protein and RNA structure, Robert (Bob) Williamson (Figure 10.4a, [61]), first in Glasgow and then in London, was using the new molecular cloning techniques to isolate their genomic DNA; this would lead to the more general application of these techniques to the many mendelian genetic disorders with no known defect at the protein level, and to the use of genetic linkage and positional cloning, as outlined below.

(a) (b)

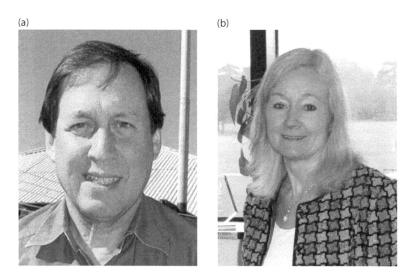

Figure 10.4 **(a)** Robert (Bob) Williamson (born 1938). Pioneer of molecular genetics in mapping and isolating human genes. (Photo courtesy of Royal Society, London. Recorded interview 09/08/2010 [61].) Bob Williamson was born in America to Scottish parents but lived in London from the age of 16, studying chemistry at University College London. Following his PhD he went to Glasgow in 1963 to work in molecular biology, particularly on the molecular basis of human haemoglobin and its disorders. In 1976 he moved to St Mary's School of Medicine, London and was responsible for the development and use of DNA polymorphisms in gene mapping, especially for cystic fibrosis and Duchenne muscular dystrophy. In 1995 he moved to Melbourne, Australia, as head of research at the Murdoch Institute, and later became Secretary of Science Policy to the Australian Academy of Science. **(b)** Kay Davies (born 1951), (recorded interview 22/02/2011 [80]) was born in Stourbridge, England, and after studying chemistry and biochemistry at Oxford University worked in Paris at Pasteur Institute. In 1980 she came to Bob Williamson's lab, where she was responsible for creation of the first X chromosome DNA library and for detection of the first genetic linkage for Duchenne muscular dystrophy to DNA markers. Moving to the Oxford Institute for Molecular Medicine in 1984, she has continued to work on neuromuscular disorders and on fragile X syndrome, among other conditions, and is now head of the Oxford Centre for Gene Function. (Photo courtesy of Kay Davies and Genetics and Medicine Historical Network.)

At the practical level these molecular studies on haemoglobin and its disorders led the way in allowing prenatal diagnosis, especially in the first trimester by chorionic villus sampling, as illustrated for thalassaemia in the interview with Bernadette Modell [70], quoted earlier in Chapter 5.

Among numerous contributions from America on haemoglobin, the work of YW Kan, related more to sickle cell disease than to thalassaemia, had a particular impact in showing how DNA based analysis could be used practically in prenatal diagnosis (Kan and Dozy, 1978). As Bob Williamson relates, most of the workers in the field came together at an intensive workshop in Crete in 1978, where:

> Y-W was talking on day 4 or day 5 and he didn't say a word until day 4 or 5 and then he described the critical linkage experiment, showing the polymorphism that's in linkage disequilibrium with haemoglobin S. And it was stunning and everyone realised the minute he said it exactly what it meant. There is a certain revisionism of history around this. A number of us, including David Weatherall and myself, went up to Y-W and just congratulated him. It was seriously, probably the most important thing I have heard in the whole of my scientific career. The Kan and Dozy paper explained it beautifully. Solomon and Bodmer realised, were the first to realise, the extent to which this allowed the superimposition of a genetic map and a physical map. And so-called reverse genetics, positional cloning, is really about the superpositioning of a genetic and a physical map on each other. And so all of a sudden, because of cloning, we had a very large number of positionally located sequences of which we could prepare large amounts and which we could distribute to one another and at the same time, we also had, we were beginning to develop the family resources, and the DNA resources to look at it. So Kan and Dozy really were the people who suddenly made the whole of genetics accessible to molecular technology through that one advance.

Interview with Bob Williamson [61]

At that point (around 1980) there were only a few other genetic disorders whose molecular basis was sufficiently well understood to allow the relevant gene to be isolated through knowledge of its protein and RNA. The next key step in human molecular genetics, probably the most important of all from the viewpoint of medical genetics, was the recognition of the abundant variation in DNA which could be identified by a combination of new techniques and which would lead in time to the isolation of most of the genes responsible for human mendelian disorders.

Most of these new techniques (Table 10.2) were first introduced in America, including the discovery and use of restriction enzymes and the polymorphisms

Table 10.2 New techniques in the development of human molecular genetics

USA
Restriction enzymes and RFLPs
DNA amplification in phage
Polymerase chain reaction (PCR)
Pulsed field gel electrophoresis
DNA libraries

UK
Southern blotting
Sanger sequencing
Chromosome sorting and chromosome specific DNA libraries
DNA fingerprinting

they could detect (RFLPs), the development of DNA 'libraries', the use of the polymerase chain reaction (PCR) to amplify DNA, and of pulsed field gel electrophoresis to isolate long stretches of DNA. But some were primarily UK inventions, notably Ed Southern's 'Southern' blotting and 'Sanger' sequencing (see Chapter 11), which would form the basis for DNA sequencing in the Human Genome Project, as well as for most clinically applied molecular genetic analysis, and which would win Frederick Sanger a second Nobel Prize. Automated chromosome sorting, devised by Bryan Young in Glasgow, would also play a valuable role in isolating chromosome specific DNA that could form the basis for isolating DNA sequences and RFLPs on the X chromosome, leading to the first DNA-based linkage for Duchenne muscular dystrophy by Kay Davies and Bob Williamson in London (Murray et al. 1982). The discovery of DNA fingerprinting by Alec Jeffreys is described further in Chapter 11.

The contributions of Bob Williamson's lab in attracting a large series of outstanding workers, some basic scientists and others with a clinical background, into the positional cloning of a wide series of disorders, cannot be overestimated. Many, including our own Cardiff unit, were based in medical genetics, as were others from across Britain and many other European countries, with the result that molecular genetics rapidly became an essential part of the laboratory basis of medical genetics as a whole and did not remain the domain of just a few large basic research institutes. This was aided by the fact that for positional cloning genetic linkage analysis was initially essential, and this in turn required resources of DNA from carefully studied families, both being factors that medical genetics centres were well positioned to provide. Bob Williamson's enthusiastic and inclusive approach was a key factor in boosting UK medical genetics research and bringing it into a world leading position for a wide range of disorders over the 1980s and early 1990s.

The profound and lasting effects of working in the Williamson lab are well illustrated in the interviews with two outstanding molecular geneticists, Kay

Davies and Gillian Bates, who worked there during the early years of their careers in the 1980s. First Kay Davies:

PSH: Can I ask you, what was it like working with Bob in those early years?

KD: It was manic because he had so much energy. I mean he'd start at 6 o'clock in the morning and just keep going. But the good thing was that you could walk into his office and say, 'I need a new lambda phage' or whatever it was to do the experiment, and by the afternoon he'd found someone who'd got it. And it might be in Cambridge; it might be in Edinburgh, but he was so well connected he could find a collaborator to do anything; so it was very enabling. He had lots of energy. And for Bob, everything was going to work; he was the eternal optimist.

PSH: I've always been amazed at, not just Bob's enthusiasm, but also at the number of really outstanding people who worked for a while with him, and whom he kind of launched off into their own careers, and have done fantastic things in their own right.

KD: It's an outstanding number, actually, but that's because once he lets you go, he doesn't ever let you go completely: he's ringing you up all the time, telling you what you should be doing next. And it's not just because I'm female; he does it to everybody. He does it with Pete Scambler and Brandon Wainwright, you know, and Brandon's in Australia, and Peter, as you know, is in GOS [Great Ormond Street Hospital] now. So he does it with everybody.

PSH: Yes.

KD: That's called extensive mentoring and it's incredibly useful. And he is forever saying... he never says you shouldn't do something, but he's always saying, 'Yes, you can do this. Try for this.'

Interview with Kay Davies [80]

The interview with Gillian Bates, best known now for her work on Huntington's disease (see Chapter 11) reinforces this:

PSH: It is amazing. There's a lot of people who have gone on to do great things, all in a way cut their teeth in that lab, even though, as you say, there wasn't a huge amount of what you might call direct supervision.

GB: I think it was being thrown in at the deep end. Bob was very inspiring and I think if you had potential then you could show it in Bob's system. So people who might not have necessarily excelled in the same way, found their capabilities. I mean I know that was true to a certain extent for me. I was terribly, terribly shy and terrified of giving talks. Bob would just throw you into things and then you found out you could do them. He also gave quite good advice too. Not necessarily experimental details, but how to give a talk and how to prepare yourself and go about things and build up your confidence. He was always telling us how good we were and that we would be running science. So for people he believed in and thought had potential, he was forever telling them not to under-sell themselves and I think that really was quite good.

Interview with Gillian Bates [57]

A further factor, mentioned by Bob Williamson himself in his interview [61], is generosity, in terms of allowing people to take their projects with them when they leave:

I'm very proud of the people who trained with me and where they have gone. It's a terrific bunch and they have done incredibly well. I think I am an enthusiast myself and if you are an enthusiast you attract enthusiasts. I love working with bright people and I'm reasonably good at spotting bright people. I commented already that I think that anyone who is a leader in this kind of area and in an advancing scientific field, has to combine this with generosity and the generosity in my case meant that many of these people actually took their projects with them.

Interview with Bob Williamson [61]

FROM GENE LINKAGE TO GENE ISOLATION

While mapping a disease-related gene with DNA markers gave immediate practical applications in genetic prediction, it gave no information in itself on the nature of the particular gene and on the defects involved in genetic disease, in contrast to the story told above for haemoglobin. Initially the progress from linkage to isolation of the gene itself was slow, taking 10 years intensive work by an international multi-group collaboration in the case of Huntington's disease. But where large scale gene deletions or rearrangements, at times involving several adjacent genes, were involved, the process could be speeded up. Clinical geneticists played an important role here in recognising rare patients with a combination of disorders, some of which had already been identified by chromosome studies as showing visible small deletions or translocations. New techniques such as pulsed-field gel electrophoresis for manipulating long sequences of DNA, and the detection of linkage disequilibrium, where association of the disorder with a particular allele of a DNA polymorphism indicated that the disease gene itself was adjacent, also helped.

The upshot was that during the 1990s and subsequently a series of important disease-related genes were actually isolated, finally allowing the molecular pathology of the many mendelian disorders that had previously been inaccessible and little understood to be analysed. This meant that these diseases now reached the point of understanding gene dysfunction at the protein level, which had been largely present from the beginning for disorders of haemoglobin, opening up new possibilities for downstream research on whatever systems were principally involved, be it muscle, brain or anything else.

A major difference between the disorders whose gene was isolated by positional cloning and those where a known protein was the starting point was that the workers involved usually had little or no clue until the very last minute what the nature of the protein defect might be. Having used DNA-based technology throughout the often prolonged positional cloning process, the emergence of the gene sequence could suddenly show that its role might be in any one of a number of quite different areas of cell biology; this might be one with already established techniques of its own and experienced scientists working in the area, or alternatively the gene sequence might give little or no indication of the protein's function. Either way the geneticists responsible for the gene isolation found themselves in a new world with difficult choices to make. Should they convert themselves into cell biologists in a strange area requiring a radical change of orientation, or confine themselves to the detailed analysis of the gene and its mutations?

A further practical consideration was that the technology involved in gene mapping and positional cloning was largely a shared one for all genes, so that it was possible to carry out the work for several genes, often in the same chromosomal region, in parallel. But these genes might, once isolated, point in totally different directions for work on their protein nature and function, so for most groups it was possible to follow this line for only one or a very few genes. Where promising avenues of research already existed at the protein level, funding bodies and lay societies often turned to groups with established research in the relevant field, so that those who had made this possible by isolating the gene might find themselves largely bypassed.

Such sudden changes are not new in the history of science and technology, but they have occurred repeatedly and at times unexpectedly in genetics; Huntington's disease provides an example where many of the investigators involved had to radically reshape their research strategies involved when the gene and mutation responsible were finally identified after the 10-year positional cloning effort to find the gene. Chapter 11 explores a few of these discoveries in more detail.

SERVICE APPLICATIONS OF HUMAN MOLECULAR GENETICS

The new linked DNA markers were rapidly brought into service use for a range of serious genetic disorders – perhaps too rapidly in the light of a significant error rate initially from recombination between marker and disease – but it should be remembered that these were conditions for which virtually nothing in the way of prediction could be offered previously.

As technology improved, and especially as linked markers steadily gave way to the detection of specific gene mutations, clinical molecular genetics emerged as a specific diagnostic and predictive specialty, rather than a by-product of research. As with cytogenetics 20 years before, this necessitated major changes in laboratory culture as well as in technology, with the need for quality control systems and standardised protocols to ensure high standards. Among the major changes in technology were the replacement of 'Southern blotting' by PCR-based methods and the development of automated sequencing techniques, based until recently on the method devised by Sanger, as mentioned above and in Chapter 11.

The first molecular genetics laboratories to be specifically funded by the NHS in Britain, as a pilot scheme in 1985, were all in major medical genetics centres (Manchester, Cardiff and London), not in wider pathology departments. This was not just because molecular techniques had not yet entered general laboratory medicine but because of the initial need to interpret genetic linkage data and also because of the close relationship with clinical geneticists for genetic counselling, in relation to presymptomatic testing and prenatal diagnosis in such disorders as Huntington's disease and Duchenne muscular dystrophy.

The Department of Health funded a parallel project to evaluate this development but, in the event, its delayed report was overtaken by the setting up of further service laboratories across Britain, again mostly in regional medical genetics centres, so that a pattern now emerged of clinical genetics, cytogenetics and molecular genetics all functioning as essentially a single overall service. The report of Meredith et al. (1988) provides an early example of molecular genetics in a NHS setting.

A problem soon arose, though, of duplication and relatively small numbers of individual tests in some centres. The obvious solution to this was to create a nationwide consortium to cover and share out the rapidly growing number of disorders for which testing was becoming possible. Indeed, this had already been done in Scotland, which set up the 'Scottish Molecular Genetics Consortium' in 1985, giving equitable population-wide access to the service, and maintaining a high quality. Plans were underway for a comparable initiative for the rest of Britain when political events intervened; a new government introduced an 'internal market' for health, one of the first examples of politicisation of health services affecting medical genetics, as discussed in Chapter 8. This was designed to encourage different centres across the country to compete with each other rather than to cooperate, quite opposed to the philosophy of those working in the field and making a consortium approach unworkable. It took more than a decade before this damaging policy could be overcome and a new 'UK Genetic Testing Network' created.

Over the subsequent years, clinical molecular genetics has become progressively more like other laboratory services and its use as a primary diagnostic tool has opened it up to clinicians generally, as described for Huntington's disease in Chapter 6. Its applications in prenatal diagnosis and in presymptomatic testing, though, have remained closely associated with clinical genetics. Now the question is to what extent will the advent of whole genome sequencing replace the analysis of individual genes or gene panels set up for particular conditions. Widespread reorganisation of English centres is already underway to achieve this, though it remains to be seen how effective this will be. The rapidly increasing overall impact of whole genome analysis on research and services is described in Chapter 12.

STATISTICAL GENETICS AND COMPUTER DATABASES

Readers may be surprised to find this section placed in a chapter devoted to laboratory aspects of medical genetics, but in fact the concept of what is a 'lab' has changed rapidly over the past 30 years; in the same way as the microscope has largely given way to molecular techniques, so these are increasingly becoming dominated by computer based and automated approaches. These radical changes in technology can pose challenges to workers in the field, but this is nothing new. The very concept of the 'wet lab' in genetics is relatively recent; thinking back historically, Thomas Hunt Morgan's 'fly room' consisted of large numbers of Drosophila which were bred, fed and counted, yet it generated experimental results; the same could be said of the mouse genetics of Fisher and others. For population geneticists and for many medical geneticists their 'lab' can be considered to be the living human populations that they study and provide medical services for, and which spontaneously generate mutations and a range of other genetic changes, some of which have been completely unsuspected from more basic experimental organisms.

A particularly striking example is Watson and Crick's model building that led to the elucidation of the structure of DNA, which met with some disdain from experimental x-ray crystallographic colleagues such as Maurice Wilkins and Rosalind Franklin, yet was the approach which led to the key final step. Was the Cavendish basement where Crick and Watson worked and built their models a 'lab'? As Max Perutz, himself a dedicated chemist and crystallographer, tellingly remarked, 'There are many ways of doing science.'

We have already seen that statistics was an integral part of early genetics, and this has been shown most notably in the field of human gene mapping (see Chapter 12). As computers became increasingly powerful, the small but always important group of mathematical and statistical geneticists were able to develop programmes that greatly extended the possibilities for genetic linkage analysis. This applied also to gene sequencing, where computer-based analysis was essential in underpinning the human genome project.

Databases of human gene and protein sequences have been invaluable resources for studying the likely function of human genes, as have databases such as the *Human Gene Mutation Database* (Cooper et al. 1998). The important principle of making these databases readily accessible, reinforced by the human genome sequence itself being in the public domain, means that these powerful tools are available, generally through the internet, to researchers across the world for their own particular areas of work.

These approaches have also greatly influenced more clinical areas too. Clinically orientated databases include the *London Dysmorphology Database* for the diagnosis and delineation of rare and new malformation syndromes (Winter and Baraitser 2001; see also Chapter 4), and the *Cancer Chromosome Database*, originated by Felix Mitelman of Lund, Sweden (Mitelman 1983). At a more day-to-day level, what used to be large and heavy printed volumes, such as Victor McKusick's *Mendelian Inheritance in Man* and Charles Scriver's *Metabolic Basis of Inherited Disease*, have become computer-based databases, though their continuous updating makes it difficult to use them as a historical source, by comparison with the successive printed editions. As Victor McKusick (2007) said of his own *Mendelian Inheritance in Man*, which went through 12 printed editions before becoming a purely online database:

> The historian in me regrets the loss of the archival function of the print edition.

A newcomer that is proving to be of major practical value for identifying the specific molecular and genomic basis of unidentified syndromes and developmental disability of unknown cause is the *DECIFER* database linked to the DDD project (see Chapter 11).

The largest of broader databases in Britain related to genetics is the *UK Biobank*, which records phenotypic and, increasingly, genetic and genomic data on around 500,000 individuals, mostly middle-aged adults, who when prospectively studied should yield valuable data on death and morbidity from major adult-onset diseases (Bycroft et al. 2018). This project got off to a shaky start, with criticism of lack of consultation and lack of clarity as to its aims (see Chapter 7), but the resulting delay was put to good use in remedying these faults, so that it now has a robust structure to handle both its scientific and ethical aspects. Genomic developments over the past decade mean that it is likely to provide valuable data on the determinants for common diseases, though, as noted in Chapter 12, its mainly Caucasian population base may limit its application to other populations. It is essentially a research resource rather than a day to day working tool.

Complementary to *Biobank* for childhood and early life, though smaller, is the *ALSPAC (Avon Longitudinal Study of Parents and Children)* database, founded by Jean Golding, and based on a cohort of around 15,000 children born in Bristol during 1991–1992, together with their parents. These children are now nearly 30 years old and, like *Biobank* for adults, are starting to form a valuable resource for the study of both environmental and genetic factors in childhood disease.

REFERENCES

Bangham J, de Chadarevian S. 2014. Human heredity after 1945: Moving populations centre stage. *Stud Hist Philos Biol Biomed Sci.* 47:45–49.

Barr ML, Bertram EG. 1949. A morphological distinction between the neurones of the male and female, and the nucleolar satellite during accelerated nucleoprotein synthesis. *Nature.* 163: 676–677.

Brown WM, Jacobs PA, Brunton M. 1965. Chromosome studies on randomly chosen men and women. *Lancet.* 2(7412):561–562.

Bycroft C, Freeman C, Petkova D. et al. 2018. The UK biobank resource with deep phenotyping and genomic data. *Nature.* 562:203–209.

Carr DH. 1963. Chromosome studies in abortuses and stillborn infants. *Lancet.* 2:603.

Caspersson T, Zech L, Johansson C. 1970. Differential binding of alkylating fluorochromes in human chromosomes. *Exp Cell Res.* 60:315–319.

Caspersson T, Lomakka G, Zech L. 1971. The 24 fluorescence patterns of the human metaphase chromosomes: Distinguishing characters and variability. *Hereditas*. 67:89–102.

Chrustschoff GK, Berlin EA. 1935. Cytological investigations on cultures of normal human blood. *J Genet*. 31:243–261.

Chrustschoff GK, Andres AH, Ilina-Kakujewa WI. 1931. Kulturen von blutleukozyten als methods zum stadium des menslichen karyotypus. *Anat Anz*. 73:159–168.

Cooper DN, Ball EV, Krawczak M. 1998. The human gene mutation database. *Nucleic Acids Res*. 26(1):285–287.

de Chadarevian S. 2006. Mice and the reactor: The 'genetics experiment' in 1950s Britain. *J Hist Biol*. 39:707–735.

de Chadarevian S. 2018. Whose turn? Chromosome research and the study of the human genome. *J Hist Biol*. 51:631–655.

de Grouchy J, Turleau C. 1977. *Atlas des Maladies Chromosomiques* [*Clinical Atlas of Human Chromosomes*] 1st edn., Wiley, New York, 2nd edn 1984.

Denver Conference. 1960. A proposed standard system of nomenclature of human mitotic chromosomes. *Lancet*. 1:1063–1065.

Ferguson-Smith MA. 2008. Cytogenetics and the evolution of medical genetics. *Genet Med*. 10(8):553–559.

Ferguson-Smith MA. 2015. History and evolution of cytogenetics. *Mol Cytogenet*. 8:19. doi: 10.1186/s13039-015-0125-8. eCollection 2015.

Haldane JBS. 1930. *Enzymes*. London: Longman's, Green and Co.

Haldane JBS. 1954. *The Biochemistry of Genetics*. London: George Allen and Unwin.

Hamerton J. 1969; 1971. *Human Cytogenetics (vols 1 and 2)*. New York: Academic Press.

Harnden DG. 1960. A human skin culture technique used for cytological examination. *Brit J Exper Pathol*. 41:31–37.

Harnden DG. 1994. The nature of ataxia-telangiectasia: problems and perspectives. *Int J Radiat Biol*. 66(6 Suppl):S13–S19.

Harper PS. 2006. *First Years of Human Chromosomes*. Oxford: Scion Press.

Hsu TC. 1979. *Human and Mammalian Cytogenetics: An Historical Perspective*. New York: Springer-Verlag.

Jacobs PA. 2014. An opportune life: 50 years in human cytogenetics. *Annu Rev Genomics Hum Genet*. 15:29–46.

Kan Y-W, Dozy AM. 1978. Antenatal diagnosis of sickle-cell anaemia by DNA analysis of amniotic-fluid cells. *Lancet*. 2:910–912.

Lubs HA. 1969. A marker X chromosome. *Am J Hum Genet*. 21(3):231–244.

McGowan-Jordan J, Simons A, Schmid M (eds.). *ISCN 2016: An International System for Cytogenomic Nomenclature*. Basel: Karger.

McKusick VA. 2007. *Mendelian Inheritance in Man* and its online version, OMIM *Am J Hum Genet*. 80:588–604.

Meredith AL, Upadhyaya M, Harper PS. 1988. Molecular genetics in clinical practice: Evolution of a DNA diagnostic service. *BMJ*. 297:843–846.

Mitelman F. 1983. *Catalog of Chromosome Aberrations in Cancer*. Basel: Karger.

Moorhead P, Nowell P, Mellman W, Battips D, Hungerford D. 1960. Chromosome preparations of leukocytes cultured from human peripheral blood. *Exp Cell Res.* 20:613–636.

Murray JM, Davies KE, Harper PS, Meredith L, Mueller CR, Williamson R. 1982. Linkage relationship of a cloned DNA sequence on the short arm of the X chromosome to Duchenne muscular dystrophy. *Nature.* 300:69–71.

Needham J. 1931. *Chemical Embryology*, vols. 1–3. Cambridge: Cambridge University Press.

Needham J. 1954. *Science and Civilisation in China*, vol. 1. Cambridge: Cambridge University Press.

Olby R. 2003. Quiet start for the double helix. *Nature.* 421:402–405.

Pardue ML and Gall JG. 1970. Chromosomal localization of mouse satellite DNA. *Science.* 168:1356–1358.

Pearson PL, Bobrow M, Vosa CG. 1970. Technique for identifying Y chromosomes in human interphase nuclei. *Nature.* 226:78–80.

Pembrey ME, Winter RM, Davies KE. 1985. A premutation that generates a defect at crossing over explains the inheritance of fragile X mental retardation. *Am J Med Genet.* 21(4):709–717.

Perutz MF. 1998. Enemy alien. In: Perutz MF. 2003. *I Wish I'd Made You Angry Earlier: Essays on Science, Scientists and Humanity*, 2nd edn. Cold Spring Harbor, NY: Cold Spring Harbor Laboratory Press, pp. 73–106.

Puck TT. 1994. Living history biography. *Am J Med Genet.* 53:274–284.

Ratcliffe SG, Stewart AL, Melville MM, Jacobs PA, Keay AJ. 1970. Chromosome studies on 3500 newborn male infants. *Lancet.* 1(7638):121–122.

Rowley JD. 1973. A new consistent chromosomal abnormality in chronic myelogenous leukaemia identified by quinacrine fluorescence and Giemsa staining. *Nature.* 243:290–293.

Seabright M. 1971. A rapid banding technique for human chromosomes. *Lancet.* 2:971–972.

Scriver CR, Beaudet AL, Sly WS, Valle D (eds.). 2001. *The Metabolic and Molecular Bases of Inherited Disease*, 8th edn. New York: McGraw-Hill.

Sutherland GR, Ashforth PL. 1979. X-linked mental retardation with macro-orchidism and the fragile site at Xq 27 or 28. *Hum Genet.* 48(1):117–120.

Stanbury JB, Wyngaarden JB, Fredrickson DS (eds.). 1960. *The Metabolic Basis of Inherited Disease.* New York: McGraw-Hill.

Weatherall DJ. 1982. *The New Genetics and Clinical Practice.* London: The Nuffield Provincial Hospitals Trust.

Winter RM, Baraitser M. 2001. Oxford Medical Databases: London Dysmorphology Database Version 3.0. London Neurogenetics Database Version 3.0. Dysmorphology Photo Library on CD-ROM Version 3.0 http://dx.doi.org/10.1136/jmg.39.10.782-b. Oxford: Oxford University Press.

11

Discovery and research

ABSTRACT

Since the very beginnings of medical genetics, Britain has been in the forefront of the field internationally, and it remains so. Many of the important pre-war advances in human genetics, largely theoretical but often founded on clinical data, were British in origin, while most of the initial post-war developments in cytogenetics likewise came from Britain. During the second half of the twentieth century, which can be considered as the 'classical' period of medical genetics, a steady flow of discoveries, many by basic scientists in fields other than genetics, flowed into medical genetics research and also allowed new genetic services to develop. This is continuing as the field moves into a new 'genomic' phase following completion of the Human Genome Project. Close collaboration between disciplines and internationally has been a prominent feature of all this work. This chapter looks at just a few of the many research advances involving medical genetics in Britain; collectively and individually they show a remarkable array of talent, ingenuity and originality, as well as a mostly stable and responsible research governance by the funding bodies involved, such as Medical Research Council, Wellcome Trust and other major medical charities.

Of all areas of science and medicine, there can be none where research and application are closer together and more rapid than in medical genetics. In recent years the discovery of a disease-related gene has frequently enabled new applications that were previously quite impossible – Huntington's disease provides a good example for accurate diagnosis and prediction – while areas for future research are immediately opened up by the gene isolation for further study of the mutations and protein involved. Indeed, one of the increasing roles of medical geneticists in recent years has been to caution against over-hasty applications, particularly in an age when communication via the internet is virtually instantaneous, and with patients and lay societies understandably eager for progress. Outside the medical field, discoveries like DNA fingerprinting have also immediately been used in areas such as forensic science and paternity testing, as described below.

Most advances, in genetics as in other areas of science, are incremental in nature, resulting from a series of small steps made by a number of individuals or groups. But from time to time an important discovery occurs, either a new technology or a finding with a major medical or biological impact, which stands out from the general background of progress and gives us a new level of understanding.

It is difficult to single out British contributions from others in this process. Not only are most discoveries strongly collaborative internationally, but many outstanding British workers making the discoveries have been born or have had their early careers elsewhere; the refugees from fascism in the 1930s have already been mentioned, while the European Union and its major collaborative scientific programmes are a more recent example of the benefits Britain has received from the fluidity of boundaries, something sadly in the process of being damaged as I write.

Taking the field of medical genetics in its broadest and most inclusive sense, key contributions have come from an exceptionally wide range of workers; many have been from basic scientists rooted in disciplines other than genetics, while at a clinical level a wide range of medical specialties have been involved, as we have seen in Chapter 4.

Whatever one's viewpoint, it is indisputable that British scientists, both laboratory and clinically based, have had a pre-eminent role in this progress; in this chapter I focus principally on some of the people whom I have interviewed, in the hope that their role in this remarkable period of the past half century will be remembered and fully acknowledged. Table 11.1 summarises just a few of the major landmarks in an approximately chronological form; some receive more detailed mention in other chapters, as indicated in the table. The 'timeline' given in Appendix 1 attempts to place these and other discoveries in the context of the worldwide development of the field.

Table 11.1 is divided into four sections, corresponding to different, though overlapping, periods of genetics as related to medicine.

The early years of genetics generally, as we have seen, involved medicine conspicuously, and provided a firm foundation for later developments in human and medical genetics. Discoveries such as the first human genetic linkage (Bell and Haldane 1937), the first measurement of a human gene mutation rate – Haldane again (Haldane 1935), and the recognition of the potential application of linkage to genetic prediction and life insurance (Fisher 1935) are all examples of the forward thinking of geneticists in Britain at this time, especially those based at or around University College, London discussed in Chapter 1, such as Haldane, Fisher, Julia Bell, Hogben and later Penrose. Much of their work and ideas must have circulated freely among this talented group and it is remarkable what they achieved, given that they had almost no experimental techniques available to them. Even at that early stage it was clear that data on patients and families with genetic disorders, provided that it was collected and analysed properly,

Table 11.1 Some landmarks in British medical genetics-related research

The early years

1937. First human genetic linkage: haemophilia and colour blindness (Bell and Haldane 1937).

1938. Lionel Penrose's 'Colchester Study' on the causes of mental handicap.

1946. Chemical mutagenesis by nitrogen mustards shown by Charlotte Auerbach; the discovery remained unpublished during the war (Auerbach and Robson 1946).

Post-war medical genetics

1951, 1954. First autosomal genetic linkages (Mohr; Renwick and Lawler) (Chapter 12).

1953. Dietary treatment of phenylketonuria (Bickel et al. 1953).

1953. Structure of DNA (Watson and Crick 1953). (This has been included here as a reference point. It would be stretching matters to claim this work as related specifically to medical genetics!)

1956. Molecular structure of haemoglobin completed by Max Perutz and colleagues.

1959. First human chromosome abnormalities (Edinburgh, Harwell, London) 1959–1960 (see Chapter 2).

1960. Prevention of Rhesus haemolytic disease by Clarke and colleagues, Liverpool.

1960s. Ultrasound in amniocentesis (Donald, Glasgow) (Chapter 5).

1971. X-chromosome inactivation (Mary Lyon, Harwell).

1973. Neural tube defect prenatal diagnosis; raised AFP (Brock et al. Edinburgh).

1978. AFP screening for neural tube defects (Brock et al. Edinburgh).

1991. Folic acid conclusively shown to prevent neural tube defects.

Human molecular genetics in medicine

1976. Molecular basis of haemoglobin disorders (Lehmann; Weatherall).

1981. First linkage by DNA markers (Duchenne muscular dystrophy) (Davies; Williamson).

1990. Sex determination and the Y chromosome; isolation of the SRY gene (Goodfellow).

1991–1993. Unstable DNA; first trinucleotide repeat mutations (fragile X, myotonic dystrophy, HD).

1995. Isolation of *BRCA2* gene (Institute of Cancer Research, London).

The genomic era

2000. 'First draft' of human genome sequence (UK contribution led by John Sulston) (Chapter 12).

2010–2017. First use of whole genome (initially exome) sequencing for diagnosis of rare disorders and non-specific mental handicap. The Deciphering Developmental Disorders (DDD) study.

could provide information on basic biological processes which was difficult or impossible to obtain from other species.

The second period, occupying most of the second half of the twentieth century, may, with hindsight, be looked on as the 'classical age' of medical genetics and laid the foundations both for genetic services and for research leading to the understanding and prevention of many genetic disorders.

The third period, which in Table 11.1 is termed 'human molecular genetics in medicine', dates from around 1980 with the elucidation of the molecular pathology of haemoglobin disorders, extending over the following decade, thanks to positional cloning, to the great majority of mendelian conditions.

For those who, like myself, have been privileged to witness and contribute to this phase, it still seems extraordinary that we have moved from a position of near total ignorance to one of widespread (even though far from complete) understanding of many major genetic conditions over the span of a single professional lifetime. Finally, since completion of the human genome project at the turn of the century, we are seeing a succession of major discoveries based on this, though so far only a few have had significant practical applications in medicine.

I can only give a few examples here from these different periods, though others are mentioned in various other chapters. Hopefully they will give a flavour of their importance and of the skills and ingenuity of the workers involved.

DIETARY TREATMENT OF PHENYLKETONURIA

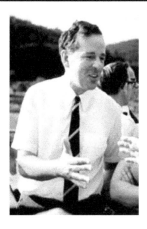

Figure 11.1 Horst Bickel (1918–2000), originator of dietary treatment for PKU while working in Birmingham UK, who later returned to work in Germany. (Courtesy of Deutsche Interessen-gemeinschaft Phenylketonurie und verwandte angeborene Stoffwechselstörungen e.V.)

1953 is a year most often remembered scientifically for the discovery of the structure of DNA, but it also marks another landmark UK discovery, the first successful treatment for a serious genetic disorder, phenylketonuria, by restricting the quantity of phenylalanine in the diet (Bickel et al. 1953). This took the form of clinical assessment following a largely phenylalanine-free diet, first at home, then in hospital, along with measurement of blood phenylalanine levels, with clinical progress closely correlated with the fall in blood phenylalanine, even though the affected child was already over two years old. The study was carried out by paediatrician Horst Bickel (1918–2000), originally from Germany, who was then working at Birmingham Children's Hospital (Figure 11.1), and is a good example of the value of carefully undertaken clinical research.

Scientifically this report may not seem particularly impressive, being based on a single patient, but it had major consequences; notably, phenyketonuria became a prototype for newborn screening, now that there was an effective therapy. It also helped to dispel the previously widespread view that genetic disorders were necessarily untreatable.

PREVENTION OF RHESUS HAEMOLYTIC DISEASE

This represents one of the earliest and most dramatic examples of population prevention for a severe, often fatal genetic disorder, resulting from a maternal-fetal interaction; indeed, so completely has the condition disappeared that it is in danger of being forgotten by those involved in wider medical genetics. The story has many fascinating elements, including the central role of an investigator, Cyril Clarke of Liverpool (see Chapter 2), who was also a practicing physician, as was his research fellow, Ronald Finn; Clarke collaborated closely with geneticists mainly involved with other species (notably Philip Sheppard, zoologist), but also with blood group geneticists (Race and Sanger), immunologists and obstetricians. The different transatlantic approaches to the field are also interesting – the Liverpool group used volunteers from the local police force for the initial experimental immunisation with anti-RhD antibody, whereas their American counterparts used prisoners!

The key paper of the Liverpool group concludes:

> Our results show quite conclusively that the administration to Rh-ve male volunteers of 10 ml of a particular anti-D has, firstly, coated a good proportion of previously injected Rh-positive cells and, secondly, as judged by radioactive tagging, caused the elimination of at least 50% of them in two days. These results are very encouraging, … [they] suggest that it may be possible to prevent most cases of Rh sensitisation, and thus in time eliminate Rh haemolytic disease.

> *From Finn et al. 1961*

Events were to prove that this prediction not only was correct, but that it would be more complete and more rapid than even the optimists could have hoped for.

Fortunately Clarke (1975) has brought together in a single volume all the key papers on the topic across the world, including the first recognition of the disorder, its pathology and immunology, as well as the key steps in its prevention, beginning in 1960, which led to its almost total elimination across most of the world within a decade. A later Witness Seminar (Zallen et al. 2004) provides personal accounts by some of those involved.

NEURAL TUBE DEFECTS: ENVIRONMENTAL FACTORS, GENETICS AND PREVENTION

Anencephaly and spina bifida, the most frequent forms of neural tube defect, have been a major challenge and topic for research by those in medical genetics since the 1950s. Rather than being a single isolated discovery, advances have come from a series of workers ranging into the allied fields of epidemiology, malformation pathology, paediatrics and nutrition. The exceptionally high frequency of the condition across much of Britain (not forgetting Ireland) by comparison with America and much of continental Europe, along with marked regional variations, prompted a search for environmental factors, but family studies, initially by Cedric Carter and Michael Laurence [13] in South Wales (Carter et al. 1968) and by Norman Nevin [26] in Belfast (Elwood and Nevin 1973), among others, showed that genetic factors were relevant too, though ruling out any clear mendelian pattern. John Edwards (1961), working with McKeown and Record in Lancelot Hogben's Birmingham unit, had already noted seasonal variation, while all studies found a marked association with deprivation and poor nutrition, the frequency being highest in the poorer parts of the country.

Norman Nevin's description of neural tube defects in Northern Ireland makes clear the extent of the problem and the contrast with the situation today:

NN: But the big challenge really coming back to Northern Ireland was the situation with neural tube defects. We had, from early work that I was doing, we had a prevalence of 1 in 100 babies born either with anencephaly or spina bifida, indeed like South Wales we had one of the highest incidence in the United Kingdom and indeed in the world, so that was a big challenge. So one of the first things I started to do, having had the experience with Cedric Carter collecting pedigrees and documenting the information, was to carry out first of all an epidemiology study. How common were these problems?

Now the advantage of Northern Ireland is a population in those days of 1.5 million and very good records. The children with spina bifida who would eventually have to have surgery would have to come to the one paediatric hospital for surgery. Children born with neural tube defects, there are only about 5 major obstetric hospitals and I had good liaison with all the people there, so we did a very good ascertainment of the neural tube defects and then we moved into the study of the families and we collected pedigrees of all these families and then published them to try and work out what were the recurrence risks of neural tube defects. In those days, that was the early seventies, we were having families with 3 and 4 children with neural tube defects and today we just don't see that at all. It is one of the very positive developments that has come out from clinical genetics.

PSH: Did you find a lot of stratification? I'm thinking again, the South Wales situation was that up the valleys, where there was a lot of deprivation, again there was a frequency of up to 1%, whereas in Cardiff and some of the more prosperous areas, much lower. Did you find those same differences, or was it more widely spread?

NN: No, I found exactly the same sort of differences, because I can remember that taking the data and looking at them in terms of what was the old registrar general's social classification 1–5, and when you break into that stratification there is no doubt that social classes 4 and 5 had the highest incidence of neural tube defects, whereas social classes 1 and 2 had the lowest incidence of neural tube defects. So quite clearly in those early days there was evidence that in the underprivileged areas of poverty, you had the highest prevalence of those abnormalities.'

Interview with Norman Nevin [26], 2004

Suspicion had rested on folic acid deficiency during pregnancy from the time of an early but non-significant trial in South Wales by Michael Laurence, but was only fully proven after a multicentre trial, coordinated by the MRC (MRC Vitamin Study Research Group 1991), confirmed a marked reduction in birth frequency of neural tube defects with preconceptional folate supplementation; an earlier trial of multivitamins based on the work of Smithells in Leeds (Smithells et al. 1980) was also successful but unable to distinguish which was the key agent.

In the meantime, the studies of David Brock and colleagues in Edinburgh during the mid 1970s had allowed prenatal diagnosis from raised alphafetoprotein levels in amniotic fluid (Brock and Sutcliffe 1972), followed by a combination of maternal blood AFP screening (Brock et al. 1974) and ultrasound detection as described in Chapter 5. As a result of these advances, neural tube defects are now relatively uncommon as a cause of malformations in both live births and in early pregnancy, and might be even rarer if the government were to improve the diet with supplementary folate in flour. (It finally approved this in 2018 after more than 30 years delay!)

The story of the successful prevention of neural tube defects, like that of rhesus haemolytic disease before it, provides a good example of the cross-disciplinary thinking and working that has been a strength of UK medical genetics since its beginnings, in this case involving workers in epidemiology, paediatrics, pathology and biochemistry, from different centres across Britain, in close cooperation with each other, as well as with medical geneticists.

X CHROMOSOME INACTIVATION

This provides a story where the flow of knowledge occurred mainly, at least initially, in the opposite direction, from basic experimental science to clinical consequences. The early (1949) studies of Canadian anatomists Barr and Bertram (see interview [23]) on the sex chromatin of cat neurones (Barr and Bertram 1949) had already had considerable significance for the understanding of human sex chromosome anomalies, so that by the end of the 1950s it was clear that the 'sex chromatin body' was a condensed X chromosome, but it was the work of Mary Lyon (Figure 11.2) at Harwell (interview [18]) on X-linked coat pigmentation genes in mice which formed the basis of her hypothesis (Lyon 1961) that all females (at least in placental mammals) are mosaics for the X chromosome at the cellular level, with inactivation randomly distributed, and permanent in any

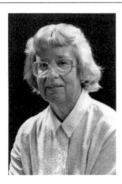

Born in Norwich, England, Mary Lyon attended Cambridge University during the war years, and after graduating, earned a PhD there with RA Fisher on mouse mutants. Her particular interest in developmental genetics led her to move to Edinburgh after the war to work with Conrad Hal Waddington on radiation genetics, where she encountered X-linked mouse mutants. In 1955 the mouse genetics group moved to Harwell to join the new MRC Radiobiology Research Unit (now the Mammalian Genome Unit) and Mary Lyon remained there for the rest of her life.

Figure 11.2 Mary Lyon (1925–2012). Recorded interview 11/10/2004 [18]. (Photo courtesy of Mary Lyon.)

somatic cell lineage once established in early embryonic life. This provided an immediate solution to the puzzling phenomenon that heterozygotes for most X-linked disorders showed a variable degree of expression of the condition.

Mary Lyon, a notably quiet-spoken and laconic person, describes this in a later (2010) interview with Jane Gitschier, who was able to draw her out more than I had in my own interview [18] with her:

Gitschier: When did you first start having this idea about the X chromosome inactivating?

Lyon: I was still studying the mutants that we had found in mutagenesis experiments. We found quite a number of mottled [mutants], and they weren't all the same. In some the affected males die as embryos; in others they are born and have white coats. The females were variegated. And I found one in which the original animal of this particular mutant was a mottled male, which was odd because males have got only one X chromosome. So why was he mottled?

So we bred from it to find whether the mottled pattern was inherited. This mouse had some daughters who looked like himself and he also had normal daughters and normal sons. So his mottled appearance was inherited. When we bred from his affected daughters, they bred as the previous mottled mutants that had been found. That is they had mottled daughters, like themselves, and also affected males, which died. So the females were behaving like ordinary mottled mice with a mutant gene on their X chromosome.

But we still had the question of the original mottled male mouse. How did he get to be mottled? Then it occurred to me that he had a mutation that had occurred in him, when he was just an embryo, when he was just a few cells, and that gave rise to one progeny group of cells with a mutant X chromosome and another group of cells with the unmutated, normal X chromosome. So this original mutant male was a mosaic of two types of cells, some with the mutated X chromosome and others with the normal X chromosome.

So then, it occurred to me that if that explanation of him having two types of cells applied to his pattern, could it not also apply to the pattern of his daughters? His daughters could have two types of cells, one with the mutant gene active and one with the normal gene active.

And that involved me in finding out about recent work on the mammalian X chromosome. One important point was that XO mice are normal fertile females, and thus a female mouse needs only one X chromosome for normal development. Furthermore, female mammals have the sex chromatin in their nuclei, and, just recently before that time, Ohno had found that the sex chromatin consisted of one highly condensed X chromosome.

So the female mouse only needs one X chromosome, and in female mice the X chromosome behaves strangely. So I put all those things together and came up with the idea of X-chromosome inactivation.

Gitschier: Before you read the literature and pieced all this together, did you already have the idea that in females only one X was active?

Lyon: Yes.

Gitschier: These mice that you are referring to: were they also the product of radiation?

Lyon: No, the original male was a spontaneous mutant.

Gitschier: Do you remember the year that original male appeared?

Lyon: 1959 or 1960.

Gitschier: You published your paper in 1961, so the pieces of the puzzle must have very quickly fallen into place. And do I take it that X-inactivation is also playing a role in the Tabby mutant?

Lyon: The striped pattern in Tabby females is indeed due to X-inactivation. It is not due to differences in pigmentation of the coat but to differences in hair texture. Tabby males have an obviously abnormal coat, which looks too sleek. Females have patches of this abnormal hair and where the patches of mutant and normal hair meet, one sees a stripe. The sizes and shapes of patches and stripes in heterozygotes for different X-linked genes depend on the way that the cells underlying the patches migrate and mingle during development.

An interesting example concerns the tortoiseshell cat. The pattern is produced by cells giving black or yellow pigment. If the cat has an autosomal gene for white spotting, patches of black and yellow are larger. This is because the spotting gene reduces the number of pigment cells and hence each precursor cell must cover a wider area and hence produces a larger patch.

From Gitschier J 2010. Speaking of Genetics: A Collection of Interviews. Cold Spring Harbor, New York: Cold Spring Harbor Laboratory Press. Quoted courtesy of Dr Jane Gitschier.

This recognition at once explained many of the long-standing puzzles surrounding human X-linked diseases, notably the variability of expression in heterozygotes, which had made the reliable detection of carriers so difficult. Not until the direct analysis of DNA became feasible would it become possible fully to overcome this problem (see Chapter 10).

In fairness to American workers and readers it should be said that the phenomenon of X-inactivation was also discovered independently by Ernest Beutler in California, by measuring enzyme levels in human females heterozygous for G6PD deficiency and showing that two populations of red blood cells existed for this, one deficient and the other with normal levels (Beutler et al. 1962).

DNA SEQUENCING

The ability to sequence DNA owes much to the inventive mind of Fred Sanger (Figure 12.3), based in the Cambridge Laboratory for Molecular Biology, who had earlier already won a Nobel Prize for sequencing the amino acid structure of a protein, insulin. Although a basic scientist without direct clinical links, his work, like that of his Cambridge Laboratory of Molecular Biology colleague Max Perutz on haemoglobin, has had profound effects later on clinical molecular genetics services as well as on molecular research generally.

Sanger's 'dideoxy' sequencing approach to nucleic acid sequencing (Sanger et al. 1977) involves the use of modified chain terminating nucleotides that are labelled by radiation or fluorescence to give DNA fragments which can be separated by electrophoresis. Separate use of each of the four modified nucleotides gives a 'ladder' pattern for A, T, G and C.

The method's value for human genes was first shown by the sequencing of the human mitochondrial genome (Anderson et al. 1981) – 16,569 DNA base pairs, by comparison with other studies sequencing just a few dozen before Sanger began work on the problem.

Not only was this method the basis of most of the DNA sequencing involved in the Human Genome Project, but it has also allowed sequencing of specific individual genes to identify pathological mutations, with automated modifications progressively simplifying and accelerating the work for clinical molecular genetics laboratories across the country (Figure 11.3).

Sanger's practical and 'down-to-earth' approach to science is well illustrated by his statement that:

Of the three main activities involved in scientific research, thinking, talking and doing, I much prefer the last and am probably best at it. I am all right at the thinking, but not much good at the talking.

(a) 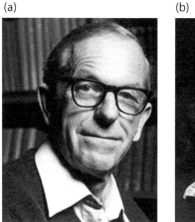 (b)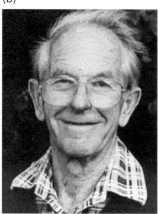

Figure 11.3 Frederick Sanger (1918–2013). Formal and informal views of a double Nobel Prize winner. **(a)** (Courtesy Torinosciencia.) **(b)** (Courtesy 'DNA from the beginning', dnaftb.org.)

Born into a medical family but deciding to follow a career in science, Sanger spent his entire career at Cambridge, completing his PhD in biochemistry there during the war years, when he was a conscientious objector. His first major achievement was to determine the structure and amino-acid sequence of the protein insulin, and after joining the newly established MRC Laboratory of Molecular Biology he focused on developing a sequencing method for nucleic acids, initially RNA and then DNA. A modest person, who decided not to continue research after reaching the then statutory retirement age of 65, but rather to concentrate on his garden, his name is appropriately commemorated in the Wellcome Trust Sanger Institute.

DNA FINGERPRINTING

Some of the numerous advances from molecular genetics techniques as applied to human genetic disorders are given in Chapters 10 and 12; many of these have involved large-scale international collaborations, but one discovery in this area, DNA fingerprinting (Jeffreys et al. 1985), not only provides an example of the originality of a single investigator and his small group, but of how such a scientist (in this case Alec Jeffreys; Figure 11.4) can have a major social impact through their awareness of wider, often controversial issues.

Many people will be familiar with the story of DNA fingerprinting, but it is worth quoting a description of the discovery in 1984 from Alec Jeffreys' interview with the author:

> ... out of the blue in 1982/83 was a report of the accidental discoveries of what we now call minisatellites or VNTRs near the

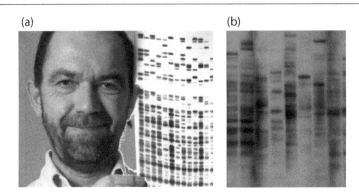

(a) (b)

Figure 11.4 **(a)** Alec Jeffreys (born 1950). Recorded interview 16/02/2010) [75]. (Photo courtesy Forensics Library.) **(b)** DNA fingerprinting; the original autoradiograph. (Courtesy of Science Museum, London.)

Born in Oxford and brought up in Luton, Alec Jeffreys had a fascination with both biology and chemistry from an early age, enhanced by his father's technical skills and enthusiasm, and inspired by teachers at his state grammar school. He studied chemistry at Oxford University, followed by a D Phil there in genetics and biochemistry with Ian Craig. A Fellowship in Amsterdam took him into molecular genetics and he then was appointed lecturer in genetics in Leicester (he admits to not knowing at the time where Leicester was!). Following his discovery of DNA fingerprinting he might have chosen to move to a larger or more prestigious centre or to become director of a large institute, but he chose to remain in Leicester, which had always supported him and continued to do so with the help of a Royal Society Professorship that freed him from all administrative duties. After embarking on what Jeffreys calls 'the great detour of my academic life', he returned to basic molecular genetics research, though always remaining keenly aware of the social aspects of his discovery, and severely critical of any potential abuse that might result from it.

insulin gene and in the alpha globin gene cluster; at that point I knew these things were real so we doubled our efforts and still got nowhere. Then the eventual clue for getting at these bits of DNA came from our gene evolution programme that we were working on. It actually came through a study of the myoglobin gene, initially in the grey seal, which provides an abundant source of messenger RNA needed to identify and clone the gene. In the human gene that we sequenced we found a minisatellite inside an intron and took one look at the sequence of the minisatellite repeat and it looked familiar and it sort of showed a similarity to the repeat sequence of the insulin minisatellite and the alpha-globin minisatellite as if there were some sequence motive associated with these tandem repeat DNAs.

So we took the human myoglobin minisatellite and went into a genomic library at very low hybridisation stringency and showed that you could indeed pull other minisatellites. We then used the sequence of those minisatellites to define a little sequence motif shared across all these different minisatellite loci. Then we thought, ok we now have a generic way of getting at minisatellites. Of course the reason for getting at these was to provide much better and more informative genetic markers for linkage mapping and other applications in medical genetics. So just to check this idea before taking this little shared core motif and using that to go into a genomic library, the obvious experiment was simply to take a repeated core probe and hybridize it to total genomic DNA to check whether it picked up multiple variable minisatellites. That was the key, almost accidental, experiment that triggered the entire field of human DNA identification.

It is worth commenting at this point that, while the discovery was indeed founded on fundamental 'blue skies' research, it was only in part serendipitous, since Jeffreys was fully aware of the importance of the molecular basis of variation as a biological topic, even if he was not expecting to find such a unique identifier of it. This is clearly shown by his immediate recognition of the wide impact of the discovery for such widely differing areas of science as taxonomy and conservation, as well as application to areas of human uniqueness and descent such as paternity and forensic science. But the human genetics aspects were in the forefront from the outset:

On the autoradiograph that we got was a set of fuzzy bar-code-like patterns coming out from the three individuals that we had on that Southern Blot. They happened to be my technician, still working in this laboratory, who in the New Year's honours list got an MBE, which is very, very good, for services to science; and also her mother and father. We could tell those three people apart, and you could see how the child's fingerprint was a composite of mum and dad's, so we could immediately see biological identification using DNA and we could see establishing family relationships. All of this was gained purely by accident on this first Southern blot.

We had a whole lot of non-human species on the blot too. So there was a mouse, a rat, a cow, a seal, a lemur, a baboon, tobacco DNA, and just about everything came up with what looked like a DNA fingerprint. It was an extraordinary moment and I think the penny dropped within seconds from that first autoradiograph coming out of the developing tank. I think my first reaction was what the hell is going on here, what a mess, and then the penny dropped. Here was DNA-based biological identification, family relationships and then all of the non-human applications, from dog paternity disputes to conservation biology, biodiversity monitoring, it was all there. It was a very exciting moment. I'd never ever planned to come up with a technology for identification; we just found it.

Fortunately this historic 'blot' (Figure 11.4b) has been preserved as part of the Wellcome Collection exhibit on Jeffreys' work; the preparation shown in Figure 11.4a is based on improved techniques.

Where less confident and forthright scientists than Jeffreys might not have ventured, though, was to recognise and take forward the social issues that the discovery raised and to tackle them directly, being prepared to be highly critical when any abuse relating to his work might seem likely. Even more unusual has been that, after what he has called 'the great detour of my scientific life', as described below, he has been able to return to and continue work in basic molecular genetics.

PSH: How did you decide which of these multiple avenues to take up first? Was it forced on you?

AJ: It was not really forced on us, but the following sequence of events meant that I was now embarking on what I call the great detour of my academic life, which was to go charging off into the world of forensic and legal medicine. So the sequence of events was that we published this in Nature, and in the paper we speculated on biological identification, though for patenting reasons we said little about the animal identification. That article was picked up by Andrew Veitch, a science correspondent with The Guardian; he wrote a lovely little piece on it that was read by a lawyer in London who represented a family involved in a very tricky immigration dispute. They'd been through all the blood group testing that basically failed to convince anybody of anything so she then wrote to me and said 'look I've heard about this new fangled DNA stuff, could you possibly help with this family?' And I thought 'ok, right this is it', we'd done a lot more work; fuzzy blobby bands had turned into something quite pretty and highly informative, so we thought 'ok this is crunch time now, you cannot possibly say no to this woman'. So that was our first case, which had a successful resolution, a young lad facing deportation reunited permanently with his family. It was a good news story, a great story. So that was the trigger and as soon as publicity came out on this case there was an avalanche of enquiries – I'd no idea of how many people were trapped in immigration disputes, they all wanted DNA testing. So that case was done in April 1985, and I think it was in June that the immigration tribunal dropped this case against this boy. By the summer of '85 we'd taken on the first paternity dispute anywhere, to my knowledge, and that then opened another flood gate, and then life went completely mad. So I desperately struggled to keep the science going, but in parallel with that, there was a huge demand from the public for DNA testing.

The wider world, like Jeffreys, soon realised that by turning uncertainty into something close to certainty, DNA fingerprinting could rescue the lives of many ordinary people from great injustice, whether this was in the area of immigration disputes or in forensic criminal cases, such as a local murder near Leicester where a man had been convicted on the grounds of his confession:

… we were just phoned up out the blue about the Enderby murder case, with a request that we do DNA typing on the forensic samples recovered. They already had the guilty party, he'd already confessed to one of the murders, so the key thing was to simply confirm his guilt, matching DNA between him and semen recovered from one of the victims. However, this person denied any involvement in a second very similar murder, so we were asked to see if we could tie him into that murder as well. So I took this on in the full expectation that we'd get nothing back. Up to that point I'd set up a collaboration with people, particularly Peter Gill, we'd done a lot of work showing that mock forensic specimens could yield typeable DNA, because not even that was obvious. I mean if you take an old blood stain, can you get DNA from it? Can you analyse it? So we'd shown during '85 that that was possible.

In '86 the forensic samples arrived here and we went through, not multi-locus DNA fingerprinting, but the single locus minisatellite profiling that we'd developed and to my astonishment we got a reading out of that; I expected to get nothing at all, and what the results showed apparently very, very clearly was that the semen from the same man was present on both victims and the DNA didn't match the profile of the person who confessed to one of the murders. My first report back to the police when we got information on the first victim showed there was a mismatch. So I remember phoning them up and saying you know we've got what appears to be a clear exclusion of the involvement of this person in respect of the first murder. Then we had to wait a long time with very small amounts of DNA, very faint profiles, and then the same profile came up with the second victim, completely mismatching the person who confessed to her murder.

So I remember phoning the police and saying I think you've got the wrong guy, or that the science is completely shot, take your choice. I won't describe the sort of Anglo Saxon response to that! At that point I really started worrying very very profoundly about whether there was some fundamental flaw in the entire science. The police were so convinced that they'd got the right guy, but anyway, there was then a meeting here, with Home Office forensic scientists, the police, myself and the final conclusion was, yes the science was fine, they'd got the wrong guy. And that saw the release of this young man in custody and so the first time DNA was used in criminal investigation was to establish innocence, not guilt. This then led to the police launching what proved to be the world's first DNA based manhunt, having got the DNA profile of the assailant. They used that to flush him out, and that did work eventually.'

The very success of forensic DNA profiling led to problems, though, with the creation in Britain of a national DNA database on which the police insisted on keeping profiles and samples from people found innocent, or who had just been witnesses. Despite serious criticism from the Human Genetics Commission and others (see Chapter 7), including Jeffreys himself, both police and government proved extremely reluctant to alter this policy.

PSH: Before we get back around from the detour, can I just ask now, you've had concerns about how this is being used in recent years, in terms of things like the DNA database. What are your feelings about that at present?

AJ: Well they were expressed fairly forcefully to the Home Affairs Select Committee when was it, last week, week before, when I went down to give evidence. They were considering the use of the National DNA Database and I attempted to stay fairly focussed on the fact that, of the five and a half million people now resident on the database, one million of them, roughly, are entirely innocent people who have been arrested but have never even been charged with anything, never mind convicted. I have always taken the view that that's basically out of order, and that view was very much reflected in a European Court of Human Rights verdict a little over a year ago that this retention is illegal and that the UK is in breach of Article 8 of the Human Rights Act which guarantees an individual to the right of a private and family life. I absolutely went along with that verdict, in fact I was involved in working with Liberty in taking that case to the European Court. So I've been despondent, I have to say, about the incredibly tardy response of the British Government. This clear verdict said that these retentions are illegal. So they are still dithering about this; current proposal is that instead of retaining innocent people DNAs indefinitely they retain them for 6 years, it strikes me as a very long time. There's no other country in the world that does that, not even Scotland. So I think my evidence to the Home Affairs committee was blunt, whether it will have any effect whatsoever, I have no idea, but I have done my bit.

More than 10 years later, matters have changed little.

Ignorance among the judiciary and expert witnesses has been another problem. Clearly accuracy and reliability at all points of the process are critical factors, not always taken into account, but the tendency to quote probabilities of one in many millions can create an illusion of certainty and lead to the ignoring of context and of other essential evidence. Fortunately, education in genetics has improved this situation, though more in the United States than in Britain.

UNSTABLE DNA AND HUNTINGTON'S DISEASE: TRINUCLEOTIDE REPEAT DISORDERS

Much of classical genetics, whether involving human genetics or other species such as Drosophila, was based on the concept of stability of the gene and the permanence of mutation once it had occurred, but there have for many years been examples from human inherited disorders that seemed to question this. The phenomenon of anticipation, raised first for myotonic dystrophy and then for Huntington's disease, in association with parent of origin effects, was at first dismissed as an artefact (Penrose 1948, Höweler et al. 1989) in the absence of any plausible biological explanation. Now we know that both disorders, along with several others, result from DNA instability, associated with expansion of trinucleotide repeat sequences in the relevant genes.

The sequence of steps leading from the original observations to the isolation of the genes involved and the molecular mechanisms responsible for DNA instability has been highly international and collaborative, with UK groups (including that of the author) involved in the international consortia for both disorders. Quite apart from the immediate consequences for understanding of the specific conditions, a remarkable number of general lessons have emerged. These include the detection of DNA instability itself as a general biological phenomenon, completely unsuspected from previous research on more basic experimental organisms; the recognition of RNA toxicity as a novel mechanism for cell damage has also led to new avenues for possible therapies.

From a historical viewpoint a valuable account of the work leading to the isolation of the HD gene has been given by Gillian Bates (2005), at that point working with Hans Lehrach in London as part of one of the two British groups in the international HD consortium, and who has also subsequently been responsible for the production of a transgenic mouse model for the disorder. More background information on the international project overall can also be found in the interviews that I was able to make with a number of the key workers, including Gillian Bates herself [57], James Gusella and Marcia McDonald in Boston [82], Michael Conneally [22], Russell Snell [83] and Allan Tobin, scientific director of the Hereditary Disease Foundation [52] during the 10-year span of the project.

At a practical level, the fact that for Huntington's disease and other members of the group we now have unique and highly accurate tests has opened up possibilities for both prediction and primary diagnosis, with ethical challenges (see Chapter 7) for how to deliver these optimally as genetic services. The success of the various aspects of this field has been largely due to the close interaction of workers with a number of different skills, laboratory and clinical, and to their ability to look across and learn lessons from each other and from different diseases in the group. This is a key lesson for those involved in medical genetics research overall, which is unlikely to disappear with the use of genomic techniques.

Once the HD gene and unstable mutation had been found, attention at once also turned to how these affected the biology of the disorder. Gillian Bates (see

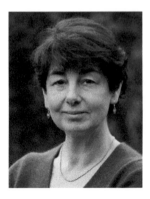

Figure 11.5 Gillian Bates, a major contributor to UK Huntington's disease research through her role in the isolation of the HD gene and creation of a transgenic mouse model. Recorded interview 21/02/2006 [57]. (Courtesy of Gillian Bates and the Genetics and Medicine Historical Network.)

Figure 11.5), by now at Guy's Hospital, focused on the production of a transgenic mouse and was able to establish a mouse line that showed a neurological phenotype (Mangiarini et al. 1996):

And then of course it took us about a year to establish the R6/2 line. They don't breed that easily, well once you know what you are doing it's fine, but when you don't know what you are doing it is not so straightforward. We didn't talk about the lines as we had no idea what we had. I mean the phenotype could have been caused by the disruption of another gene. I was very happy at the time. I didn't care what it was because I had a mouse with a phenotype and if I'd knocked out a gene that was important, then I had an interesting project. I was very happy irrespective of what it was. And I was very worried about saying it was anything to do with Huntington's because I had no idea whether it was. So it was only after we'd really managed to characterise it and were close to publishing that I presented the work. At that point, we were pretty sure that the repeat was causing the phenotype.

Interview with Gillian Bates [57]

Not only did the mouse show clinical neurological abnormalities, but in the brain there were inclusion bodies, which had been seen before but ignored:

PSH: What about the inclusions? At what point were you able to find that there were these inclusions, because they weren't really known about before were they?

GB: No, not at all. Well, we gave Steve Davies sections of brain because Steve worked in neurodegenerative disease, I mean his interests were Huntington's, Alzheimer's and Parkinson's so although he had not been working with transgenic mice, he was familiar with the structures of the brain. He performed immunohistochemistry with an anti-ubiquitin antibody, we also had an anti-huntingtin antibody (Ab1) from Marian DiFiglia. You can't miss the nuclear inclusions in the R6/2 mouse brain. You see these dots everywhere. We didn't know what they were, Steve thought it might be the nucleolus at first. They have a very good EM Unit at

UCL. Steve worked with Mark Turmaine, the head of the EM Unit and uncovered the ultrastructure of the nuclear inclusion. Again you can't miss them in the R6/2 mouse. Steve started doing some literature searches to see whether he could find anything that had a structure similar to these in other EM photographs. He turned up at my flat one Saturday morning with a book in his hand. 'I'm really excited. I've found something' and he held this book up. I said 'Oh I've got that book' because Nancy [Wexler] had given it to me just a couple of months beforehand. It was a neurology book from 1979 that had a chapter showing the ultrastructure of brain biopsies from people with HD. There was a micrograph in that chapter that looked identical to the ones from the mice.

Gillian Bates [57]

THE MALLEABLE GENOME AND EPIGENETICS

The discovery of DNA instability in Huntington's disease and other trinucleotide repeat disorders has been only one of a number of research developments to show that the genome is less 'hard-wired' than had been previously thought likely. These cannot be given adequate space here but must at least have a mention, in particular the numerous aspects of gene function that are not directly dependent on the DNA sequence of an individual gene or the genome as a whole, and which are broadly covered by the term 'epigenetics', a term first used by Conrad Hal Waddington in the 1930s. Developmental genetics as a whole has been especially involved in these wider processes, which form part of genetics just as much as do the sequences of the individual genes that underlie them. Notable examples include the role of methylation in the activation and inactivation of gene function, which is responsible for a series of human developmental abnormalities.

Likewise, chromosomes are not composed solely of DNA, and are three-dimensional structures whose function in meiosis and mitosis is influenced by a series of complex processes that include the large amount of non-coding DNA as well as individual genes, in addition to a variety of specific proteins. We are still at the early stages of beginning to understand this essential area, let alone of being able to give an adequate account of its history. In contrast with much of molecular genetics, this is a field whose three-dimensional nature requires sophisticated microscopic techniques, as shown by the studies of Wendy Bickmore and colleagues at the Edinburgh MRC Human Genetics Unit.

THE *BRCA2* GENE AND CANCER GENE ISOLATION

The field of cancer genetics research, like that of clinical cancer genetics (discussed in Chapter 4), has seen outstanding contributions from British research groups, enhanced by the fact that they have generally been part of large-scale international collaborations. The generous funding from major cancer charities and the facilities provided by their institutes has helped greatly, as has the fact that recent directors have often been geneticists, such as Walter Bodmer and David Harnden (see Figures 4.4 and 4.5b) or at least have appreciated the key role of genetics in cancer research. This makes it difficult to select a single discovery for this chapter, though. I have chosen the isolation of the BRCA2 breast cancer susceptibility gene (Wooster et al. 1995) and the researchers responsible for this, including Michael Stratton (Figure 4.5a) and his colleagues, based mainly at the Institute of Cancer Research (ICR), London.

This work, like that involving the Huntington's disease gene described above, arose from genetic linkage studies; after the BRCA1 gene had been localised by an American group, the ICR workers, also studying familial breast cancer, realised that a number of large British families were clearly not linked to the same region and in fact proved to be localised to chromosome 13. Using positional cloning techniques, including chromosomal changes involving the region, they were able to isolate the gene, opening the door not only to accurate genetic testing, but also to a series of studies, still ongoing, indicating the normal function of the gene in DNA repair and its role when mutated in the genesis of tumours. These have now continued into the genomic era and are giving important information on the somatic changes found in the much more frequent non-familial cases of breast and other cancers. The Cancer Genome Project, based at the Cambridge Sanger Institute and again led by Michael Stratton, is now taking these primarily somatic genomic studies forward on a large scale, especially in relation to identifying differing responses to therapies.

The BRCA2 discovery points to a series of general lessons that link classical human molecular genetics with the new genomics and show how important it is that the two are not artificially separated and that workers in genomics have a firm grounding in basic genetics. First is the importance of recognising genetic heterogeneity if molecular analysis is to be accurately and effectively applied in diagnosis and prediction. An incidental result of the BRCA2 work was largely to nullify the American attempts to restrict and control patenting (see Chapter 7) which were based solely on the BRCA1 discovery. A second point of general importance is the value of accurate clinical, pathological and family studies recorded in the literature as the starting point for new molecular and genomic studies, especially if archival tissue or blood samples are available, for patients who may be long deceased. A final point, already emphasised throughout this book, is the value of clinical and laboratory researchers working closely together; this applies not only to clinical geneticists but, especially in the cancer research field, to the numerous other specialties involved.

The advances described here for familial breast cancer have been paralleled for other common tumours showing a mendelian subset, such as colorectal cancer, as well as by work on rare single gene determined tumour syndromes, for most of which British medical geneticists have been prominently involved; tuberous sclerosis, neurofibromatosis, familial adenomatous polyposis and von Hippel-Lindau disease are but a few of many examples that might be given.

SEX DETERMINATION AND THE Y CHROMOSOME: THE *SRY* GENE

Ever since the original studies of human chromosome disorders in 1959, it had been clear that sex determination in humans, and in mammals in general, was due to the Y chromosome, but for the next 40 years virtually nothing was known about the gene or genes involved or how they functioned. The key person involved in this discovery was Peter Goodfellow (Figure 11.6), one of the most unusual and colourful individuals in genetics in recent years, and a visible disproof of the widely held view that such 'characters' were a feature of past times but no longer exist today.

Goodfellow's work on the molecular structure of the Y chromosome and its role in sex determination was carried out at the Imperial Cancer Research Fund laboratories in London, which were at this time directed by Walter Bodmer, with whom Goodfellow had previously worked in Oxford. His group collaborated closely with that of Robin Lovell-Badge, at National Institute of Medical Research, Mill Hill, who was analysing sexual development in transgenic mice. The Y chromosome had always been something of a 'poor relation' of the X chromosome, and little was known of

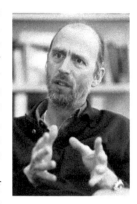

Figure 11.6 Peter N Goodfellow. Recorded interview 17/07/2014 [98]. (Courtesy Peter Goodfellow and Institute for Protein Design, Washington University.)

its gene structure or function except that there was a region of homology between X and Y involved in chromosome pairing at meiosis, the pseudoautosomal region, while information was also given by which parts were missing in rare patients with abnormalities involving the Y chromosome.

The cloning of the key region proved exceptionally arduous, with keen international competition from other groups.

> … there were three groups, myself, Jean Weissenbach and David Page, who were left with the tools and the inclination to try and clone the sex determining gene, and essentially we were all using the same approach, which was to construct a map across the Y chromosome using DNA from XX males and XY females to try and identify, classic positional cloning, the minimal region where the gene ought to be. And MIC2, which we had cloned and shown to be pseudo-autosomal and mapped it, and cloned the pseudoautosomal boundary, we knew that it was the closest marker distally to the gene, and so we started walking. And we'd identified a CPG island by using pulsed-field gel electrophoresis which we thought must be the next gene down. And it was the next gene down and it was a gene called ZFY and basically we had just isolated it when we read David Page's paper saying that he had cloned this gene and he

had been walking from below it towards it, and that he presented evidence that it was the sex determining gene.

Interview with Peter Goodfellow [98].

The interview gives a rare glimpse of the emotional side of science from the viewpoint of the 'loser' in what is often perceived as the 'winner takes all' field of gene isolation. Understandably a losing team often do not want to write about the situation in detail, while the account of the 'winners' often over-stresses the exclusivity of their discovery. In this case, though, the eventual outcome (Sinclair et al. 1990) was rather different. Peter Goodfellow continues:

I was devastated that David scooped us, and I'd had a group of five people working for two years in a chromosomal walk which was brutal, the Y chromosome is full of repeats. It was murderous, awful work, and we got scooped. I remember one of the post-docs in the lab, a guy called Paul Goodfellow, no relation, as we were sitting down crying, Paul was saying to me, 'You know there are lots of people who'd like to be failures like us.' And that was such a wise thing [laughs]. You know it's easy to feel sorry for yourself but actually there are a lot of people who would like to have been in the position of failing, that we had done, so it put it into some context. And so we sort of took a deep breath and started to think about what we would do and what experiments were worth doing when Paul said to me, 'You know, are you absolutely sure it's right?' And I said, 'It looks pretty good to me.' And he said, 'Well, there's at least one hypothesis which you can always use to test this, which is any XX male which has been created by transfer of Y material should have the pseudoautosomal region.' So if you could find pseudoautosomal region positive X chromosomes, then, the other way around, then you know that's how that was created. So basically we had a whole load of DNA from a number of collaborators and we found some patients from Marc Fellous, 15 of which we were able to show … had all the elements they should have but didn't have ZFY… So we had Y positive XX males who didn't have ZFY. And as soon as we found two patients like that we knew that it was a mistake, and there had been other indications. We'd done stuff which Jenny Graves. David Page, my lab and Jenny's lab had collaborated on looking for ZFY in marsupials and it wasn't on the Y chromosome in metatherians, so either metatherians were using a different gene or it wasn't the sex determinant gene. So it was beginning to be a bit of a feel that maybe there was something more complicated, but it was those patients from Marc Fellous that told us that the sex determinant gene hadn't been cloned. And we'd walked straight through it. Basically it was a very small gene which wasn't particularly well conserved and we had just walked through it, and we found it when we went back and looked more carefully …

During my interview series I asked everyone what they were most proud of in their career. For most experimental scientists, including Peter Goodfellow, the answer was clear, and was often something relatively early in their career, rather than later when they were well known and in charge of large teams or institutes.

> … journalists have asked me, 'What do you feel about your academic career?' and I say, 'I mapped and cloned the human sex determination gene. And for the history of time I will have done that. Robin [Lovell-Badge] and I will have our names on that cup.' And to actually put your name onto a fact which is going into the textbooks, it doesn't matter that your name's not on it but you put your little brick in the wall, you know? I made my contribution, I'm proud of that contribution.

Those workers who were more clinical often chose a more incremental achievement, or even protested, over-modestly, that they had not really done anything that they deserved to be remembered by! But actually all the people that I interviewed, and virtually all the workers in medical genetics that I have known, whether clinical or laboratory based, *have* made a significant contribution of some kind, most often in collaboration with others and, as Peter Goodfellow said, 'have put their little brick in the wall' of human knowledge.

THE GENOMIC ERA AND MEDICINE

It is neither practical nor helpful to try to separate completely the molecular genetic advances already mentioned from those based on the analysis of whole genomes, as can be seen in the cancer genetics research outlined above, which was already flourishing before the genomic era, but has accelerated subsequently.

The major role of the UK in the international Human Genome Project itself is described in the next chapter, while the beginnings of service applications of genomics techniques were outlined in Chapter 10. It was mentioned there that most of these remained in the future, and a cautious, even sceptical attitude was taken to any applications in the short term for discovering and influencing the susceptibility to common diseases. The proven value, though, of genomic approaches to the molecular basis of very rare disorders and of mental handicap of unknown cause, was also emphasised there, while its importance in analysis of cancer genomes has been touched on above, so to illustrate and conclude this selection of major advances and discoveries, I have chosen one example from this area, the Deciphering Developmental Disorders (DDD) study and its linked database *DECIPHER*.

This ongoing project, based at the Wellcome Trust Sanger Institute but involving medical genetics centres across the UK, and now internationally, was coordinated initially by Helen Firth, clinical geneticist, followed by Matthew Hurles, and has tackled the hitherto intractable problem of the molecular basis of mental handicap of unknown cause. In many ways it comes full circle back to Penrose's 1938 Colchester study, which by meticulous clinical and genetic study had taken the broad group lumped together as 'mental retardation' and shown that it was composed of numerous distinct forms with different causes. But Penrose was limited by an almost total lack of laboratory methods to identify these causes in any detail. Even chromosome analysis was impossible then, as were most biochemical techniques, though he was able to identify the first few British cases of phenylketonuria. That the gene was composed of DNA would remain unknown for another 15 years.

Over the following decades the remaining 'core' of mental handicap with no known cause was slowly chipped away at by a variety of approaches – chromosomal, biochemical and molecular analysis, in conjunction with careful clinical studies of dysmorphic and other clinical features. Yet all too many families remained without a specific diagnosis to guide genetic counselling and prognosis. The advent of genomics has changed this and a series of techniques – comparative genome hybridisation (CGH), exome sequencing and full genome sequencing – has allowed identification of genetic changes in a large number of specific genes in many such patients.

The 'DDD' study itself recruited samples from around 13,000 UK patients with mental handicap of unidentified cause, from UK regional medical genetics centres; almost 40% have been shown to have a specific molecular defect, a remarkably high proportion given that these patients had already been investigated intensively by a range of genetic tests. Around three-quarters of the molecular changes found had arisen *de novo*, allowing parents to be reassured that recurrence is very unlikely. Not only has this provided the families with a specific diagnosis for the first time, but neurobiologists are also being provided with a wealth of genes, many of them entirely unknown previously, which clearly play an important role in brain function, and which will themselves form the starting point for a large number of long-term research projects. These results have mostly come so far from 'exome sequencing', involving the expressed and functional parts of the genome, and omitting the majority which is unexpressed and where interpretation of changes may be more difficult.

In addition to its research value, The DDD project's linked *DECIPHER* database, now with over 200 centres internationally, is providing a valuable tool for clinical geneticists and other clinicians investigating specific patients requiring a diagnosis. Anonymised genetic (and genomic) data, along with phenotypic information, can be read by anyone, but new data can be entered only by experienced clinical geneticists.

The DDD study provides a series of lessons for genomics in the future: it wisely enlisted the cooperation of medical genetics centres around the UK, utilising – and recognising – their clinical diagnostic skills, their resources of patients and samples, and their willingness to collaborate – a far cry from the attitudes of the 'internal market' of the 1990s promoted by the government of the time, where such collaboration was disapproved of. It has also shown how much more valuable is a study where clinical-laboratory collaboration is built in from the outset, rather than added on to an initial 'lab only' approach. It is greatly to be hoped that these and other lessons will be incorporated into other new and future genomic studies.

The examples given in this chapter are just a few of many that I might have chosen, but I hope that they will have given at least an indication of the importance and the exciting nature of the discoveries. They also show the exceptional originality and talent of these and other workers in the field of medical and human genetics overall during the past 70 years. Undoubtedly their example has encouraged many others across the world to 'put their little brick in the wall of human knowledge', to the lasting benefit of us all.

REFERENCES

Anderson S, Bankier AT, Barrell BG. et al. 1981. Sequence and organization of the human mitochondrial genome. *Nature*. 290(5806):457–465.

Auerbach C, Robson JM. 1946. Chemical production of mutations. *Nature*. 157:302.

Barr ML, Bertram EG. 1949. A morphological distinction between the neurones of the male and female, and the behaviour of the nucleolar satellite during accelerated nucleoprotein synthesis. *Nature*. 163:676–677.

Bates GP. 2005. History of genetic disease: The molecular genetics of Huntington disease – A history. *Nat Rev Genet*. 6(10):766–773.

Bell J, Haldane JBS. 1937. The linkage between the genes for colour-blindness and haemophilia in man. *Proc R Soc B* 123:119–150.

Beutler E, Yeh M, Fairbanks VF. 1962. The normal human female as a mosaic of X-chromosome activity: Studies using the gene for G-6-PD-deficiency as a marker. *Proc Natl Acad Sci USA*. 48:9–16.

Bickel H, Gerrard J, Hickmans EM. 1953. Influence of phenylalanine intake on phenylketonuria. *Lancet*. 265:812–813.

Brock DJ, Bolton AE, Scrimgeour JB. 1974. Prenatal diagnosis of spina bifida and anencephaly through maternal plasma-alpha-fetoprotein measurement. *Lancet*. 1:767–769.

Brock DJ, Sutcliffe RG. 1972. Alpha-fetoprotein in the antenatal diagnosis of anencephaly and spina bifida. *Lancet*. 2:197–199.

Carter CO, David PA, Laurence KM. 1968. A family study of major central nervous system malformations in South Wales. *J Med Genet*. 5(2):81–106.

Clarke CA. 1975. *Rhesus Haemolytic Disease. Selected Papers and Extracts*. Lancaster: MTP Medical and Technical Publishing Co. Ltd.

Edwards JH. 1961. Seasonal incidence of congenital disease in Birmingham. *Ann Hum Genet*. 25:89–93.

Elwood JH, Nevin NC. 1973. Anencephalus and spina bifida in Belfast (1964–1968). *Ulster Med J*. 42(2):213–222.

Finn R, Clarke CA, Donohoe WT. et al. 1961. Experimental studies on the prevention of Rh haemolytic disease. *Br Med J*. 1:1486–1490.

Firth HV, Wright CF, DDD Study. 2011. The Deciphering Developmental Disorders (DDD) study. *Dev Med Child Neurol*. 53(8):702–703

Fisher RA. 1935. Linkage studies and the prognosis of hereditary ailments. *Transactions of the International Congress on Life Assurance Medicine*. London, pp. 615–617.

Fitzgerald TW, Gerety SS, Jones WD, van Kogelenberg M. 2015. Deciphering Developmental Disorders Study. Large-scale discovery of novel genetic causes of developmental disorders. *Nature*. 519:223–228.

Gitschier J. 2010. *Speaking of Genetics: A Collection of Interviews*. Cold Spring Harbor, New York: Cold Spring Harbor Laboratory Press.

Haldane JBS. 1935. The rate of spontaneous mutation of a human gene. *J Genet*. 31:317.

Höweler CJ, Busch HFM, Geraets JPM, Niermeijer MF, Stahl A. 1989. Anticipation in myotonic dystrophy: Fact or fiction? *Brain*. 112:779–797.

Jeffreys AJ, Wilson V, Thein SL. 1985. Hypervariable 'minisatellite' regions in human DNA. *Nature*. 314:67–74.

Lyon MF. 1961. Gene action in the X-chromosome of the mouse (*Mus musculus* L). *Nature*. 190:372–373.

Mangiarini L, Sathasivam K, Seller M et al. 1996. Exon 1 of the HD gene with an expanded CAG repeat is sufficient to cause a progressive neurological phenotype in transgenic mice. *Cell*. 87(3):493–506.

MRC Vitamin Study Research Group. 1991. Prevention of neural tube defects: Results of the Medical Research Council vitamin study. *Lancet*. 338(8760):131–137.

Penrose LS. 1948. The problem of anticipation in pedigrees of dystrophia myotonica. *Ann Eugen*. 14:125–132.

Sanger F, Nicklen S, Coulson AR. 1977. DNA sequencing with chain-terminating inhibitors. *Proc Nat Acad Sci USA*. 74(1977):546–567.

Sinclair AH, Berta P, Palmer MS, Hawkins JR, Griffiths BL, Smith MJ, Foster JW, Frischauf AM, Lovell-Badge R, Goodfellow PN. 1990. A gene from the human sex-determining region encodes a protein with homology to a conserved DNA-binding motif. *Nature*. 346(6281):240–244.

Smithells RW, Sheppard S, Schorah CJ, Seller MJ, Nevin NC, Harris R, Read AP, Fielding DW. 1980. Possible prevention of neural-tube defects by periconceptional vitamin supplementation. *Lancet*. 1(8164):339–340.

Watson JD, Crick FHC. 1953. Molecular structure of nucleic acids: A structure for deoxyribose nucleic acid. *Nature*. 171: 737–738.

Wooster R, Bignell G, Lancaster J. et al. 1995. Identification of the breast cancer susceptibility gene BRCA2. *Nature*. 378:789–792.

Zallen DT, Christie DA, Tansey EM (eds.). 2004. The Rhesus Factor and Disease Prevention. *Wellcome Witnesses to Twentieth Century Medicine*, vol. 22. London: Wellcome Trust.

12

Mapping and sequencing: From gene to genome

ABSTRACT

Mapping the genome began soon after it was recognised that genes were physically located on the chromosomes, with co-located 'linked' genes found for Drosophila in America in 1913 and for the mouse in Britain shortly afterwards. The first human gene linkage was found in 1937 between colour blindness and haemophilia on the X chromosome by Bell and Haldane, and from 1951 an increasing number of other gene linkages were discovered using blood groups and other inherited protein variations as markers. Between 1973 and 1991 a series of international human gene mapping workshops were held which saw a detailed map of disease genes and genetic markers established on all chromosomes, boosted by the discovery of abundant inherited variation in DNA itself. From 1985 the Human Genome Project, with Britain playing a major role, was able to sequence increasing stretches of the human genome, being essentially completed in 2003. This has led to the new and still-fluid field of 'genomics', with sequencing techniques applied to numerous research projects and increasingly to genetic services, particularly for single gene disorders, though its efficacy for most common diseases and for wider medicine has still to be fully established.

The mapping of genes has been a central part of genetics ever since it was recognised that genes had a linear arrangement on the chromosomes. It is now over a century since Alfred Sturtevant (1913), working with Thomas Hunt Morgan in America, produced the first gene map for the Drosophila X chromosome – only 6 points, but a map nonetheless. Independently and almost simultaneously in Britain JBS Haldane showed the first genetic linkage in a mammal (the mouse); Haldane was still a student, but publication was held up by World War I, in which his co-author

Alexander Sprunt was killed and Haldane himself seriously wounded. Haldane had to write to his friend and colleague William Bateson:

If I am killed, could you kindly give my sister help if she wants it.

Fortunately Haldane survived, and the paper eventually appeared in the *Journal of Genetics* (Haldane et al. 1915), probably the only paper, Haldane noted, to be published from the battlefield. Readers may like to note that Haldane's sister and second co-author became the well-known author Naomi Mitchison.

It is thus not surprising that 20 years later Haldane, together with Julia Bell (see Figures 1.11 and 1.9), should have recognised the first human genetic linkage, between haemophilia and colour blindness on the X chromosome (Bell and Haldane 1937), setting the stage, after the further interruption of World War II, for a long and steady period of progress in human gene mapping, much of it based at or around the Galton Laboratory in London.

Early human gene mapping was surrounded by a series of difficulties that did not bother those working with experimental species, such as Drosophila, which could be bred as wished and where large numbers reduced the need for complex statistics, but it did have one considerable advantage: already by 1950 there was an abundance of well-documented family data on rare inherited disorders, much of it brought together in Julia Bell's monumental *Treasury of Human Inheritance*, as described in Chapter 1. But the chance of a single family having two such disorders was minimal, so the problem initially was to find variable 'marker loci' following clear mendelian inheritance which could be tested against the segregation of a mendelian disorder or against other markers.

The first significant genetic markers were the blood groups, whose variations were already under study on account of their practical importance in transfusion medicine. When Robert Race, who had been evacuated to Cambridge as part of RA Fisher's 'serum group', returned after the war to London as head of the newly formed MRC Blood Group Unit, he collaborated with Lionel Penrose and colleagues at the Galton Laboratory to develop the search for genetic linkage, as mentioned in Chapter 2, and formed a key part of the circle of talent surrounding the Galton Laboratory at University College, London; later the unit, now under his colleague and wife Ruth Sanger, relocated to the same purpose built laboratories at Wolfson House, making the links even closer. (Race and Sanger are pictured in Figure 2.3; see also Bangham 2014).

There were by now several other blood groups in addition to the original ABO and Rhesus systems. The first positive finding actually came from Copenhagen, though, where Jan Mohr [51] had set up a blood group laboratory in the institute of Tage Kemp, after a year spent with Penrose in London; this was linkage between the Lutheran blood group and the secretor system (Mohr 1951). Mohr also tested his markers against a number of inherited disorders and came close to finding linkage with one of them, myotonic dystrophy, his hint of linkage only being confirmed 20 years later by others (Renwick et al. 1971, Harper et al. 1972).

Soon two more autosomal disease loci were mapped; the condition nail-patella syndrome was found to be linked to the ABO blood group locus by Renwick and Lawler (1955) at the Galton Laboratory (Figure 12.1); many records of this work can be found in the archives of Renwick and other Galton workers at University College, London.

(a)

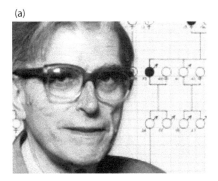

(b)

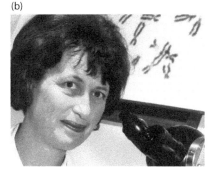

Figure 12.1 Two early workers on human gene mapping at the Galton Laboratory, responsible for detection of some of the first autosomal disease linkages. **(a)** James H Renwick (1926–1994). Renwick also introduced the first multipoint computer programme for detecting genetic linkage. (Courtesy of University of Glasgow Archives Service.) **(b)** Sylvia Lawler (1922–1996), who subsequently worked on cancer cytogenetics at Institute of Cancer Research. (Courtesy of Institute of Cancer Research, London.)

Meanwhile in America Newton Morton (1956), who was later to relocate to Britain together with his wife, Patricia Jacobs), found the harmless blood condition elliptocytosis to be linked to the Rhesus blood group locus in one large family, but not in some others, thus providing a practical demonstration of genetic heterogeneity which was to be followed by many other examples. Of course, these early findings of linkage (apart from those involving the X chromosome) did not truly 'map' the conditions, since the work gave no indication of which chromosome was involved.

Detecting genetic linkage from family material that was often fragmentary and limited required detailed mathematical and statistical analysis to extract every scrap of information. This had already been shown in Bell and Haldane's 1937 haemophilia paper, and in Penrose's 'sib pair' approach, but methods for linkage analysis were developed further by Cedric (CAB) Smith at the Galton Laboratory (see Chapter 2), and by Newton Morton, then in America, the two collaborating closely so that, according to Morton, it was often impossible to say which of the two was the primary originator of the idea. James Renwick was the first to develop a multipoint linkage programme (Renwick and Bolling 1971), which was followed by a steady series of computer programmes that could extract the maximum possible amount of information from a pedigree.

It was clear from the beginning that if widespread human gene mapping was to be achieved, a much greater range of markers was needed than could be provided by blood groups alone. Fortunately, the development of biochemical techniques such as starch gel electrophoresis, invented by Oliver Smithies, UK-born, though located in Canada for much of this work (Smithies 1955), began to identify genetic variation in a wide range of human proteins, the work being greatly developed by Harry Harris in London. These markers included red cell enzymes and a number of serum proteins, so that family samples could now be tested against a panel of these, along with blood groups, to give the hopeful investigator a reasonable, if still small, chance of finding linkage with one of them, as well as a larger chance of excluding linkage with certain parts of the genome, which Galton Laboratory worker Peter Cook, only half in jest, called 'desperation mapping'. Penrose's successors in the Galton Chair, Harry Harris, Elizabeth Robson, David Hopkinson and Sue Povey (Figure 12.2), all made the

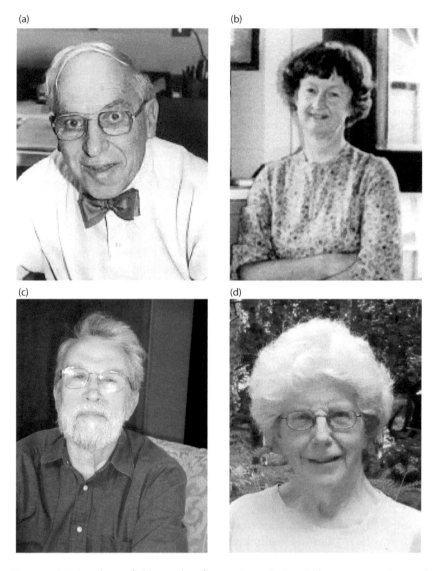

Figure 12.2 Leaders of the study of genetic variation in human proteins and successive heads of the Galton Laboratory and the MRC Human Biochemical Genetics Unit. **(a)** Harry Harris (See also Chapter 2). (Courtesy Royal Society, London.) **(b)** Elizabeth Robson. (Courtesy Sue Povey.) **(c)** David Hopkinson (born 1935). **(d)** Sue Povey (1942–2018). (c and d courtesy of Genetics and Medicine Historical Network and European Society of Human Genetics.)

analysis of inherited variation in human proteins their main field of study. The widespread recognition of this work is reflected in Robson being chosen to give the inaugural lecture on the topic at the first International Human Genetics Congress in Copenhagen in 1956.

The next development to boost human gene mapping was the discovery by Henry Harris [67] (no relation to Harry Harris) and John Watkins in Oxford (1965) that hybrid cell lines could be made between mouse and human cells in cultures treated by Sendai virus, and that these tended to lose the human chromosomes in a selective and predictable manner. This work was further developed in America (Weiss and Green 1967) and used for gene mapping particularly by Frank Ruddle and colleagues at Yale University.

This approach allowed a correlation to be made between the loss of a particular chromosome or chromosome region with loss of a particular protein, providing a location for the underlying gene and any other genes already known to be linked to it. It was at this point that a true physical map for human genes began to emerge, so that workers could envisage an eventual, if distant goal of a complete map of the human genome.

THE HUMAN GENE MAPPING WORKSHOPS

By now the initially small number of workers involved in human gene mapping was becoming a specific research community, international but closely knit, with workers from a variety of backgrounds including blood grouping, biochemical genetics, statistics and medical genetics. It was also now becoming clear that it was essential to have some internationally agreed system for nomenclature and for general coordination of the field, such as had been achieved for chromosomes by the Denver Conference in 1960 (see Chapter 10), and more recently by the international histocompatibility antigen (HLA) workshops. The upshot was the series of alternate yearly Human Gene Mapping Workshops, held between 1973 and 1991, beginning in Yale (Ruddle et al. 1974) and finishing in London, which provided a prelude to the subsequent Human Genome Project. Fortunately not only were the details of the individual workshops fully published at the time, but a recent Witness Seminar has allowed many of those directly involved, especially those from the UK, to share their wider memories (Jones and Tansey 2015, Jones 2016). My interview with Sue Povey [71] also gives a valuable picture of the later years of the Galton Laboratory, as well as illustrating some of the difficulties faced by the 'nomenclature committee', particularly with some investigators who resented the name of 'their' gene being changed. In this respect matters had changed little since the Denver conference 30 years earlier.

Like the international HLA workshops before them, the Human Gene Mapping Workshops were small, informal, 'hands on' and intensely interactive, with raw and mostly unpublished data synthesised on the spot by the participants. Each group of chromosomes — later each individual chromosome — had its own small 'committee' and the genetic map for a chromosome could be seen visibly growing in front of one's eyes. Initially the number of mapped loci was too small even to draw an actual map, but gradually the extent and density of mapping increased

(Figure 12.3), to the point that each chromosome had its own map, until finally there was too much information to place on a readable map.

Several notable features stand out from the perspective of someone like myself whose primary interest and involvement in this field was in the medical aspects: first was the progressive increase in data related to specific diseases, helpfully collated by Victor McKusick into a series of regularly updated maps showing the morbid anatomy of the human genome (McKusick, 1988); many of these points on the disease map were the beginning of intensely mapped, and later sequenced, 'islands' of DNA that would eventually form a significant proportion of the total genome, as noted below and shown for the X chromosome in Figure 12.3a.

A critical point was reached at the Oslo workshop in 1981, halfway through the series, when DNA polymorphisms entered the scene as markers, and almost immediately began to predominate over the established protein markers. Their abundance across the entire genome raised the possibility, first outlined by Walter Bodmer and Ellen Solomon, but developed more fully by Botstein et al. (1980), of using them to construct a complete human gene map. This, in turn, meant that inherited diseases were no longer essential to give the framework of the map and, had it not been for the involvement of a number of clinically orientated workers and the recognition of the important medical goals of constructing the map, medical geneticists might have ceased to play a major role. Fortunately the workshop structures were both sufficiently robust and flexible enough by this point to accommodate the new influx of molecular geneticists, who adapted rapidly to the very different community of 'gene mappers' who had until then formed its core. Also, many of the basic molecular scientists (notably in the UK Bob Williamson and Kay Davies, already described in Chapter 10 and Figure 10.4) were strongly medically motivated. Perhaps the greatest strain for those involved in the workshops was placed on the computing and informatics staff who had to bear the main burden of supporting the infrastructure of the workshops and handling the copious and exponentially increasing data. Their problems and vital role are well described in the Witness Seminar mentioned above.

Up to the advent of DNA polymorphisms, workers involved in gene mapping had not seriously considered that mapping a gene onto a specific chromosome might actually lead to its isolation. The few human genes isolated thus far, such as those for globin, had been characterised from a previous knowledge of protein structure and RNA; for most genes involved with genetic disorders, next to nothing was known about their primary protein product, so the concept of 'positional cloning', where one did not need this information but could isolate the gene from knowledge purely of its chromosomal position, and by analysis initially of adjacent DNA, was a revolutionary one. Like many revolutions, this often took more time than was initially anticipated – 10 years from the first mapping of the Huntington's disease gene on chromosome 4 to its eventual isolation was an early example (see Chapter 11 and the interview [82] with James Gusella and Marcy McDonald) but the use of new technologies, such as pulsed field gel electrophoresis for manipulating long stretches of DNA, steadily

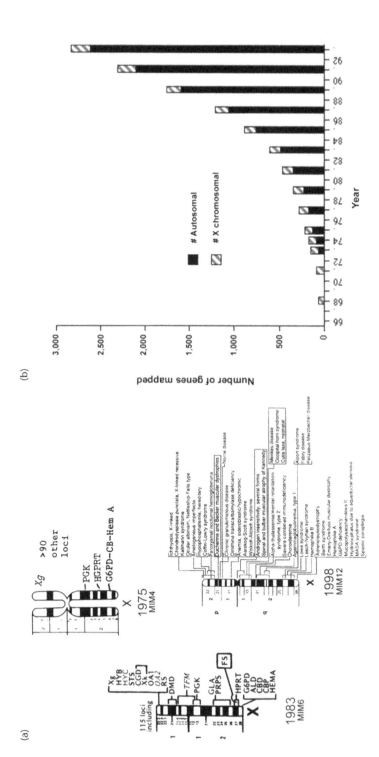

Figure 12.3 Progress in gene mapping. (a) Maps of the human X chromosome as recorded in successive editions of McKusick's *Mendelian Inheritance in Man* (b) Growth in the number of mapped human genes over the course of the human gene mapping workshops. (From McKusick 2004, courtesy of Blackwell Publishing.)

shortened this interval. So did the use of rare chromosome rearrangements in affected patients, typically deletions or X-autosome translocations, which could localise and provide a 'shortcut' to the gene itself, as was the case for Duchenne muscular dystrophy (Lindenbaum et al. 1979, Kunkel et al. 1985, Ray et al. 1985).

Progress in both the mapping and the isolation of human genes, in particular disease-related genes, now accelerated steeply, as can be seen in the tables forming a part of McKusick's *Mendelian Inheritance in Man* (1966–1998) and its online successor *OMIM,* as well as in his other gene mapping articles (see Figure 12.3b).

By 1991, however, the year of the final Human Gene Mapping workshop in London, it had become almost impossible to sustain informal workshops that attempted to cover the entire genome, so the focus moved to single chromosome workshops, under the auspices of the new Human Genome Organisation (HUGO). By this time, too, the Human Genome Project was beginning to gain momentum, principally in America, with large-scale sequencing in a small number of centres becoming the principal technology, and a consequent 'top down' approach very different from that of the gene mapping community, which was composed of numerous smaller collaborating groups.

GENE MAPPING AND DISEASE CHARITIES

For most of those involved with it, the mapping of human genes was a primarily scientific endeavour, with advancing our knowledge the main goal. But even from the earliest years a further factor was the hope that this knowledge might benefit the patients and families whose disease genes were being mapped, and this was perhaps the main factor that led to the support of families providing samples and to their lay societies playing a major role in the funding of specific mapping projects. A further factor helping this process was that the technology was shared across essentially all mendelian diseases, with first the protein markers and then DNA polymorphisms being applicable regardless of the nature of the condition, meaning that the mapping of an extra disease could be taken on as a project without prohibitive costs.

A number of the major lay societies were strong supporters of gene mapping initiatives, sensing that, once a gene relevant to 'their' disease was localised, this represented an important step towards its isolation and hopefully towards therapy. Disease associations in the UK that made significant contributions include the Cystic Fibrosis Foundation, the Muscular Dystrophy Campaign and the Tuberous Sclerosis Society. Many patients also gave key samples that helped the mapping process. These efforts, as mentioned above, progressively produced 'islands' on the genome that became extensively mapped, and later sequenced; it could even be argued that these might have eventually coalesced to give a sequence of the entire genome if there had been no overall Human Genome Project. At any rate, these initiatives deserve greater recognition than they have received.

Perhaps the final achievement of human gene mapping, before its transformation into genome sequencing, occurred neither in Britain nor in America, but in

France, where the combined efforts of a major genetic disease charity (AFM, the French Muscular Dystrophy Association) and a highly successful 'telethon' fundraising initiative, allowed a team led by Jean Weissenbach to construct in 1991 the first detailed whole human genome map (Weissenbach et al. 1992), which can be looked on as the culmination of over 50 years of progress since the original discovery by Bell and Haldane in 1937 of genetic linkage between haemophilia and colour blindness.

It is interesting as a side note that despite gene mapping giving way to sequencing over the final years of the twentieth century, the visual image that most people still have of the human genome, as pointed out by Hogan (2016), is one of a 'map' of chromosomes, usually banded or painted, rather than of a 'book' containing numerous pages of DNA sequence data. Perhaps this can be looked on as a posthumous victory for the microscope!

APPLICATIONS OF THE HUMAN GENE MAP

Even before serious gene mapping efforts had begun, early workers such as Haldane, Bell and RA Fisher had recognised that genetic linkage might provide prediction for major late-onset disorders such as Huntington's disease. Fisher even spoke to a meeting of the British insurance industry on the topic in 1935, while in their 1937 paper showing linkage between haemophilia and colour blindness, Bell and Haldane noted:

> If however, to take a possible example, an equally close linkage were found between the genes determining blood group membership and that determining Huntington's chorea, we should be able, in many cases, to predict which children of an affected person would develop the disease, and advise on the desirability or otherwise of their marriage.

It took 50 years for this to become a reality, but the effects have proved to be as profound as Bell and Haldane had anticipated, if not more so, as has been described in Chapter 7.

THE HUMAN GENOME PROJECT: SEQUENCING THE HUMAN GENOME

I do not propose to devote a large amount of space in this book to details of the Human Genome Project itself, even though it has arguably been the most important event in biology since modern science began. In part this is because it has been well publicised and written about previously from various perspectives (e.g.: Jordan 1993, an account of the early phases; Sulston and Ferry 2002, the best account from a UK viewpoint), while Wellcome Trust, Cold Spring Harbor Laboratory and other bodies are currently active in ensuring that its historical record is preserved. In fact, when starting my own historical studies around 2002, I found that the Human Genome Project and 'eugenics' were the only two topics related to human and medical genetics which most science historians, with a few notable exceptions, were aware of, almost all of the twentieth century work in the field of human and medical genetics being a complete blank. Fortunately this unawareness of genetics in medicine among historians is now well in the past, but I shall try to outline here just some of the main steps in what can be considered a truly epic project, focusing especially on those where British workers have played a particularly prominent role.

The beginnings of the human genome project

There is no doubt that the Human Genome Project as a formal endeavour began in America, and that its structure and subsequent development were also largely American in terms of both individuals and organisations involved. Perhaps surprisingly, the initial organisation to propose it was not the National Institutes of Health (NIH) but the Department of Energy (DoE), which had traditionally been involved with 'big science', as in the Manhattan Project, and which already had connections with genetics through radiation hazards and the Japan atomic bomb survivors study. NIH soon woke up, though, to the potential medical aspects of the project, and meetings were held in 1985 under the auspices of each of the two bodies.

A key decision at the Cold Spring Harbor 1985 meeting resulted from a presentation by Victor McKusick on the human gene map; most of those at the meeting had no idea of its existence, let alone that it was developing so rapidly, as recounted by McKusick (2006). It was thus decided to support mapping activities as part of the early phase of the Human Genome Project's estimated 20-year duration, while sequencing would form the main activity of the later part. This proved a wise decision, since it not only ensured that the expertise of the gene mapping community would be included in the project, but greatly helped its costs and speed during the later part as sequencing techniques improved and costs began to fall dramatically.

As the new sequencing technology became faster and more powerful, the sequencing efforts became concentrated into a few US centres and one in the UK — that in the Wellcome Trust's new Cambridge Sanger Centre (see Figure 3.23b), led by John Sulston (Figure 12.4).

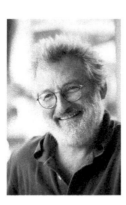

Figure 12.4 The UK and the Human Genome Project. John Sulston (1942–2018), leader of the UK contribution to the Human Genome Project and sequencer of the first multicellular organism genome (the worm *C. elegans*). (Courtesy of Wellcome Library.)

The UK influence and contribution to the Human Genome Project

While in France the Paris initiative had essentially completed the human gene map, as noted above, the group of John Sulston completed the gene sequence of the Nematode worm *Caenorhabditis elegans*, forming part of the foundations for the now internationalised Human Genome Project, officially under the aegis of HUGO, which was steadily progressing on a chromosome-by-chromosome basis.

Sulston's influence was particularly important in the decision to make all data emerging from the project immediately available on the internet – the 'Bermuda agreement' – thus providing the foundations for others to embark on numerous downstream projects, as well as projecting a positive image for a 'big science' endeavour to an initially sceptical public (Sulston and Ferry 2002).

For the UK, the biggest impact came towards the end of the Human Genome Project in its final phase, when the Wellcome Trust, using funds realised by the sale of its original pharmaceutical investments, was able to give massive support to Sulston's work that allowed his team to increase their part of the international effort, and to fend off late competition from the private company Celera, under Craig Venter, that had threatened to derail the previous steady progress. In the event, the UK contribution amounted to one third of the total sequence, including the entire X chromosome. An overall 'draft' sequence was ready for public presentation by 2000, published the following year (International Human Genome Consortium 2001, Venter et al. 2001), while the complete high-quality sequence was achieved in 2003 (International Human Genome Consortium 2004).

As its early supporters had foreseen, the completion of the Human Genome Project proved to be not just the end of an era, but the beginning of a series of new chapters, most of which are still very much in progress. Table 12.1 summarises a few of these, while some of the early medical applications of genomics, as the

Table 12.1 Some important 'downstream' initiatives resulting from the Human Genome Project

Genomic basis of mental handicap and developmental disorders; (e.g.: the DDD study)
Normal human genome variation (HAPMAP project)
Comparative genomics and evolutionary biology
Cancer genome project
Sequencing of important crop plants and domestic animals
Taxonomy
'Symbiotic' genomes; e.g.: human microbiome
Conservation biology
Ancient DNA and human origins
Geographical studies, e.g.: The 'People of British Isles' project

overall field can be collectively termed, have been described in Chapters 10 and 11; the consequences stretch far beyond genetic disorders or medicine as a whole and are already having a major impact in such fields as agriculture, wildlife conservation and taxonomy.

The UK part of the Human Genome Project, thanks to the Wellcome Trust investment, had been located mainly at what is now the Sanger Institute (aptly named after Fred Sanger), just outside Cambridge. Initially its activity was focused on the Human Genome Project itself, but after the successful completion of this, the Wellcome Trust wisely decided not to disband the collection of expertise and equipment that had been built up, but to put it to good use for supporting a variety of research projects, especially those involving genome sequencing, that the availability of the human gene sequence had now made possible. An especially valuable contribution has been to diffuse genomic technology out to other centres in Britain and internationally through a range of practical courses on both the laboratory aspects and on the informatics approaches that have become increasingly central to the field.

Among the many 'downstream' projects launched over the past 15 years are some that are more medically orientated and have attracted clinical skills, previously somewhat lacking in the earlier, technology-based phase; these have brought the Sanger Institute and its activities increasingly into contact with more classical medical genetics research and practice, to the mutual advantage of both. The examples given here focus on these medically important areas, but other fields have benefited equally.

GENOMICS IN MEDICAL GENETICS RESEARCH

The dramatic and continuing fall in the cost of DNA sequencing has made it something that now can be done on a large scale and has allowed research projects to be initiated which could not even have been considered previously. Table 12.1 has already listed just a few of these, but before considering them in more detail it is worth pausing briefly to consider the origins and meaning of the term 'genomics', since this is increasingly being used indiscriminately, reminiscent of what happened to the word 'eugenics' a century previously.

The term 'genome' has been in use for many years to designate the total complement of genetic material in an organism or a cell, but the word 'genomics' is much more recent. It seems to have been first used in relation to a new scientific journal focused on gene mapping launched in 1987, with Victor McKusick and Frank Ruddle as co-editors. Their original choice for a title was *Genome*, but it was found that this was already in use as the title of the Canadian Genetics Society journal, so the new journal was instead called *Genomics*. This flourished in a modest way; Victor McKusick wrote an editorial for its tenth anniversary (McKusick 1997) noting the origin of its title, but by this time gene mapping was giving way to gene sequencing and the term 'genomics' became adopted for the entire field of genetics based on the analysis of the genome overall, rather that of individual genes. It is not entirely clear to me why this new term was actually needed – the original word 'genetics' was elastic enough to encompass the new developments — but it became fashionable and has now firmly stuck, though those outside the field often seem very vague as to what it actually means when they use it.

This is only partly resolved if one looks at some supposedly authoritative definitions, a few of which are quoted below. Some are clear and reasonable, such as:

Genomics is an interdisciplinary field of science focusing on the structure, function, evolution, mapping, and editing of genomes. A genome is an organism's complete set of DNA, including all of its genes.

Wikipedia

Or:

…a branch of biotechnology concerned with applying the techniques of genetics and molecular biology to the genetic mapping and DNA sequencing of sets of genes or the complete genomes of selected organisms, with organizing the results in databases, and with applications of the data (as in medicine or biology)

Merriam-Webster Dictionary

But perhaps most surprising and least accurate is the definition by a World Health Organisation committee, which appears to exclude 'genetics' from any role outside 'heredity' and 'the single gene':

WHO definitions of genetics and genomics:

Genetics is the study of heredity.
Genomics is defined as the study of genes and their functions, and related techniques.

The **main difference** between genomics and genetics is that genetics scrutinizes the functioning and composition of the single gene whereas genomics addresses all genes and their inter relationships in order to identify their combined influence on the growth and development of the organism.

Many geneticists, basic as well as medical, must be surprised (and possibly somewhat aggrieved) to learn from this that much of what they have been doing all their careers is no longer regarded as 'genetics'! In relation to clinical applications, perhaps 'genome-wide' or 'whole genome' are clearer terms than 'genomic' to use for this category of investigations.

Turning now to some of the achievements of the new field, regardless of the name that one may prefer, a notable example is the analysis of the X chromosome (for whose sequencing the Sanger Institute was mainly responsible) in a large series of individuals with serious mental handicap of unknown origin, based at the Sanger Institute but with participants across the UK, and with close links with comparable studies in the Netherlands. This identified the involvement of several hundred different specific genes as responsible for patients with this complex and previously unresolvable phenotype. The project led into the wider Deciphering Developmental Disorders (DDD) study already described in Chapter 11 and the results are confirming what geneticists such as Penrose had shown in his Colchester Study (see Chapter 1) over 80 years ago, that most severe cases of mental handicap result from such specific disordered genes, many of them X-linked, in contrast to milder mental handicap, that represents the 'tail end' of a quantitative distribution of intelligence in the population.

The same progress is starting to occur for other body systems and one outcome is the progressive filling out of the molecular pathways that had already begun to be recognised prior to the genome sequence being completed, which are brought together in the late Charles Epstein's handbook *Inborn Errors of Development* (Epstein et al. 2004).

The use of whole exome sequencing is now moving into diagnostic use, not just for severe mental handicap but for rare and unidentified syndromes generally, as described below. How it will fit in with or replace current diagnostic approaches is still not entirely clear, but it seems likely to be one of the first areas where 'genomic medicine' will become part of regular medical practice rather than just an aspiration.

Returning to the wider consequences of the Human Genome Project, another major and international 'downstream' project involving the human genome, with medical importance even though primarily biological, is the now largely completed Human Variome Project, analysing sequence variation between different human populations. It is clearly essential when looking for disease-causing sequence abnormalities to be as sure as possible whether or not a finding is indeed causative; a knowledge of population differences is a vital part of this, particularly now that minorities with different ethnic origins are represented in most developed countries, not confined to their place of origin.

At a research level these studies are now possible in much larger sample numbers than was originally the case, and have linked with research that is based on the analysis of the whole genome sequences of ancient DNA, with results that are already starting to revolutionise the fields of anthropology and archaeology, and especially of human evolution, as graphically described by Reich (2018). Studies of human genetic variation have a long and distinguished tradition in British human genetics through the classical work of blood group researchers such as Arthur Mourant (1904–1994) and others (see Mourant et al. 1976). The more recent techniques are also allowing the fine detail of the British population to be analysed in a way that the earlier workers could only have dreamed of (Bodmer, 2015). Not surprisingly, the work involving ancient DNA has especially caught the public imagination with the discovery that most of us carry a small proportion of Neanderthal genes (Paabo 2015) and that interbreeding between different groups of early humans has been a regular feature of our past.

Other medically relevant genomic studies include the analysis of cancer genomes, now becoming of practical importance and discussed below; while the potential importance of bacterial genomes such as the intestinal flora and major pathogens shows that non-human genomes should not be forgotten; sequencing the genomes of many important plant and animal species will undoubtedly be relevant to our health, too. Likewise in taxonomy generally, many of the previous conclusions based on phenotypic evidence will need to be thoroughly reassessed. It is tragic that all these spectacular advances for different species should be occurring just as we are ourselves causing the greatest mass extinction event for many millions of years.

Genomics and common diseases

In the years immediately following the completion of the Human Genome Project, there was considerable hope that it would lead to identification of genes involved in susceptibility to common disorders of later life, such as coronary heart disease, diabetes and schizophrenia. It was already clear by this point that genetic linkage analysis, so successfully applied to the rarer monogenic disorders and the mendelian subsets of common disorders, was not going to be helpful for common disorders as a whole, but the possibility that there might be association of particular alleles at specific susceptibility loci seemed an attractive one, which might be detected now that there was universal and relatively uniform coverage of the genome with DNA polymorphisms.

Unfortunately these early hopes were not fulfilled to any great extent, and most initial findings proved difficult to reproduce apart from some associations with markers already known to be causally related to the particular disorder (e.g.: diabetes with polymorphisms at the insulin locus). Reasons for these largely negative initial findings included inadequate sample size, variation between different populations, but chiefly the rarity or absence of genes of large individual effect, once the mendelian disease subsets had been removed. The number of truly 'oligogenic' (as opposed to heterogeneous) disorders has proved small (Hirschsprung disease is a notable example), but for the most part common disorders are proving to be determined by large numbers of different genes, each of relatively small effect, along with a range of environmental variables. Lessons have been learned which mean that firmer gene associations are now being recognised, some of which will hopefully help to identify important environmental factors and also parts of the complex biological pathways involved, but simple cause-and-effect relationships are unlikely. To what extent a useful 'predictive polygenic score' can be produced by combining the very large number of individual associations remains uncertain, particularly in the light of the extensive variation between populations regarding this. Currently more substantial associations and predictions using over a million polymorphisms are being claimed for such conditions as coronary heart disease, but it is still unclear whether these will throw light on aetiology of the condition or provide helpful risk prediction.

While this outcome may have been disappointing for those hoping to find genes of large effect, it was not surprising, and has been helpful in confirming what most geneticists in the pre-molecular era had suspected.

GENOMICS IN CLINICAL PRACTICE

It is now 20 years since the joint US–British announcement in the year 2000 that sequencing of the human genome – or at least a 'rough draft' of it – had been achieved. It is clear from what has been said above that this landmark achievement has hugely increased our understanding of human biology and of much else, but what about the medical gains that had been promised, largely in order to obtain funding for the project? It is important to take a close look at this and to attempt to untangle the very real advances that have been achieved from the excessive hype, which it must be said has been promoted not just by politicians and the media, but by some research workers and medical policy makers, in Britain as well as in America. It is far too early to try to be definitive on this, but the importance of the field and the fact that extensive public funds are being designated for it (and hence being diverted from elsewhere) makes it important to make an attempt.

It is good to begin with the undoubted successes, two of which can be clearly identified: the diagnosis of rare diseases, especially congenital malformations, and the analysis of cancers.

The use of whole exome sequencing to identify new causes of severe mental handicap and malformation syndromes has already been mentioned in this chapter and in Chapters 10 and 11 in the context of research, such as the DDD study, but has now reached the point where it is becoming part of medical genetics services. This is impacting on how such diagnostic services should be used; reduction in costs of sequencing mean that it can now be considered as 'front line' testing rather than a last resort after chromosome analysis and testing for abnormality in specific individual genes has drawn a blank. A further important question is the extent to which whole genome testing should replace the use of specific gene testing or the panels of genes known to be involved in particular disorders. These decisions are far from simple and are likely to vary according to the particular situation. It will be most important that the valuable expertise built up in molecular diagnostic laboratories over the past 30 years is not ignored or lost as a result of premature reorganisation and centralisation.

These laboratory-related issues in turn raise questions about who should request genomic testing; should it be opened up to all clinicians, or indeed even wider, or should it be combined with the clinical diagnostic expertise of specialists such as clinical geneticists? It is worth looking back a few years at how comparable situations have resolved themselves; when chromosome analysis first became possible, those receiving samples found a much greater frequency of abnormal results in samples from the few expert clinical geneticists of the time than in samples from general paediatricians. Thirty years later the new molecular genetics laboratories had a similar experience with testing for fragile X syndrome, while surgeons and oncologists encountered it when genes for breast and colorectal cancer were isolated. These situations gradually settled without any firm 'rules' being needed, important factors being close links between the laboratories, clinical geneticists and referring clinicians, but also the careful audit of data allowing patterns of good practice and clinical guidelines to evolve.

The situation for genomic tests is likely to be comparable – in this respect whole genome analysis could be regarded as a more sophisticated form of chromosome analysis –and it is important that from the beginning detailed data should be collected which can allow sensible use of these new and powerful approaches. Such data are now starting to become available (e.g. Taylor et al. 2015) and, as expected, show that the maximal benefit of whole genome sequencing requires the careful coordination of clinical, clinical genetic and laboratory skills; interestingly in this collaborative study there was no clear benefit from genome sequencing in common diseases, even when extreme in terms of severity or age at onset.

As the volume of whole genome sequencing increases it is likely that economies of scale and need for quality control will require a degree of laboratory centralisation, but this might well change yet again as the technology becomes simpler, perhaps even 'trivial' at some point in the future. Again, lessons can be learned from historical experience with cytogenetics. It is certainly important that the value of personal links between laboratory and clinical workers in the field should not be ignored or underestimated in the interpretation of results. Most important, as noted above, will be the collection of detailed evidence on how genomic analysis is actually working out in practice. Fortunately, the UK is well placed to lead the way in this process provided it is coordinated through the NHS, not farmed out to the commercial sector.

CANCER GENOMICS

An account has been given in Chapter 4 of the way in which clinical cancer genetics has evolved, largely as a part of medical genetics and stimulated by the recognition of both specific cancer syndromes and the important subset of common cancers following mendelian inheritance. These are due primarily to constitutional genetic changes and testing of the actual tumours has not usually been involved. Most common cancers carry a low genetic risk to relatives and genes involved in constitutional susceptibility are generally of small individual effect, so their analysis remains mostly a research activity at present, not a service.

By contrast, the somatic changes in genes occurring in the tumours themselves are proving increasingly relevant to determining which treatment regimes are optimal; this is where whole genome analysis is starting to become a service tool. Naturally this is a field where clinical geneticists are much less involved than they are in the familial cancers and for constitutional genetic testing, and oncologists, surgeons and haematologists are the main clinicians concerned. The common technology may mean, though, that laboratory centres best share this work with other sequencing activities. Actually, the situation is not a new one since many cytogenetics laboratories have over past decades undertaken chromosome analysis both for tumours, including leukaemias, and for constitutional defects. The main impact of these technological changes is likely to be on more general pathology laboratories, particularly histopathology, where the diagnostic techniques have until now been primarily based on microscopy. As with medical genetics laboratory services, a shift from microscopy to molecular and sequencing techniques is a fundamental one in terms of the skills required from the staff involved and the organisation of laboratory services generally. These changes provide a valuable opportunity for historians to document them as they are occurring and to interview those involved.

OTHER SERVICE APPLICATIONS OF GENOMICS

Once we have considered these two important examples where genomic research is becoming genomic healthcare, we enter much more uncertain territory. This is especially the case for susceptibility to common disorders generally, the field where genome analysis has repeatedly been promoted as that which will most justify the use of genomic approaches to medicine. We saw earlier in this chapter how even extensive genome-wide association studies (GWAS) often failed to find strong and reproducible disease associations. While persistence in these and more sophisticated searches can be justified as a research approach to finding the biological basis for these frequent and burdensome disorders, using them in a clinical service setting for determining the susceptibility of individuals is an entirely different matter.

To start with, the risk alterations involved even for robustly associated markers, individually or as part of a whole genome analysis, are mostly small — a few percent as compared with those of 25% or 50% encountered for mendelian disorders, though claims of more extensive risk alteration are now being made on the basis of using very large numbers (over a million) of polymorphisms, as noted above. Even more importantly, it is unclear whether or not there is any real demand, or expected benefit, from finding that susceptibility is slightly increased or lowered for any particular condition. It may be suggested that this will give people opportunities for altering their 'lifestyle', but long before genomic testing existed it had been recognised that most people were extremely reluctant to change their lifestyle even if obvious and powerful risk factors were already known (smoking habits and diet are clear examples). Public health physicians and other clinicians, including medical geneticists, have all recognised that, apart from identifying the highest risk groups, notably the mendelian subsets of common disorders, it is more effective to apply a measure to the population as a whole rather than to just a portion of it with a modestly raised risk. Much of the current promotion of these additive 'polygenic scores' appears to be driven by commercial US-based companies whose primary aim is to increase business rather than to improve health.

Medical geneticists have encountered this situation in relation to genetic counselling, too, where demand for this service is mainly in relation to mendelian and other disorders where there is a reasonable chance that risk can either be greatly reduced or greatly raised, and much less for the common disorders of later life. Of course, for common disorders the population baseline risk is high anyway, so complete exclusion of risk is impossible.

At this point it is relevant to look ar some of the drawbacks and hazards of whole genome testing, especially if this were to be done on a population scale. These have already been raised in Chapter 7 in relation to testing for specific genes and apply equally or even more to genomic tests. The 2003 UK Health Department 'white paper' on genetics (see Chapter 8) suggested, presumably seriously, that whole genome screening should be considered for all newborns, using the blood sample already being collected for testing for phenylketonuria and a few other serious but treatable genetic disorders. Although this 'barcoding of babies' (as it became known) did not find favour then, it has surfaced again with the feasibility and declining cost of whole genome screening, raising a raft of ethical issues involving consent (or lack of it), privacy (access of third parties such as insurers and employers), and discrimination. Quite what the benefits might be remain unclear at the present.

The privacy of personal information generally, including health information, has been shown recently to be extremely insecure, so it is easy to imagine that existing information on a person's genome could be misappropriated or misused. This possibility already exists with such repositories as the UK forensic DNA database, where the ethical dangers were largely ignored (see Chapter 7) until pointed out by the Human Genetics Commission. Lionel Penrose, prescient as always, pointed out in his inaugural lecture, over 70 years ago and a year after the Japanese atomic explosions, both the dangers and a possible solution.

> The general problem of mental health is among the most important problems confronting the human race. We do not, in civilised countries, willingly entrust persons judged to be insane or mentally defective with dangerous weapons such as knives and firearms. Now that weapons are constructed capable of instantaneous annihilation of large populations, the question of ensuring the intelligence and mental stability of people entrusted with the power of decision has become extremely significant.
>
> *Penrose 1946*

If politicians were to be made the first to undergo systematic genome screening this might perhaps help to curb any premature enthusiasm they might have for applying this to the rest of the population. A very recent (2019) example of this has just occurred in England, with the expected results of misinterpretation and confusion!

PHARMACOGENETICS AND PHARMACOGENOMICS

It has long been recognised that there is extensive genetic variation in response to a number of drugs, leading in some cases to major reactions, while in others a different dosage may be required. Over 50 years ago this became a major topic for research by workers such as Werner Kalow (1962, 2005) and human geneticists Friedrich Vogel and Arno Motulsky, who coined the term 'pharmacogenetics'. In Britain, the work was taken up by David Price Evans (Evans et al. 1960), working with Cyril Clarke in Liverpool, where I myself remember in the 1960s patients being tested prior to starting antituberculous therapy to see if they were 'fast' or 'slow' acetylators of the drug isoniazid.

Following the human genome project, the field has been rebranded as 'pharmacogenomics' and the earlier work largely forgotten or ignored, but the situation has not essentially changed, though a wider aim has been promoted of 'personalised' or 'precision' medicine in relation to individualised drug and other therapy. So far though, with the exception of some cancer-related therapies, mentioned above in this chapter, this remains an aspiration rather than a clear service. Pharmaceutical companies have also been wary of attempts to subdivide a single market, while the very concept of every patient being given a specifically tailored drug or dose leads to the possibility of increased prescribing errors, currently the biggest cause of adverse drug effects.

All in all, genomics remains at present, with a few important exceptions, at the research stage rather than a major part of clinical medicine; this may well change in future, but a lot more research is needed first, along with critical evaluation of any new proposed service applications. This is also, broadly, the conclusion of a recent report from the Public Health Genomics Foundation (see Chapter 8).

Attempting to look ahead at the future of genomics is rash, given the speed of change in technology and the rapid fall in costs of most applications. I try to address this in the final chapter, but if this technology is to support our needs in medicine, rather than to drive the field regardless of need, then we shall have to be vigilant that it does not harm the clinical and laboratory practices in medical genetics that have grown up and been well validated over the past 30 or more years.

REFERENCES

Bangham J. 2014. Blood groups and human groups: Collecting and calibrating genetic data after World War Two. *Stud Hist Philos Biol Biomed Sci.* 47 Pt A:74–86.

Bell J, Haldane JBS. 1937. The linkage between the genes for colour-blindness and haemophilia in man. *Proc R Soc Lond B.* 123:119–150.

Bodmer WF. 2015. Genetic characterization of human populations: From ABO to a genetic map of the British Isles. *Genetics.* 199: 267–279.

Botstein D, White RL, Scolnick M, Davis RW. 1980. Construction of genetic linkage map in man using restriction fragment length polymorphisms. *Am J Hum Genet.* 32:314–331.

Epstein CJ, Erickson RP, Wynshaw-Boris A (eds.). 2004. *Inborn Errors of Development: The Molecular Basis of Clinical Disorders of Morphogenesis.* New York: Oxford University Press.

Evans DAP, Manley KA, McKusick VA. 1960. Genetic control of isoniazid metabolism in man. *Brit Med J.* 2: 485–491.

Fisher RA. 1935. Linkage studies and the prognosis of hereditary ailments. *Transactions of the International Congress on Life Assurance Medicine.* London, pp. 615–617.

Haldane JBS, Sprunt AD, Haldane NM. 1915. Reduplication in mice. *J Genet.* 5:153.

Harper PS, Rivas ML, Bias WB, Hutchinson JR, Dyken PR, McKusick VA. 1972. Genetic linkage confirmed between the locus for myotonic dystrophy and the ABH-secretion and Lutheran blood group loci. *Am J Hum Genet.* 24:310–316.

Harris H [Henry], Watkins JF. 1965. Hybrid cells derived from mouse and man: Artificial heterokaryons of mammalian cells from different species. *Nature.* 205:640–646.

Hogan AJ. 2016. *Life Histories of Genetic Disease: Patterns and Prevention in Medical Genetics.* Baltimore: Johns Hopkins University Press.

International Human Genome Sequencing Consortium. 2001. Initial sequencing and analysis of the human genome [PDF]. *Nature.* 409: 860–921.

International Human Genome Sequencing Consortium. 2004. Finishing the euchromatic sequence of the human genome. *Nature.* 431: 931–935.

Jones EM, Tansey EM (eds.). 2015. *Human Gene Mapping Workshops c1973-c1991. Wellcome Witnesses to Contemporary Medicine,* vol 54. London: Queen Mary University of London.

Jones EM. 2016. A witness seminar on the history of the human gene mapping workshops. *Gene.* 589:123–6.

Jordan B. 1993. *Travelling around the Human Genome.* Paris: John Libbey.

Kalow W. 1962. *Pharmacogenetics: Heredity and the Responses to Drugs.* London: WB Saunders.

Kalow W. 2005. Pharmacogenomics: Historical perspective and current status. *Methods Mol Biol.* 311:3–15.

Kunkel LM, Monaco AP, Middlesworth W, Ochs HD. 1985. Specific cloning of DNA fragments absent from the DNA of a male patient with an X chromosome deletion. *Proc Natl Acad Sci U S A.* 82:4778–4782.

Lindenbaum RH, Clarke G, Patel C, Moncrieff M, Hughes JT. 1979. Muscular dystrophy in an X; 1 translocation female suggests that Duchenne locus is on X chromosome short arm. *J Med Genet.* 16:389–92.

McKusick VA. 1966. *Mendelian Inheritance in Man: Catalogs of Autosomal Dominant, Autosomal Recessive, and X-Linked Phenotypes,* 1st ed. Baltimore: The Johns Hopkins University Press. (12th edition, 1998.)

McKusick VA. 1988. *The Morbid Anatomy of the Human Genome: A Review of Gene Mapping in Clinical Medicine.* Chevy Chase, MD: Howard Hughes Medical Institute.

McKusick VA. 1997. Genomics: Structural and functional studies of genomes. *Genomics.* 45:244–9.

McKusick VA. 2006. A 60-year tale of spots, maps and genes. *Annu Rev Genomics Hum Genet.* 7:1–27.

McKusick VA. 2007. Mendelian inheritance in man and its online version, OMIM. *Am J Hum Genet.* 80(4):588–604.

Mohr J. 1951. Estimation of linkage between the Lutheran and Lewis blood groups. *Acta Pathol Microbiol Scand.* 29:339–344.

Morton NE. 1956. The detection and estimation of linkage between the genes for elliptocytosis and the Rh blood type. *Am J Hum Genet.* 8:80–96.

Mourant AE, Kopec AC, Domaniewska-Sobczak K. 1976. *The Distribution of the Human Blood Groups and Other Polymorphisms.* Oxford: Oxford University Press.

Paabo S. 2015. The diverse origins of the human gene pool. *Nat Rev Genet.* 16: 313–314.

Penrose LS. 1946. Phenylketonuria: A problem in eugenics. *Lancet.* 1:949–953.

Ray PN, Belfall B, Duff C, Logan C, Kean V, Thompson MW, Sylvester JE, Gorski JL, Schmickel RD, Worton RG. 1985. Cloning of the breakpoint of an X;21 translocation associated with Duchenne muscular dystrophy. *Nature.* 318:672–5.

Renwick JH, Bolling D. 1971. An analysis procedure illustrated on a triple linkage of use for prenatal diagnosis of myotonic dystrophy. *J Med Genet.* 8:399–406.

Renwick JH, Lawler SD. 1955. Genetical linkage between the ABO and nail-patella loci. *Ann Hum Genet.* 19:312–331.

Reich D. 2018. *Who We Are and How we Got There: Ancient DNA and the New Science of the Human Past.* Oxford; Oxford University Press.

Ruddle FH, Bootsma D, McKusick VA. et al. (eds.). 1974. New Haven Conference, 1973; First International Conference on Human Gene Mapping. *Cytogenet Cell Genet.* 13:1–216.

Smithies O. 1955. Zone electrophoresis in starch gels: Group variations in the serum proteins of normal human adults. *Biochem J.* 61:629–641.

Sturtevant AH. 1913. The linear arrangement of six sex-linked factors in *Drosophila*, as shown by their mode of association. *J Exp Zool.* 14:43–59.

Sulston J, Ferry G. 2002. *The Common Thread.* London: Bantam Press.

Taylor JC, Martin HC, Lise S. et al. 2015. Factors influencing success of clinical genome sequencing across a broad spectrum of disorders. *Nat Genet.* 47: 717–726.

Venter JC, Adams MD, Myers EW. et al. 2001. The sequence of the human genome. *Science.* 291(5507):1304–1351.

Weiss MC, Green H. 1967. Human-mouse hybrid cell lines containing partial complements of human chromosomes and functioning human genes. *Proc Natl Acad Sci U S A.* 58:1104–1110.

Weissenbach J, Gyapay G, Dib G. et al. 1992. A second-generation linkage map of the human genome. *Nature.* 359:794–801.

13

Medical genetics and genetics in medicine: Now and future

Throughout this book I have used both the terms 'medical genetics' and 'genetics in medicine', often indiscriminately. But these words reflect a deeper meaning in terms of how one thinks about genetics and how one uses it in one's practice, regardless of whether this is clinical or laboratory based. I believe that the balance and counterpoint between these two terms and the approaches that underlie them have been critical and essential to the development of the field as reflected in its history, and that this balance will be equally important in determining its future.

By 'genetics in medicine' most people mean the incorporation of genetic technology and genetic thinking in medical practice overall, whatever speciality may be concerned. We have seen that this stretches back in time over many years, and that physicians took a keen interest in the familial nature of disorders they encountered long before there was any sound explanation for their observations. This was the case both for rare disorders and for common diseases, as was appreciated as far back as 1814 by Joseph Adams in his distinction between 'disposition' and 'predisposition' and also, nearly a century later, by those taking part in the 1908 Royal Society of Medicine 'Debate on Heredity and Disease'.

The term 'medical genetics' began its life with a meaning little different from 'genetics in medicine', and with particular application to the teaching of genetics to medical students. Madge Macklin in America may have been the first to use the term regularly during the 1930s. Over the second half of the twentieth century, though, it progressively came to denote the emergence of a new medical speciality, based on origins in established fields such as adult internal medicine and paediatrics, but with particular characteristics and identity that subsequently resulted in separate training programmes and permanent posts. Over the same period, laboratory techniques such as chromosome and later molecular genetic analysis, with their roots in basic research, developed codes of practice and identities in their service applications that allowed them to become part of 'medical genetics' as an overall discipline. A comparable evolution of specific non-medical, genetic counsellors has also occurred, so that medical genetics as a field of practice is now a multidisciplinary profession, something that those within it have supported and greatly welcomed.

For most of the twentieth century medical practitioners in general felt that, while genetics was clearly important for an increased understanding of disease and in allowing patients with genetic disorders to be recognised and at times referred to medical genetics specialists, it was not something integral to their own regular practice. There were a few exceptions, such as haematologists involved in haemophilia and haemoglobinopathies, but for most common diseases 'genetics in medicine' was an area of research aimed at increasing understanding of these complex conditions, rather than of practice, while 'medical genetics' denoted a separate speciality, including both research and also service applications.

To a large extent this still remains true, despite exhortations from health policy makers and politicians that genetics should be 'mainstreamed' into primary care and overall hospital medicine. Despite the advent of genomics, and increasing use of the term to cover many areas which are no different essentially to the activities covered by medical genetics in its various forms, this has so far made little difference outside a few specific areas, nor is it likely that it will do so until there is much more evidence that new genomic activities are actually beneficial rather than just technically feasible. Meanwhile, repeated surveys have shown that existing specialist medical genetics services are valued by patients, families and clinicians, so it is greatly to be hoped that enthusiasm among policy makers for the new and mostly still unproven benefits of genomics will not damage or divert resources away from the more established but equally innovative services and research fields characterising medical genetics.

In fact, medical geneticists themselves have been the most active proponents for the 'mainstreaming' of their field, recognising from the outset that they are able to deal themselves with only a fraction of the need for genetic services. In both their practice and their writings they have emphasised that genetic knowledge and genetic thinking are essential for all workers in medicine if they are to recognise and deal satisfactorily with the genetic issues that arise throughout medical practice.

Over the past 60 or more years a series of technological advances has increasingly allowed families at high genetic risk to take positive action to avoid or at least minimise this, but this has at the same time increased the chances of harm occurring if potential dangers are not recognised. This is especially the case for the wider aspects of genetic testing, where initial use by medical geneticists has pioneered patterns of good practice that have subsequently been passed on to clinicians generally, who might have otherwise been unaware of the potential problems.

The end result until now has been that Britain has had a good record of how it has handled most of the difficult and sensitive issues arising from genetic aspects of medicine. It has also resulted in an efficient and economical use of scarce resources, avoiding wasteful and at times unnecessary use of tests, genetic or otherwise. It is unlikely that the basic situation will need to change much as new genomic approaches to testing come into practice.

Looking ahead a few more years, the possibility that everyone will have their complete genome sequenced at some point in their life needs to be considered realistically, even though at present most would consider this unnecessary and undesirable; this might be at birth, in relation to employment or insurance, or as a prelude to a medical consultation. It is quite possible that they will not have consented to this, have any control over access to the information, or even know that it has been done. An important role here for those recording the history of the field is to ensure that changes leading in this direction, whether or not they actually occur, are fully and accurately documented, analysed and linked to past events that could provide evidence on any harm or benefit that could result from the new developments. A further role is to point out to people those lessons that have been learned (or in some cases not learned) from issues in the past, so that comparable problems do not occur again.

Where will medical genetics as a specialty fit in among other parts of medicine as genetics (including genomics) increasingly forms an integral part of wider medical practice? In theory it might be thought that this process would reduce the need for specialist medical geneticists and genetic counsellors, but the experience of the past 30 years has shown that the demand for both genetic counselling and wider clinical genetics services has steadily increased, with new activities more than balancing those that have been handed on to paediatricians, obstetricians and other clinical specialties. Education of these colleagues will also form (and indeed already is) an increasing part of the work of the medical geneticist.

Thus the future evolution both of medical genetics, and of genetics in wider medicine looks promising, particularly in Britain, with its universal healthcare under the National Health Service and its strong tradition of close links between research and service aspects, and between laboratory and clinical workers. If one looks broadly at how the field has developed since the end of the last world war, the remarkable power of the science involved has been matched by generally sensible and beneficial applications. New and controversial developments have been fully and widely discussed, especially by authoritative bodies like the Human Genetics Commission and the Nuffield Council on Bioethics; patients and the public have been consulted and listened to, while abuse and unwise applications have mostly been avoided. Sensationalism and false claims, made at times by both the media and professionals, have usually been corrected at an early stage. Just as important is that availability of any new proven advances has on the whole been equitable and based on need, rather than commercially driven. Provided that these trends continue, and are allowed to evolve naturally, I think that the future for both medical genetics and genetics in wider medicine should continue to be a bright one.

PROBLEMS IN THE EVOLUTION OF UK MEDICAL GENETICS

I have focused mostly in this book on what may fairly considered as advances and successes, but It would be wrong to regard the development of medical genetics in

Britain over the past half century as being without its problems, at times serious. Some of these problems have been due largely to external factors, but others have been more intrinsic.

Among the extrinsic factors, several have been of a general social and political nature. First has been the widespread connection in the political and public mind between genetic services and abortion over the half century since this became available. In fact, as described in Chapter 5, the attitude of most medical geneticists to abortion on grounds of genetic risk has been a cautious and responsible one and it is likely that considerably more pregnancies have been saved than lost as the result of interaction with a clinical geneticist or genetic counsellor. When it comes to general screening programmes for fetal abnormality, medical geneticists have been among the strongest critics of those programmes that seem to be mainly public health or eugenic in nature rather than aligned with the wishes of individual women and couples.

Despite this, the perception has persisted of the link, and for many years resulted in the then UK Health Department staying away from any clear policy on medical genetics as a whole in case of adverse political effects (see the discussion in the Clinical Genetics Witness Seminar described in Chapter 8).

A serious early problem with long-lasting effects, mentioned in Chapter 2, was the sharp contraction in funding for university posts and departments, starting in the mid 1970s, just as medical genetics was expanding across the country. This meant that by comparison with the longer established medical-scientific specialties such as anatomy and physiology, there was a lack of well-staffed and supported departments of medical genetics, and few academic training posts outside the MRC units. While it is fortunate that increasing numbers of NHS posts were created at that time, the end result was (and remains) an unbalanced situation, with a number of highly able academically inclined workers diverted into posts that carried a progressively increasing service and administrative load.

Matters were worsened for medical genetics by the introduction of the 'internal market' for NHS services (see Chapter 8), forcing different centres into artificial competition with each other when the success of the field as a whole was largely the result of collaboration. This was later abandoned (and never occurred in Scotland, which had already built its consortium model for genetic testing), but it required persistent effort and opposition from workers in medical genetics and their professional societies to ensure that what had been created with great effort over the previous 30 years was not wilfully destroyed. Yet another problem, still continuing, has been the increased distancing over the past two decades of the University and NHS systems from each other, and the loss of flexibility between them that had been such a key factor in the early years of medical genetics.

Readers from other UK medical specialties will of course recognise these and similar problems from their own experiences, and the fact that medical genetics has survived and flourished in the face of numerous difficulties is a testament to the cohesiveness of its community, both clinical and laboratory, and to a combination of resilience, ingenuity, opportunism and the forging of strong links with key policy makers. The whole saga would make an excellent project for detailed objective analysis by someone less closely involved than myself!

Not all of the difficulties encountered by the new field of medical genetics as it developed can be blamed on external factors, so it is worth a glance at some internal issues, though as an 'insider' my views are perhaps of limited value. Looking back to the early years of human genetics, the strongly mathematical and statistical nature of much of the work, while allowing much progress despite a lack of experimental techniques, undoubtedly deterred many clinicians, though fortunately the next generation of clinical geneticists, as seen particularly by those emerging from the first training posts, were able to build bridges with other medical specialties.

The older academic centres, notably Oxford, Cambridge and Edinburgh, the best endowed with both funds and talent, which with their major research achievements should have led progress in medical genetics overall, have sadly been among the slowest to do so, for a variety of reasons – including personal difficulties, inter-academic rivalries and an at times dismissive attitude to the field of medical genetics generally; these attitudes have to an extent been contagious due to the extensive wider influence of these centres. By contrast, most 'regional' universities have had strongly positive relationships with their medical genetics centres, as have many of their corresponding university teaching hospitals.

It would be wrong to overemphasise these and other difficulties, which are probably no greater than those occurring in other developing areas of science and medicine. In fact, if one looks at the achievements of the past 50 years in terms both of scientific advance and of benefits to patients and families, it would be hard to find another area where comparable advances have taken place so rapidly. A glance at the websites of the various centres shows that the field has expanded greatly since their founding, with overall staffing having risen from just a handful of people to often over a hundred in major centres. Correspondingly, the number of clinical staff in regional NHS centres, which 30 years ago were often single-handed, is often now in double figures, while this applies even more to genetic counsellors.

It would also be hard to find a field that has been more collegiate in terms of mutual help between different centres and individuals, something that has made it a pleasure for almost everyone, myself included, to have spent a career working in it. A high proportion of the thought and forward planning at local, national and international levels has resulted from extensive 'out of hours' efforts by its members; as in most fields, such 'goodwill' is a precious, though fragile commodity that often receives less recognition than it deserves.

MEDICAL GENETICS AND THE OVERALL STRUCTURE OF MEDICINE AND SOCIETY

The developments that we have seen in the science and medicine of genetics need to be seen in the context of the equally striking changes in society as a whole which have been occurring over this time. Back in 1950 and before, the overall pattern of disease was dominated by infections, poor nutrition and other major environmental factors; genetic disorders were inconspicuous outside a small number of families. The attitude to sick, premature or malformed newborns was often fatalistic and family size was large. Contraception was inadequate and abortion illegal. Patients were reluctant to ask questions about genetic aspects of a family disorder and at times concealed information due to perceived stigma. Medical professionals frequently had no answers to give anyway, while lay societies for genetic disorders barely existed.

The present time shows marked contrasts with the past for all these aspects, though they still persist in the less well educated. For example, my own experience in seeing families with Huntington's disease over many years has been one of increasing openness regarding the disorder from those at risk for it, with a widespread willingness to share even such sensitive details such as predictive test results, which professionals have always treated with the greatest caution in regard to confidentiality. Might such openness extend to the outcomes from whole genome screening, especially if it were widespread or universal in the population? This may largely depend on how much people trust their government and policy makers, the former being currently held in generally poor esteem in Britain and many other countries. Social scientists and others need to begin to document these aspects now.

Readers may have noted a number of places throughout this book where I have commented 'this topic deserves a detailed historical analysis', or words to that effect. I made the same comment in my earlier 2008 book *A Short History of Medical Genetics* and gave a table of suggested projects there (p. 478). Since few of these seem to have been taken up so far, I give an updated (and enlarged) list in Table A2.6. This would be sufficient to occupy productively a small army of workers!

WHAT HAS MEDICINE IN GENERAL LEARNED FROM MEDICAL GENETICS?

As genetic approaches progressively become a greater part of wider medical practice, it is important to look at what skills and knowledge have already been transferred from medical genetics. This is often considered principally in terms of technology, and this is indeed of the highest importance, as has been discussed in Chapter 12, but 'genetic thinking' is just as, if not more, important. Table 13.1 lists just a few essential aspects of genetic medicine, regardless of who practices it; most of these have been mentioned in previous chapters. Not all of these have yet been fully incorporated or even widely recognised in wider practice.

POSTSCRIPT

Genetics and medicine – A personal note

Readers of this book may feel, probably rightly, that I have already given more than enough space to my personal views, but since one of the pleasures of writing a book, as opposed to a scientific paper, is to be able to include things that might have been removed by a more objective referee, I shall conclude with this personal note, which I think may reflect the feelings of others as well as myself.

During the making of my interview series, I repeatedly encountered people who stressed how much they had loved their career in medical genetics, and

Table 13.1 'Genetic Thinking': Some of the genetic approaches that have passed or are passing into wider medical practice

Avoidance of a directive approach

Uncertainty in relation to genetic risk; how to quantify and handle it

Provision of a written record of genetic consultation for the patient/family

Awareness of risks and needs of the extended family

Necessity of adequate time for genetic counselling and communication generally (Chapter 6)

Recognition of the wider issues of genetic testing (Chapter 7); ability to consent, e.g. testing of children; sharing of information within the family and with third parties

Complexity and potential pitfalls of genetic (and genomic) testing, especially for common diseases (e.g. normal variants, population differences, importance of clinical context, inadvertent testing)

what a privilege it had been to have taken part in its development during such exciting years. Some of these people were laboratory scientists, others clinicians, but they shared, as do I, this love of the field and of their own work. Here are a few examples, dating from the earliest years to recent times.

Caroline Berry on Paul Polani:

> When I went to visit the unit, he was a great enthusiast. I remember he showed me around the department and it was awfully interesting and exciting and he said 'here we breathe genetics', and we did.

David Weatherall on Cyril Clarke:

> ... what he taught me was an enquiring mind, it was a kind of hopping around enquiring mind. He was interested in everything. And this enormous enthusiasm; when he had this conversation with Philip Sheppard who worked with him on butterflies and this idea that there might be something in genetics for medicine, ... an extraordinary kind of enthusiasm evolved and that was really quite infectious, the whole place was buzzing. Crazy ideas some of them but, you are right, he was one of that old generation of physician naturalists, really you know, he was in a curious way a bit of a polymath.

Muriel Lee, technician to Patricia Jacobs:

> ... it was exciting, it really was. And to this day, although I have been retired over a year, to this day it still gives me great pleasure to look down the microscope and actually see a metaphase cell. I mean it is just, I still find that exciting, you know.

Caroline Berry again gives one of the main reasons why those involved were so enthusiastic:

PSH: It's been an extraordinarily exciting period to work in genetics. Have you ever had any regrets or wishes that you had chosen anything else?

CB: No, no. I used to say that people needed to change their job every seven years so that they didn't get stale, but with genetics the job changed so much there was no need to change, the job changed.

PSH: Yes, and you had to change with it.

Interview with Caroline Berry

To which I might add that in my experience, not only did the job change but that, as a clinician, every patient one saw presented different challenges in the use of one's skills and experience, so that I was able to continue to encounter entirely new problems until the day I retired from active clinical practice.

I share the feelings of those I have quoted above, not only from the viewpoint of a clinician, but also through having seen how in many ways research advances have been of direct help to patients and families where one previously could offer little.

A number of Paul Polani's paediatric colleagues expressed their disappointment when, soon after the war, he entered medical genetics full time, after being a highly skilled paediatrician (and children's surgeon) during the wartime years.

Cyril Clarke managed to continue practicing general internal medicine in combination with medical genetics throughout his career, though his enjoyment and sense of 'fun' came principally from his genetics research.

David Weatherall, in my interview with him, questioned whether the clinical geneticist could feel fulfilled if one was not responsible for treating one's own patients. I think that he may have been asking indirectly about my own experience.

… many clinical geneticists really had very limited clinical practices in a sense and perhaps they would make the diagnosis and prognostications, but then perhaps hand over to the specialist in that general area. I think that has always been one of the problems with clinical genetics in a sense, but as it's abutting more and more across into general medicine, there is still, I think there's an enormous place for specialists in clinical genetics, but I often wonder how satisfying that life is for the ones who are very much more patient orientated.

I have thought about this a lot over subsequent years, and have concluded that after 50 years in medical genetics, with the first 30 spent in general medicine too, any worthwhile contributions that I may have made have been almost entirely in medical genetics, though having a thorough general medical background has helped greatly. In fact, I am in no doubt that I have practiced considerably more, and more varied, clinical medicine through genetics than I ever did in general internal medicine. Certainly if I compare the amount of 'organic pathology' encountered over the years during genetic consultations, including genetic counselling, with that seen in my unselected general medical clinics that I continued for many years, it was far more in the former, though I suspect that many of my general medical patients with no obvious pathology benefited from my being able to take the time to listen to their largely non-medical problems.

Many clinical geneticists working in the area of dysmorphology find that they develop an intuitive sense of recognition for particular disorders. I myself have found a comparable, almost subconscious recognition when seeing patients with very early or mild stages of Huntington's disease or of myotonic dystrophy, to name two late-onset conditions with which I have been involved with over many years, even to the point of having patients referred for diagnosis by experienced neurologists! I do not think that reflects special abilities in myself, but rather having had the opportunity to see many families and affected patients, perhaps several hundred for each of these disorders, previously, whereas most neurologists would have seen only a handful over their whole career.

Have I missed the responsibilities for treatment provided by acute general medicine? Perhaps I would have done if I had left it earlier, but after 30 years I had already found that most active acute therapeutic measures were best left to more junior staff, with my own occasional interventions increasingly being to restrain what seemed sometimes to be excessive enthusiasm. In any case, most therapy is now a team responsibility and there is increasing scope for involvement of the clinical geneticist in this; Table 13.2 gives some important examples.

Table 13.2 Some genetic disorders where medical geneticists now play a major role in management and therapy, usually as part of a multidisciplinary group

Muscular dystrophies
Huntington's disease
Familial colorectal and breast cancer
Tuberous sclerosis
Neurofibromatosis
Marfan syndrome
Bone dysplasias
Phenylketonuria and other 'inborn errors'

So my broad conclusion, like that of virtually all the colleagues who I have interviewed or worked with over many years, is that medical genetics has been an immensely rewarding and satisfying field of medicine and of science to have worked in, and that it has indeed been a privilege to have been able to do this over a professional lifetime. I have seen it change greatly and it will doubtless continue to do so, but I see no inherent reason why it should not remain as rewarding for future generations as it has been for my own, and that this should be true also for the increasing number of more general clinicians who are adopting aspects of genetic medicine into their own fields of practice.

Appendix 1: A timeline for genetics and medicine in Britain

Modern medical genetics as a well-defined field of medicine has developed so rapidly since its beginnings three-quarters of a century ago that it is often forgotten how far back in time its roots and origins go. It can be reasonably argued that genetics overall was based in considerable measure on problems of human inheritance and inherited disease, and studies of this, especially in Britain, extend back long before the twentieth century acceptance of mendelism. Thus medical genetics, when thought of in the widest sense, is perhaps the oldest area of genetics, and certainly not the recent addition that it is sometimes portrayed as.

This 'timeline' gives some of what I consider to be the main landmarks along this lengthy course. Not all of these can be considered to be directly part of 'medical genetics', even in the broadest definition, but they are all relevant to it in one way or another. I have also included some more general 'world events' that have particularly impacted on the development of the field.

The timeline is based on that originally used for the Genetics and Medicine Historical Network website (www.genmedhist.org/timeline) over 15 years ago and tries to put contributions that are mainly, or at least substantially, British (left-hand column) in the context of developments primarily made elsewhere (right-hand column). It must be emphasised, though, that the field has been from the outset exceptionally international and collaborative, one of its great strengths, as I hope that I have made clear throughout this book.

The selection of advances for this timeline is inevitably arbitrary and fragmentary, especially for the period since 2000, which has seen a rapid acceleration of progress in the genomics field.

Contributions mainly (or substantially) from the UK	Contributions mainly from outside the UK
1651 William Harvey's book *De Generatione Animalium* studies the egg and early embryo in different species and states: 'Ex ovo omnium' (all things from the egg).	
	1677 Microscopic observations of human sperm (Leeuwenhoek).
1699 Albinism and its familial nature noted in the 'Moskito Indians' of Central America (Wafer).	
	1735 Linnaeus' *Systema Naturae*. First comprehensive classification of plants and animals.
	1751 Maupertuis proposes equal contributions of both sexes to inheritance and a 'particulate' concept of heredity.
	1753 Maupertuis describes polydactyly in the Ruhe family, and gives the first estimate of likelihood for it being hereditary.
1794 John Dalton describes colour blindness in himself and others; he finds it limited to males.	
1800 Erasmus Darwin (Grandfather of Charles Darwin) publishes *Zoonomia*; progressive evolution from primaeval organisms was recognised by him.	
	1803 Haemophilia in males and its inheritance through females described (Otto, USA).
	1809 Inherited blindness described in multiple generations (Martin, USA).
	1809 Lamarck (France) supports evolution (including human), based on inheritance of acquired characteristics.

(Continued)

Contributions mainly (or substantially) from the UK	Contributions mainly from outside the UK
1814 Joseph Adams' book defines the concepts of 'predisposition' and 'disposition'; 'congenital' and 'hereditary', corresponding to later mendelian and multifactorial categories.	
1852 First clear description of Duchenne muscular dystrophy by Edward Meryon.	
1853 Haemophilic son, Leopold, born to Queen Victoria in England.	
1858 Charles Darwin and Alfred Russel Wallace; papers on Natural Selection read to Linnean Society of London.	
1859 Charles Darwin publishes *On the Origin of Species*.	
	1865 Gregor Mendel's experiments on plant hybridisation presented to Brunn (Brno) Natural History Society.
	1866 Mendel's report formally published.
1868 Charles Darwin's 'provisional hypothesis of pangenesis'. This, together with collected details of inherited disorders, published in *Animals and Plants under Domestication*.	
	1871 Friedrich Miescher isolates and characterises 'nucleic acid'.
	1872 George Huntington describes 'Huntington's disease'.
	1882 First illustration of human chromosomes (Walther Flemming).
	1885 Concept of 'continuity of the germ plasm' (August Weismann).
	1887 Theodor Boveri shows constancy of chromosomes through successive generations.

(Continued)

Contributions mainly (or substantially) from the UK	Contributions mainly from outside the UK
	1888 Waldeyer coins the term 'chromosome'.
	1888 Weismann presents evidence against inheritance of acquired characteristics.
1889 Francis Galton's *Law of Ancestral Inheritance*.	
	1891 Henking identifies and names the 'X chromosome'.
1894 William Bateson's book *Material for the Study of Variation*.	
	1896 EB Wilson's book *The Cell in Development and Inheritance*.
1899 Archibald Garrod's first paper on alkaptonuria.	
	1900 Mendel's work rediscovered (de Vries, Correns and Tschermak).
	1901 Karl Landsteiner discovers ABO blood group system.
1901 Archibald Garrod notes ocurrence in sibs and consanguinity in alkaptonuria.	
1902 Bateson and Saunders' note on alkaptonuria as an autosomal recessive disorder. Bateson and Garrod correspond.	
1902 Garrod's definitive paper on alkaptonuria as an example of 'chemical individuality'.	
1902 Bateson's book *Mendel's Principles of Heredity. A Defence* supports mendelism against attacks of the biometricians.	
	1902 Chromosome theory of heredity proposed by Theodor Boveri and by Walter Sutton.
	1903 American Breeders Association formed. Includes section of eugenics from 1909.

(Continued)

Contributions mainly (or substantially) from the UK	Contributions mainly from outside the UK
	1903 Lucien Cuénot in France shows Mendelian basis, and multiple alleles, for albinism in mice.
	1903 Castle and Farabee (Boston) show autosomal recessive inheritance in human albinism.
	1903 Farabee shows autosomal dominant inheritance in brachydactyly.
	1905 Nettie Stevens and EB Wilson separately show inequality of sex-chromosomes and involvement in sex determination in insects.
1905 Bateson coins the term 'genetics'.	
1906 First International Genetics Congress held in London.	
1908 Garrod's Croonian lectures on 'inborn errors of metabolism'.	
1908 Royal Society of Medicine, London, 'Debate on Heredity and Disease' gives first major interaction between geneticists and clinicians.	
1908 Hardy (England) and Weinberg (Germany) independently show relationship and stability of gene and genotype frequencies ('Hardy Weinberg equilibrium').	
1909 Bateson's further book *Mendel's Principles of Heredity* documents a series of human diseases following mendelian inheritance.	
1909 Karl Pearson initiates *Treasury of Human Inheritance.*	
	1909 Wilhelm Johannsen, Copenhagen, introduces term 'gene'.

(Continued)

Contributions mainly (or substantially) from the UK	Contributions mainly from outside the UK
	1910 Thomas Hunt Morgan (New York) discovers X-linked 'white eye' *Drosophila* mutant.
	1910 Eugenics Record Office established at Cold Spring Harbor (USA) under Charles Davenport.
	1911 EB Wilson's definitive paper on sex determination shows X-linked inheritance for haemophilia and colour blindness.
	1912 Winiwarter (Belgium) proposes diploid human chromosome number as approximately 47. First good quality human chromosome analysis.
1912 First International Eugenics Congress (London).	
	1913 Alfred Sturtevant, student with Morgan, constructs first genetic map of *Drosophila* X-chromosome loci.
	1913 American Genetics Society formed as successor to American Breeders Association.
	1914 Boveri proposes chromosomal basis for cancer.
1914 (Outbreak of World War I)	
1915 JBS Haldane and colleagues publish first mammalian genetic linkage in mouse (publication delayed by the war).	
1916 Relationship recognised between frequency of a recessive disease and of consanguinity (F Lenz).	
	1916 Calvin Bridges shows nondisjunction in *Drosophila*.
	1918 Anticipation first recognised in myotonic dystrophy (Fleischer, Germany).
1918 RA Fisher shows compatibility of mendelism and quantitative inheritance.	

(Continued)

Contributions mainly (or substantially) from the UK	Contributions mainly from outside the UK
	1919 Hirszfeld and Hirszfeld show ABO blood group differences between populations, based on military personnel.
1919 Genetical Society founded in UK by William Bateson.	
1922 Inherited eye disease volumes of *Treasury of Human Inheritance* (Julia Bell) published.	
	1923 Painter recognises human Y chromosome; proposes human diploid chromosome number of 48.
	1927 Hermann Muller shows production of mutations by X-irradiation in *Drosophila*.
	1927 Compulsory sterilisation on eugenic grounds upheld by courts in America (*Buck v. Bell*).
	1928 Stadler shows radiation induced mutation in maize and barley.
1928 Griffiths discovers 'transformation' in Pneumococcus.	
	1929 Blakeslee shows effect of chromosomal trisomy in Datura, the thorn apple.
1930 RA Fisher's book *Genetical Theory of Natural Selection*.	
	1930 Beginning of major Russian contributions to human cytogenetics.
1930 JBS Haldane's book *Enzymes* attempts to keep biochemistry and genetics connected.	
1931 Archibald Garrod's second book *Inborn Factors in Disease* provides the foundation for modern concepts of multifactorial inheritance.	

(Continued)

Contributions mainly (or substantially) from the UK	Contributions mainly from outside the UK
1931 UK Medical Research Council establishes specific Research Committee on Human Genetics (Chairman JBS Haldane).	
1933 Lionel Penrose discovers maternal age effect in Down syndrome.	1933 Nazi eugenics law enacted in Germany.
	1934 Fölling in Norway discovers phenylketonuria.
1934 *Treasury of Human Inheritance* volume on Huntington's disease (Julia Bell) published.	
	1934 OL Mohr's book *Genetics and Disease*.
	1934 Mitochondrial inheritance proposed for Leber's optic atrophy (Imai and Moriwaki, Japan).
1935 First estimate of mutation rate for a human gene (haemophilia; JBS Haldane).	
1935 RA Fisher (amongst others) suggests use of linked genetic markers in disease prediction.	
1937 First human genetic linkage - haemophilia and colour blindness (Bell and Haldane).	
	1937 Moscow Medical Genetics Institute closed; director Levit and others arrested and later executed. Destruction of Russian genetics begins.
	1937 7th International Genetics Congress, Moscow, cancelled on Stalin's instructions.
1937 Max Perutz begins crystallographic studies of haemoglobin in Cambridge.	
1938 Lionel Penrose publishes *The Colchester Survey* on genetic basis of mental handicap.	

(Continued)

Contributions mainly (or substantially) from the UK	Contributions mainly from outside the UK
1939 7th International Genetics Congress held in Edinburgh on the eve of outbreak of war. 'Geneticists' Manifesto' issued.	
1939 (Outbreak of World War II)	
	1939 Cold Spring Harbor Eugenics Record Office closed.
	1939 Rh blood group system discovered (Landsteiner and Wiener).
	1941 Beadle and Tatum produce first nutritional mutants in *Neurospora* and confirm 'one gene – one enzyme' principle.
1941 Charlotte Auerbach discovers chemical mutagens in Edinburgh (not published until the end of the war).	
	1943 Nikolai Vavilov, leader of Russian genetics, dies in Soviet prison camp.
	1943 First American genetic counselling clinic.
	1943 Mutation first demonstrated in bacteria (Luria).
	1944 Schrödinger's book *What is Life?* provides inspiration for the first molecular biologists.
	1944 Oswald Avery shows bacterial transformation is due to DNA, not protein.
1945 Lionel Penrose appointed as head of Galton Laboratory, London and founds modern human genetics as a specific discipline.	
	1945 (Hiroshima and Nagasaki atomic explosions)
	1945 Genetic study of effects of radiation initiated on survivors of the atomic explosions (JV Neel, director).

(Continued)

Contributions mainly (or substantially) from the UK	Contributions mainly from outside the UK
1946 Penrose's inaugural lecture at University College, London uses phenylketonuria as paradigm for human genetics. 1946 John Fraser Roberts begins first UK genetic counselling clinic in London.	
	1946 Sexual processes first shown in bacteria (Lederberg). 1948 Total ban on all orthodox genetics (including human and medical genetics) teaching and research in Russia. 1948 American Society of Human Genetics founded. HJ Muller, President. 1949 *American Journal of Human Genetics* initiated. Charles Cotterman, first editor.
1949 JBS Haldane suggests selective advantage of sickle cell heterozygotes due to malaria resistance.	1949 Linus Pauling and colleagues show sickle cell disease to have a molecular basis. JV Neel shows it to be recessively inherited. 1949 Barr and Bertram (London, Ontario) discover the sex chromatin body. 1950 Curt Stern's Book *Human Genetics.* 1950 Frank Clarke Fraser initiates Medical Genetics at McGill University, Montreal.
1951 Fred Sanger sequences first protein (insulin).	1951 Linus Pauling shows triple helical structure of collagen. 1951 HELA cell line established from cervical cancer tissue of Baltimore patient Henrietta Lacks. 1952 First human inborn error shown to result from enzyme deficiency (glycogen storage disease type 1, Cori and Cori).

(Continued)

Contributions mainly (or substantially) from the UK	Contributions mainly from outside the UK
1952 Rosalind Franklin's x-ray crystallography shows helical structure of B form of DNA.	
1953 Bickel et al. initiate dietary treatment for PKU.	
1953 Watson and Crick discover double helix structure of DNA.	1953 Enzymatic basis of PKU established (Jervis).
	1953 Specific chair in Medical Genetics founded in Paris (first holder Maurice Lamy).
	1954 Allison proves selective advantage for sickle cell disease in relation to malaria.
	1955 Sheldon Reed's book *Counseling in Medical Genetics*.
	1955 Oliver Smithies develops starch gel electrophoresis for separation of human proteins.
	1955 Fine structure analysis of bacteriophage genome (Benzer).
	1956 Tjio and Levan show normal human chromosome number to be 46, not 48.
	1956 First International Congress of Human Genetics (Copenhagen).
	1956 Amniocentesis first validated for fetal sexing in haemophilia (Fuchs and Riis).
1957 Vernon Ingram shows specific amino acid change in sickle cell disease.	1957 Full Medical Genetics departments opened in Baltimore (Victor McKusick) and Seattle, Washington (Arno Motulsky).
	1958 First HLA antigen detected (Jean Dausset, Paris).
1959 Harry Harris' book *Human Biochemical Genetics*.	
1959 Max Perutz completes structure of haemoglobin.	

(Continued)

Contributions mainly (or substantially) from the UK	Contributions mainly from outside the UK
1959 First human sex chromosome abnormalities identified in Turner syndrome (Ford et al.), Klinefelter syndrome (Jacobs and Strong).	1959 Trisomy 21 identified in Down syndrome (Lejeune, Gautier and Turpin, Paris).
1960 Trisomies 13 and 18 identified (Patau et al., Edwards et al.)	
Paternal age effect for new dominant mutations (Blank; Apert syndrome).	
First full UK Medical Genetics Institute opened (under Paul Polani, Guy's Hospital, London).	1960 First edition of *Metabolic Basis of Inherited Disease* (Stanbury et al.).
	1960 Role of messenger RNA recognised.
	1960 First specific cytogenetic abnormality in human malignancy (Nowell and Hungerford, 'Philadelphia chromosome').
	1960 Chromosome analysis on peripheral blood allows rapid development of diagnostic clinical cytogenetics (Moorhead et al.).
	1960 Denver conference on human cytogenetic nomenclature.
	1960 First Bar Harbor course in Medical Genetics, under Victor McKusick.
1961 Prevention of rhesus haemolytic disease by isoimmunisation. (Cyril Clarke and colleagues, Liverpool).	1961 Cultured fibroblasts used to establish biochemical basis of galactosemia (Krooth and Weinberg), establishing value of somatic cell genetics.
	1961 'Genetic Code' linking DNA and protein established (Nirenberg and Matthaei).
1961 Mary Lyon (Harwell, UK) proposes X-chromosome inactivation in females.	
	1963 Population screening for PKU in newborns initiated (Guthrie and Susi).

(Continued)

Contributions mainly (or substantially) from the UK	Contributions mainly from outside the UK
1964 Ultrasound used in early pregnancy monitoring (Donald, Glasgow).	
1964 First journal specifically for medical genetics (*Journal of Medical Genetics*).	
	1964 Genetics officially restored as a science in USSR after Nikita Khrushchev dismissed.
	1964 First HLA Workshop (Durham, North Carolina).
1965 Human-rodent hybrid cell lines developed (Harris and Watkins, Oxford).	1965 High frequency of chromosome abnormalities found in spontaneous abortions (Carr, London Ontario).
	1966 First chromosomal prenatal diagnosis (Steele and Breg).
	First edition of McKusick's *Mendelian Inheritance in Man*.
	Recognition of dominantly inherited cancer families (Lynch).
	1967 Application of hybrid cell lines to human gene mapping (Weiss and Green).
	1968 First autosomal human gene assignment to a specific chromosome (Duffy blood group on chromosome 1) by Donahue et al.
	1969 First use of 'Bayesian' risk estimation in genetic counselling (Murphy and Mutalik).
	1969 First Master's degree course in genetic counseling (Sarah Lawrence College, New York).
1970 Identification of interphase human Y chromosome by fluorescence techniques (Pearson, Bobrow and colleagues).	1970 Fluorescent chromosome banding allows unique identification of all human chromosomes (Zech, Caspersson and colleagues).
	1970 First restriction enzyme discovered (Hamilton Smith, USA).
	1971 'Two hit' hypothesis for familial tumours, based on retinoblastoma (Knudson).

(Continued)

Contributions mainly (or substantially) from the UK	Contributions mainly from outside the UK
1971 Giemsa chromosome banding suitable for clinical cytogenetic use (Seabright).	
	1971 First use of restriction enzymes in molecular genetics (Danna and Nathans).
	1972 Population screening for Tay Sachs disease in Baltimore (Kaback and Zeiger).
1973 Prenatal diagnosis of neural tube defects by raised alpha fetoprotein (David Brock, Edinburgh).	
	1973 First Human Gene Mapping Workshop (Yale University).
1975 DNA hybridisation using 'Southern blot' filter (Edwin Southern).	
1977 First DNA sequencing, by dideoxy method (Frederick Sanger).	1977 Human beta-globin gene cloned.
	1978 Prenatal diagnosis of sickle cell disease through specific RFLP (Kan and Dozy).
	1978 First mutation causing a human inherited disease characterised (beta-thalassaemia).
1978 First birth following in vitro fertilisation (Steptoe and Edwards).	
	1979 Vogel and Motulsky's textbook *Human Genetics, Problems and Approaches*.
1980 Primary prevention of neural tube defects by preconception multivitamins (Smithells et al.).	
	1980 Detailed proposal for mapping the human genome by RFLPs (Botstein et al.).
1981 Human mitochondrial genome sequenced by Sanger's group in Cambridge (Anderson et al.).	

(Continued)

Contributions mainly (or substantially) from the UK	Contributions mainly from outside the UK
1982 Linkage of DNA markers on X chromosome to Duchenne muscular dystrophy (Murray et al.).	
	1983 First autosomal linkage using DNA markers for Huntington's disease (Gusella et al.).
	1983 First general use of chorionic villus sampling in early prenatal diagnosis.
1984 DNA fingerprinting discovered (Alec Jeffreys, Leicester).	
1985 Application of DNA markers in genetic prediction of Huntington's disease.	
	1985 First initiatives towards sequencing of entire human genome (US Dept of Energy and Cold Spring Harbor meetings).
	1986 Polymerase chain reaction (PCR) for amplifying short DNA sequences (Mullis).
	1987 Duchenne muscular dystrophy gene cloned (Kunkel).
	1988 International Human Genome Organisation (HUGO) established.
	1988 US Congress funds Human Genome Project.
	1989 Cystic fibrosis gene isolated.
	1989 First use of preimplantation genetic diagnosis.
	1990 First attempts at gene therapy in immunodeficiencies.
	Fluorescent in situ hybridisation introduced to cytogenetic analysis.
	1991 Discovery of unstable DNA and trinucleotide repeat expansion (fragile X).
1992/1993 Myotonic dystrophy and Huntington's disease genes and mutations identified by international consortia, including British groups.	1992 Isolation of *PKU* (phenylalanine hydroxylase) gene (Woo and colleagues).

(Continued)

Contributions mainly (or substantially) from the UK	Contributions mainly from outside the UK
	1992 First complete map of human genome produced by French *Généthon* initiative (Weissenbach et al.).
1993 Tuberous sclerosis (*TSC2*) gene isolated (UK-led European consortium).	
	1994 *BRCA1* gene for hereditary breast-ovarian cancer identified (Myriad genetics).
1995 *BRCA2* gene isolated (Institute of Cancer Research, London).	
1996 'Bermuda Agreement' giving immediate public access to all Human Genome Project data (John Sulston the main proponent).	
1997 First cloned mammal ('Dolly the sheep'); Roslin Institute, Edinburgh.	1997 Tuberous sclerosis (*TSC1*) gene isolated.
1998 First total sequence of model multicellular organism *C. elegans*	
1998 Isolation of human embryonic stem cells.	
	1999 Sequence of first human chromosome (22).
2000 'Draft sequence' of human genome announced jointly by International Human Genome Consortium and by Celera.	2000 Gene therapy for inherited immune deficiency (SCID).
	2002 Discovery of microRNAs.
2003 Complete sequence of human genome achieved.	
First major UK government initiative in medical genetics ('Our Inheritance, our Future').	
2004 Cancer genome project initiated (Wellcome Trust Sanger Institute).	
2005 Haplotype map of the human genome (HAPMAP project).	

(Continued)

Contributions mainly (or substantially) from the UK	Contributions mainly from outside the UK
	2006 Prenatal detection of free fetal DNA in maternal blood clinically feasible.
2007 Wellcome Trust case control study. Genome-wide association studies give first robust findings in common disorders.	
2008 New Solexa sequencing allows rapid, large scale genome sequencing.	2008 First specific individual human whole genomes sequenced.
Retinal gene therapy for Leber's congenital amaurosis.	
2010 1000 genomes project analyses extent of genome variation.	2010 Neanderthal DNA detected in most human genomes.
2010 Correction of mitochondrial disorder by preimplantation nuclear transfer.	
2011 Deciphering Developmental Disorders (DDD) project initiated. Whole exome sequencing found to be clinically valuable in detecting the molecular basis of mental handicap of unknown cause.	
2012 100,000 genomes sequencing project begun.	
2014 First major report from DDD study consortium.	2014 Netherlands-led study of genome sequencing in developmental disorders (parallel to DDD study).
	2015 Gene editing using CRISPR techniques introduced experimentally.
	2016 Detailed sequence analysis of protein coding genome (exome).
2018 100,000 genomes project completed.	

Source: Based on the timeline of the Genetics and Medicine Historical Network (www.genmedhist.org/timeline).

Appendix 2: Recording the history of British medical genetics

When I first began to take a serious interest in preserving and recording the history of medical genetics, around the year 2002, it was not with the intention of this becoming a major field of my own research, but because I could see that it needed doing, and doing urgently. I could also see that nobody else appeared to be doing it or planning to do it. Historians at that time, to my surprise and great disappointment, appeared, with a very few exceptions, to be largely unaware of and not interested in the overall field of modern human and medical genetics, preferring to focus on eugenics, which they often seemed to consider as the same as medical genetics. Turning to my fellow geneticists, laboratory and clinical, I found that, while many were interested and keen that the work should be done, most were too busy (including those officially 'retired') to take an active role themselves.

It was thus clear to me that if the history of human and medical genetics was to be saved for posterity, I would have to make a start myself. Fortunately, I had recently passed over the burden of being head of an active academic and service department to able colleagues, so I had more time available; also, with retirement approaching (compulsory at age 65 in those days) I was beginning to hand on my long-running research activities, involving Huntington's disease and myotonic dystrophy among other topics, so I could hope, in theory at least, for still more time then.

The upshot was that I founded the Genetics and Medicine Historical Network (Genmedhist) in 2003 to bring together anyone interested in the field worldwide, whether historians, geneticists or others. With a website (www.genmedhist. org), a newsletter and a series of broad aims (Table A2.1), it seemed better to embark on these activities collectively rather than in isolation. Fifteen years on it is encouraging to find that, for Britain at least, most of these original aims have been achieved. I have written about this elsewhere (Harper PS 2014. The origins of the Genetics and Medicine Historical Network. *Genmedhist Newsletter* 18:5–9), so in this Appendix, I shall give only a brief account of what has been done — and what still remains for the future.

Table A2.1 The Genetics and Medicine Historical Network: aims and achievements, 2003–2018

Genmedhist website (www.genmedhist.org), 2003-present. Curated by Cardiff University, 2003–2015; by ESHG, 2015- present.

Identification and cataloguing of important record sets. 14 major sets identified and catalogued (see Table A2.3).

Newsletter/Bulletin. 17 issues between 2003 and 2014.

Recorded interviews. 51 UK workers interviewed (part of international series of 100 interviews). See Table A2.4.

International workshops on genetics, medicine and history. Series of seven workshops between 2003 and 2017 (see Table A2.2 and Figure A2.1).

Genetics and Medicine Historical Library. Now approaching 4000 volumes.

First, the website, www.genmedhist.org: This has provided the cement that has helped to coordinate the other activities and it is fortunate that Cardiff University was able to host it for its first 12 years, and that European Society of Human Genetics (ESHG) has been prepared to continue this subsequently. Likewise, the *Genmedhist Newsletter*, archived on the website, (www. genmedhist.org/newsletters) provided a valuable forum for the Network's first 10 years.

In terms of creating and maintaining personal links between historians and geneticists, the series of seven international workshops on genetics, medicine and history (Table A2.2) really opened the eyes of all involved to the range of historical work that was beginning to occur, and to the value of collaborations between the humanities and scientists.

Table A2.2 International workshops on genetics, medicine and history, 2003–2017, organised by the Genetics and Medicine Historical Network

Date	Place	Theme
2003	Birmingham, UK	Launching the Genetics and Medicine Historical Network
2005	Brno, Czech Republic	Preserving the records of human genetics
2007	Barcelona	Genetics, history and public understanding
2010	Gothenburg	Early history of human molecular genetics
2012	Nuremberg	The biological future of man: continuities and breaks in the history of human genetics, before and after 1945
2015	Glasgow	Human gene mapping; oral history of human genetics
2017	Copenhagen/ Lund	50 years of human genetics in Europe: discoveries, challenges and the foundation of the European Society of Human Genetics

(a)

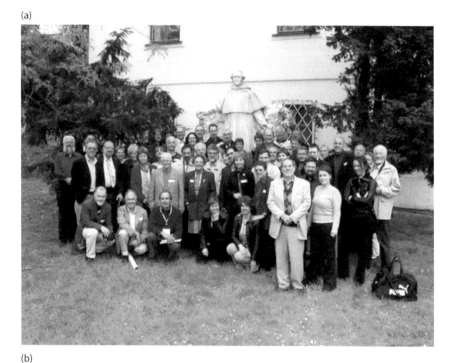

(b)

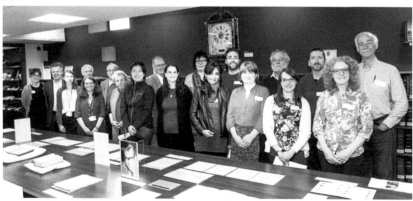

Figure A2.1 International workshops in genetics, medicine and history. **(a)** Second workshop at Mendel's Abbey St Thomas, Brno, 2005. **(b)** Archive exhibits on Pontecorvo, Ferguson-Smith and Renwick at the 6th (Glasgow) Workshop 2015. (Courtesy Genetics and Medicine Historical Network and European Society of Human Genetics.)

With hindsight it would have been good if all of the workshops had been published individually, but a valuable volume containing many of the contributions has now been produced (Petermann et al. 2017), and of course others have been published in a range of journals. The website also contains programmes and reports on the different workshops (www.genmedhist.org/workshops).

RECORDS OF INDIVIDUAL WORKERS IN GENETICS AND MEDICINE

The principal body responsible for the archiving of the scientific records of post-war workers has until recently been the National Cataloguing Unit for the Archives of Contemporary Scientists (NCUACS), formerly based at Bath University. When I first made contact with this unit they had catalogued almost no geneticists' records, the exceptions being Arthur Mourant (blood group scientist and anthropologist) and Cyril Clarke (see Chapter 2), but a collaboration initiated with the unit director Peter Harper (no relation to the author) and senior archivist Timothy Powell resulted in the preservation and cataloguing of a series of important sets of records, listed in Table A2.3.

Sadly, Bath University closed the unit on financial grounds while this project was in progress, but funding from Wellcome Trust allowed two archivists from the unit to complete the work over the following two years at Cardiff University.

Table A2.3 Major records sets of workers in genetics and medicine

Name	Principal field of work	University or other body where records are located
Walter Bodmer	Population genetics; cancer genetics	Oxford, Bodleian Library
John Edwards	Human genetics	Birmingham University
Malcolm Ferguson-Smith[a]	Cytogenetics; medical genetics	Glasgow University
George Fraser	Human genetics	London, Wellcome Library
Hans Grüneberg[a]	Mouse/human genetics	Wellcome Library
JBS Haldane[a]	Human and general genetics	University College, London
Harry Harris	Human biochemical genetics	University College, London; University of Pennsylvania
Henry Harris	Cancer biology and genetics	Oxford University
Alec Jeffreys	Human molecular genetics	Wellcome Library
Anne McLaren	Developmental genetics	Wellcome Library
Arthur Mourant[a]	Blood group genetics	Wellcome Library
Lionel Penrose[a]	Human genetics	University College, London
Robert Race/Ruth Sanger[a]	Blood group genetics	Wellcome Library
James Renwick[a]	Human gene mapping	Glasgow University
Cedric AB Smith	Statistical genetics	University College, London

[a] Indicates that there is digitised material on Wellcome Library 'Codebreakers' website, https://wellcomelibrary.org/collections/digital-collections/makers-of-modern-genetics/

Several further important sets of paper-based records have been catalogued by other bodies recently, notably those of Walter Bodmer, now at the Oxford Bodleian Library, and of Anne McLaren, at Wellcome Library, so it seems likely that most of the major paper-based UK sets have been identified and preserved; ensuring the preservation and archiving of electronic records, including email correspondence, remains a major challenge, although my own experience shows that it is feasible with careful planning.

The policy of NCUACS was always to return catalogued records to the relevant university for permanent archiving rather than try to create a single comprehensive national archive, a wise policy that has begun to result in archivists across Britain undertaking detailed work on the geneticists whose records they care for.

Apart from these relatively recent records, there are extensive archives at University College, London and Wellcome Library, for such earlier workers as JBS Haldane, Lionel Penrose and Harry Harris, extending back to Karl Pearson and Francis Galton; we thus have a near continuous record of work at the Galton Laboratory during the century of its existence, apart from the records of RA Fisher, which are mainly at University of Adelaide (he emigrated to Australia near the end of his life). There are also notable recent gaps for some important individuals where significant records appear not to exist, such as Paul Polani and Cedric Carter.

The role of the Genetics and Medicine Historical Network in relation to written records has been mainly as a linking agent for UK archives, by first identifying important record sets that the Bath cataloguing unit could work on, then sustaining its work through Cardiff University during the difficult period following the unit's closure, and finally encouraging the Wellcome Trust to support the cataloguing and archiving of further important human genetics records, both of individuals and of organisations, through the Wellcome Library, British Library, Bodleian Library and others. The end result is that we now have a fairly complete collection of the main substantial record sets of British human and medical geneticists (Table A2.3). But looking to the future it may, as mentioned, be more difficult to ensure this for the current and future generations of workers whose records, especially correspondence, are almost exclusively electronic.

Recorded interviews have probably been my own main contribution to the initiative, and out of a total of 100 interviews worldwide in my own series I have been able to undertake around 50 of these with UK workers (Table A2.4), almost all of which are freely accessible on the Genmedhist website (www.genmedhist. org/interviews). Much of the information given in this book has been based on them. Historians seem to be divided in their opinions on the value of oral history generally, but allowing for the fallibility and subjectiveness of memory, I personally have found little to suggest major bias or inaccuracy. Most importantly, these personal accounts capture much background and other information that is unpublished and which would otherwise be irretrievably lost when the individual dies, as has since happened for a number of those who I interviewed. Fortunately the list given in Table A2.4 represents a sizeable proportion of the first generations of British medical geneticists, including many of the more 'ordinary', yet still important workers in the field. Other European countries are now taking steps to ensure that the pioneers in their own countries are interviewed. But as with all

Table A2.4 Recording the history of medical genetics: interviews by the author with key UK workers in the field

Name	Number	Place	Field of work
Baraitser, Michael	33	London	Neurogenetics; dysmorphology
Bates, Gill	57	London	Human molecular genetics; Huntington's disease
Berry, Caroline	20	London	Clinical genetics
Berry, RJ (Sam)[a]	31	London	Population genetics
Blank, Eric[a]	–	Sheffield	Medical genetics
Bobrow, Martin	24	Oxford; London; Cambridge	Medical genetics
Bodmer, Walter	68	Oxford	Human population genetics; cancer genetics
Burn, John	100	Newcastle	Medical genetics
Clarke, Angus	96	Cardiff	Clinical genetics; social and ethical issues
Davies, Kay	80	Oxford; London	Human molecular genetics
Delhanty, Joy	25	London	Human cytogenetics; preimplantation diagnosis
Donnai, Dian	63	Manchester	Clinical genetics; dysmorphology
Edwards, Anthony	29	Cambridge	Human population genetics
Edwards, John[a,b]	14	Oxford; Birmingham	Medical genetics
Emery, Alan	48	Manchester; Edinburgh	Medical genetics; neuromuscular disorders
Evans, H John[a,b]	04	Edinburgh	Human cytogenetics
Evans, Edward[b]	15	Harwell	Cytogenetics
Evans, Kathleen[a]	–	London	Genetic counselling
Farndon, Peter	97	Birmingham	Clinical genetics; genetic education
Ferguson-Smith, Malcolm[b]	03	Glasgow; Cambridge	Cytogenetics; human gene mapping
Fraser, George	32	Oxford	Medical genetics; cancer genetics
Goodfellow, Peter	98	London; Cambridge	Human molecular genetics

(Continued)

Table A2.4 (*Continued*) Recording the history of medical genetics: interviews by the author with key UK workers in the field

Name	Number	Place	Field of work
Hamerton, John[a,b]	21	London; Winnipeg	Human cytogenetics; prenatal diagnosis; gene mapping
Harnden, David[b]	08	Edinburgh; Manchester	Human cytogenetics; cancer genetics
Harper, Peter (interviewed by Angus Clarke)	16	Cardiff	Medical genetics
Harris, Henry[a]	67	Oxford	Cancer genetics
Harris, Rodney[a]	59	Manchester	Medical genetics
Hastie, Nick	11	Edinburgh	Human molecular genetics
Hopkinson, David	81	London	Human biochemical genetics
Hughes, Helen	90	Cardiff; Toronto	Clinical genetics; dysmorphology
Hulten, Maj[b]	10	Stockholm; Birmingham	Human cytogenetics
Jacobs, Patricia[b]	06	Edinburgh; Honolulu; Southampton	Human cytogenetics
Jeffreys, Alec	75	Leicester	Human molecular genetics
Jenkins, Trefor	69	Johannesburg	Human population genetics; medical genetics
Johnston, Alan[a]	74	Aberdeen	Clinical genetics neural tube defects; malformation pathology
Laurence, K Michael[a]	13	Cardiff	
Laxova, Renata	55	Brno; London; Madison	Clinical genetics
Lee, Muriel[b]	12	Edinburgh	Human cytogenetics
Lyon, Mary[a]	18	Harwell	Mammalian genetics
Medvedev, Zhores[a]	58	Obninsk; London	Radiation genetics; cell aging
Mittwoch, Ursula	07	London	Human developmental genetics
Modell, Bernadette	70	London	Thalassaemias

(*Continued*)

Table A2.4 (*Continued*) Recording the history of medical genetics: interviews by the author with key UK workers in the field

Name	Number	Place	Field of work
Morton, Newton[a]	34	Honolulu; Southampton	Human population and mathematical genetics
Nevin, Norman[a]	26	Belfast	Clinical genetics
Pembrey, Marcus	62	London	Clinical genetics
Polani, Paul[a,b]	01	London	Medical genetics; human cytogenetics
Povey, Sue[a]	71	London	Human biochemical genetics; gene mapping
Read, Andrew	64	Manchester	Clinical molecular genetics
Roberts, Derek[a]	02	Newcastle	Human population genetics; medical genetics
Sampson, Julian	91	Cardiff	Clinical genetics; cancer genetics; tuberous sclerosis
Searle, Anthony[a]	19	Harwell	Radiation genetics; cytogenetics
Snell, Russell	83	Cardiff; Auckland	Human molecular genetics; HD
Strong, John	–	Edinburgh	Endocrinology
Weatherall, David[a]	30	Liverpool; Oxford	Thalassaemias
Williamson, Robert	61	Glasgow; London; Melbourne	Human molecular genetics

Note: The total of 55 interviews includes some who spent part of their career in other countries.

[a] Deceased.

[b] Recorded interview audiofile as well as transcript available on the Genmedhist website (www.genmedhist.org/interviews). The website also lists other recorded interviews from outside the UK, while the full series of 100 interviews is discussed in Harper (2017).

The interview number is that corresponding to the full interview series as given on the website and in Harper (2017). Background material on all interviews is archived with the History of Human Genetics Project at Cardiff University.

aspects of history, time passes with remarkable speed and there is now another generation of workers retiring whose contributions will be just as important to record as the earlier ones, so ideally there needs to be a rolling programme to interview them. Who will undertake or coordinate this?

A complementary approach to oral history has been the use of 'Witness Seminars', where a small group of workers previously involved in an important specific field hold a recorded group discussion. Britain has been especially fortunate in having had historian Tilli Tansey to lead and coordinate an extensive

Table A2.5 Witness seminars covering medical genetics and related topics

2003	Genetic screening
2004	The rhesus factor and disease prevention
2010	Clinical genetics in Britain: origins and development
2013	Clinical cancer genetics: polyposis and familial colorectal cancer c.1975–c.2010
2014	Clinical molecular genetics in the UK c.1975–c.2000
2015	Human gene mapping workshops c.1973–c.1991

series of these, initially under the aegis of Wellcome Trust, then under Queen Mary University of London; six of these have been on various aspects of genetics (Table A2.5). Not only do these give the benefit of ensuring that multiple viewpoints are represented, but meticulous editing and annotation has allowed permanent volumes, both printed and internet based, to be produced for each seminar.

OTHER IMPORTANT SOURCES

Primary sources

The main sources that I have used for this book are the interviews (mainly conducted by myself) and the record sets of early workers in the field, mentioned above, but there is a considerable amount of other primary material available. I have tried to give the specific source used at the relevant place in the text, but mention here several that are of particular significance.

ROYAL COLLEGE OF PHYSICIANS (LONDON)

1. Minutes and other material of the College Committee on Medical Genetics. This is a valuable and comprehensive record that gives a detailed picture of how clinical genetics was evolving between the committee's beginning in 1984 and its subsuming into the Joint Committee on Medical Genetics Services in 2001. Valuable attached documents in the archive include a series of reports discussed by the committee. The material has not yet been digitised.
2. Lives of Fellows of the Royal College of Physicians ('Munk's Roll'). This remarkable document, now available online (munksroll.rcplondon.ac.uk), stretches back over 300 years and is an invaluable source of biographical detail, especially on the numerous clinical geneticists who do not have obituaries in medical journals or newspapers, but are almost all Fellows of the College.
3. Reports on medical genetics published by the College. These valuable and often influential reports are mentioned in Chapter 8 (Table 8.1) and elsewhere. While not specifically archived by the College itself, copies of most of them are available as hard copy in the Human Genetics Historical Library.
4. Transcripts of recorded interviews arranged by the College in conjunction with Oxford Brookes University. This series includes several with workers involved with genetics, some of whom also appear in my own later interview series.

They are mainly based in Oxford and London and include Walter Bodmer, Kay Davies, Henry Harris, Anne McLaren, Paul Polani and David Weatherall.

NATIONAL ARCHIVES, KEW, LONDON

This very extensive archive contains the records of most UK government and other official bodies. A digitised catalogue (www.nationalarchives.gov.uk) is available, but original documents can be viewed by arrangement. I did not try to make a systematic search of the National Archives, but there must be a considerable amount of material relevant to genetics and medicine scattered through records of the MRC and Department of Health. Of particular importance for medical genetics is the web archiving of reports from now defunct committees such as the Advisory Committee on Genetic Testing (ACGT) and the Human Genetics Commission (HGC). Also of relevance to early medical genetics are the minutes of the MRC Human Genetics Committee (File FD1/3267), which met between 1932 and 1939 (see Chapter 1).

PROFESSIONAL AND SCIENTIFIC SOCIETIES

The records of these societies are of real interest and importance in giving a picture of how a scientific or medical field is evolving, as described in Chapter 9. The programmes of meetings, membership lists and even business details and accounts all help to document this. Most interesting are the early years around the formation of the society, when it is still relatively informal and its role still fluid; unfortunately these years are often the time when documentation is least complete. Sets of minutes may move around and sometimes be lost as society secretaries change, while if a society merges or ceases to function, no arrangements may have been made for proper archiving. The use of email and the electronic nature of most reports and documents now adds to the fragility of the situation and the difficulty of preserving a complete record.

Genetics is probably no different from other areas in these respects, but it is fortunate that its oldest society, the Genetical Society, has had a well-organised archiving system from the outset.

Genetical Society (now Genetics Society)

Founded in 1919 by William Bateson, this is one of the oldest societies relating to genetics in the world (though not quite the oldest, which is probably the Mendelian Society of Lund, Sweden, founded in 1909). The Society's records from the beginning (see Chapter 9) are housed in the archive of the John Innes Institute, Norwich (https://www.jic.ac.uk), of which Bateson was Director, along with Bateson's Library and other records. (Copies of the Bateson material are with the American Philosophical Society in Philadelphia.) The Society's meetings have covered a number of medical genetics topics.

Clinical Genetics Society

The early records of this (see Chapter 9) moved with successive secretaries, but, largely due to the efforts of Peter Farndon, have mostly been reassembled, with copies in the Cardiff-based *British Human Genetics Archive*. Valuable material includes early correspondence on the founding of the Society, programmes of meetings and membership lists.

British Society for Human Genetics (BSHG); now British Society for Genetic Medicine (BSGM).

This has likewise been mentioned in Chapter 9.

WEB-BASED AND VIDEO RESOURCES

Genetics and Medicine Historical Network (Genmedhist). Website: www.genmedhist. org (See above) This resource, created in 2003 by the author and colleagues, is now hosted by European Society of Human Genetics (ESHG) since 2015, having originally been under Cardiff University. The complete website was scanned by the British Web-archiving Service prior to transfer and an archival printed copy was also made, these also containing material specific for Cardiff-based work that was not considered relevant to the new ESHG-hosted version.

Wellcome Library

The Wellcome Library's website, 'Codebreakers: Makers of Modern Genetics' has grown over the past decade into a major resource of information relating to human genetics. Initially focused on the Human Genome Project, where Wellcome Trust was the principal UK funder (see Chapter 12), it has developed a progressively wider remit, including human gene mapping, and has now digitised much of the material contained in the older record sets listed in Table A2.2, with a number of images and also an illustrated timeline. It remains primarily focused on basic research and especially on Wellcome Trust-related initiatives and on the pioneers of molecular biology.

Wellcome Library has now also digitised many of its own books, and a list of those on or relevant to genetics that can be accessed in full is given on the 'Codebreaker' website (https://wellcomelibrary.org/collections/digital-collections/makers-of-modern-genetics/). It also houses the former Eugenics Society archives (see Chapter 1).

Sources relevant to MRC units involved with research on human and medical genetics

Considerable archival material is available in the library of the MRC Human Genetics Unit in Edinburgh, which I consulted during the writing of my earlier book *First Years of Human Chromosomes* (Harper 2006). So far, unfortunately, it has not been formally catalogued, something that deserves urgent attention. Sadly, very little early information seems to be available for the Harwell unit or its workers, though some might be found in the overall MRC records.

A valuable website on the Edinburgh University and Agricultural Research Council Research units now gives detail of general genetics research in Edinburgh over the past century (https://collections.ed.ac.uk), including such workers as Conrad Hal Waddington and Douglas Falconer, both highly relevant to human and medical genetics.

Recorded interviews by myself that are relevant to these MRC units, (available at www.genmedhist.org/interviews) include those with:

Patricia Jacobs [06]
Muriel Lee [12]
John Strong (not recorded but notes available)
David Harnden [28]
H John Evans [04]
Nicholas Hastie [11]

And for the Harwell MRC unit:

Mary Lyon [18]
Anthony Searle [19]
Edward Evans [15] (material on Charles Ford)
John Edwards [14] (collaborations with Harwell)
John Hamerton [21] (material on Charles Ford, also on Paul Polani and the Guy's
    Hospital unit)

For the Oxford Stevenson MRC unit:

John Edwards [14]
Martin Bobrow [24]
Norman Nevin [26]
Derek Roberts [02]

For John Fraser Roberts and Cedric Carter at Institute of Child Health, London:

Marcus Pembrey [62]
Norman Nevin [26]
Michael Baraitser [33]
John Burn [100]
Kathleen Evans (interview not recorded but notes available)

Witness seminar series: Makers of Modern Biomedicine

This series, pioneered and organised by Professor Tilli Tansey of University College London and Queen Mary University of London, has covered some of the most important areas of medical genetics, as shown in Table A2.5. The transcripts are available both on the Web (www.histmodbiomed.org) and as printed books, and are thoroughly annotated and also illustrated, making them both valuable historical documents and enjoyable to read.

Video archive of European human and medical geneticists

Professor Hans Galjaard (Rotterdam) has made, over many years, a series of visual records of international (including UK) workers in the field, beginning as cine film, then videotape, with an edited version finally created as a DVD, a copy of which is held in the Human Genetics Historical Library.

A number of other film records have been made of early workers and of international congresses that include images of UK workers.

Secondary sources

The principal UK-based human and medical genetics journals have been described in Chapter 9. Journal articles and reviews cited in the book are referenced in the text where relevant and are not included here, but the following books bring together a considerable amount of historical material:

Rushton AR. Genetics and Medicine in Britain, 1600–1939. *This valuable book gives the most detailed account of pre-World War II observations on the topic, but does not cover the past 80 years, thus excluding virtually all modern medical genetics.*

Petermann HI, Harper PS Doetz S. 2017. *History of Human Genetics: Aspects of its Development and Global Perspectives.* Springer International.

Harper PS. 2008. *A Short History of Medical Genetics.* New York, Oxford University Press. (2nd edition, online, 2013). This book covers medical genetics from an international perspective, but inevitably deals only briefly with most British work and workers – hence the need for the present book.

Harper PS. 2006. *First Years of Human Chromosomes.* Oxford. Scion Press. A considerable part of the key research in human cytogenetics was undertaken by UK workers and is covered, along with work from other countries, in more detail than can be done in the brief account given here in Chapter 10.

Harper PS (ed.). 2004. *Landmarks in Medical Genetics: Classic Papers with Commentaries.* Oxford: Oxford University Press. Many of the papers in this collection are difficult to find in their original journals.

Several general accounts of the development of genetics, general and human, have appeared in recent years. They are all valuable but being mainly American based are of limited direct use as sources for British work and so have not been cited in individual chapters. They include:

Lindee S. 2005. *Moments of Truth in Genetic Medicine.* Baltimore: The Johns Hopkins University Press.

Comfort N. 2012. *The Science of Human Perfection: How Genes Became the Heart of American Medicine.* New Haven, CT: Yale University Press.

Mukherjee S. 2016. *The Gene: An Intimate History.* London: Vintage.

Hogan AJ. 2016. *Life Histories of Genetic Disease: Patterns and Prevention in Medical Genetics.* Baltimore: Johns Hopkins University Press.

WORTHWHILE PROJECTS FOR THE HISTORY OF MEDICAL GENETICS

The list given in Table A2.6 is based on a corresponding one in my previous book, *A Short History of Medical Genetics* (Harper 2008). I have included it here since most of the projects suggested there still need to be done more than 10 years later! I feel strongly that a number of these would be suitable for students or graduates

Table A2.6 Worthwhile projects for the history of medical genetics

- Successive advances in medical genetics as reflected in books and specialist journals
- The development and role of lay societies in medical genetics research, applications and policies
- The influence of medical charities' (major and minor) funding of human and medical genetics research, especially gene mapping and isolation
- The transition from laboratory research to laboratory services, as seen in clinical cytogenetics and clinical molecular genetics
- The effects of war and persecution, especially World War II and its aftermath, on the international development of human genetics
- National and international networks in the delineation and diagnosis of genetic syndromes and in molecular genetic testing
- The balance between competition, collaboration, and cooperation in the development of human molecular genetics
- The development and subsequent rejection of attempts to patent and restrict the use of human gene sequences
- Popular literature for the general public on human and medical genetics
- Medical genetics and genetic disorders as portrayed in the media
- NHS developments in medical genetics – the UK Health Department's views as recorded in its archives
- Why was familial hypercholesterolaemia so neglected as a common and treatable genetic disorder?
- Detailed historical analysis of the background and effects of the Human Genetics Commission and Nuffield Council on Bioethics
- Analysis of and reasons for perceived distancing between basic and applied geneticists
- Effects on the development of medical genetics on the separation of University and NHS systems
- Variation between medical specialties in the use of and interaction with medical genetics
- Analysis of the value and preservation of adequate time in a genetic counselling session
- Gender shifts in clinical and laboratory staff working in medical genetics
- The value of personal and other links with NHS management, and the harm if destroyed
- Ethical issues associated with population screening for genetic disorders
- Genomics and its consequences for wider medical laboratory practice; e.g. histopathology

working in the history of science field, but potential supervisors do not seem to agree, while scientific or clinical workers rarely have access to research students. Recently retired workers are perhaps the best placed to undertake relevant projects, since they have time and freedom, as well as expertise in a particular field over a professional lifetime – and they do not have to be paid!

Index

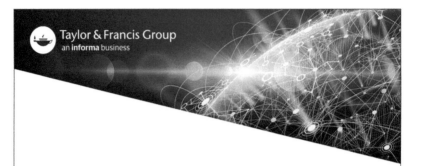

T - #0357 - 071024 - C8 - 234/156/16 - PB - 9780367178093 - Gloss Lamination